(BI3145G

RECEIVED
BETH ISRAEL MEDICAL CENTER

APR 18 1978

DIRECTOR, AMBULATORY
HEALTH SERVICE

RECENT ADVANCES
IN GASTROENTEROLOGY

IAN A. D. BOUCHIER

MD FRCP(Lond) FRCP (Edin)
Professor of Medicine,
University of Dundee,
Department of Medicine,
Ninewells Hospital and Medical School,
Dundee DD1 9SY

RECENT ADVANCES IN GASTROENTEROLOGY

EDITED BY
IAN A. D. BOUCHIER

NUMBER THREE

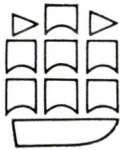

CHURCHILL LIVINGSTONE
Edinburgh London and New York
1976

CHURCHILL LIVINGSTONE
Medical Division of Longman Group Limited

Distributed in the United States of America by
Longman Inc., 19 West 44th Street, New York,
N.Y. 10036, and by associated companies,
branches and representatives throughout
the world.

© LONGMAN GROUP LIMITED 1976

All rights reserved. No part of this publication
may be reproduced, stored in a retrieval system,
or transmitted in any form or by any means,
electronic, mechanical, photocopying, recording
or otherwise, without the prior permission of
the publishers (Churchill Livingstone,
23 Ravelston Terrace, Edinburgh, EH4 3TL)

ISBN 0 443 01319 5

Library of Congress Catalog Card Number 76-21318

Printed in Great Britain

PREFACE

The expansion in knowledge relating to clinical and basic gastroenterology continues unabated. The difficult task for the Editor has been one of selection and how to meet the varying demands of the wide readership of this series. Fortunately much of the new development in physiology, biochemistry and pathology has had a direct bearing on patient care; the clinician and the laboratory specialist have developed good lines of communication and both are in a strong position to appreciate the potential and the problems created by the rapid proliferation of information.

The choice of subject has been conditioned on the one hand by those fields of particular growth and on the other by an attempt to reflect as many interests as possible as may be accommodated within a volume of this size. Thus paediatric gastroenterology, hitherto rather neglected but currently exhibiting healthy growth, claims a fair amount of space. Gastrointestinal hormones is another area of rapid expansion which was covered in the previous edition but none the less requires further elaboration. The topic has been introduced in a more clinical fashion by a description of hormone-secreting tumours of the gastrointestinal tract. The influence of exogenous agents on the gut is important and both alcohol and laxatives have been the subjects of much recent research. An understanding of the consequences of the loss of large areas of functioning absorptive surface has resulted in a more rational approach to therapy and considerable improvement in mortality and morbidity rates. One important development has been the enunciation of scientific principles for parenteral nutrition. The study of the gastro-oesophageal junction is another topic where the joint efforts of physiologists and clinicians have led to a better, though still slightly confused, understanding of normal function, and paved the way for more effective therapy. Bile acid metabolism, for so long a rather esoteric area of biochemical research, has achieved clinical respectability. No modern gastroenterologist can afford to be without some understanding of the role of bile acids in gastrointestinal physiology and the manner in which they may be manipulated diagnostically and therapeutically.

The authors have been chosen because of the acknowledged expertise in their subjects. I am grateful to them for their unstinted cooperation. Their contributions are a splendid testimony to the many exciting ways in which gastroenterology has developed in the past decade.

IAN A. D. BOUCHIER

Dundee, 1976

CONTRIBUTORS

CHARLOTTE M. ANDERSON MD MSc FRACP FRCP
Professor of Paediatrics and Child Health, Director of the Institute of Child Health, University of Birmingham, Birmingham B16 8ET

R. A. BROWN MD
Department of Surgery and Division of Gastroenterology, McGill University and Montreal General Hospital, Montreal, Quebec

P. W. BRUNT MD MRCP
Department of Medicine, University of Aberdeen

PETER B. COTTON MD MRCP
Consultant Physician, Middlesex Hospital, London W1N 8AA

JOHN H. CUMMINGS MSc MB MRCP
MRC Dunn Nutrition Unit, Milton Road, Cambridge

J. W. DUTTON MD
Department of Surgery and Division of Gastroenterology, McGill University and Montreal General Hospital, Montreal, Quebec

C. F. HAWKINS MD FRCP
Consultant Physician to United Birmingham Hospitals, Lecturer in Clinical Medicine to University of Birmingham, Queen Elizabeth Hospital, Birmingham 15

K. W. HEATON MD FRCP
Senior Lecturer in Medicine, University Department of Medicine, Bristol Royal Infirmary, Bristol BS2 8HW

A. M. HOARE MA MB BCh MRCP
Senior Registrar, Queen Elizabeth Hospital, Birmingham 15

WILLIAM H. LIPSHUTZ MD
Assistant Professor of Medicine, Hospital of the University of Pennsylvania, Head, Section of Gastroenterology, Department of Medicine, Pennsylvania Hospital, Philadelphia, Pennsylvania

CONTRIBUTORS

RONALD A. MALT AB MD(Harvard) FACS
Professor of Surgery, Harvard Medical School, Chief of Gastroenterological Surgery, Massachusetts General Hospital, Boston 02114, USA

GEORGE B. McDONALD MD
Instructor in Medicine, Veterans Administration Hospital and University of Washington, Seattle, USA

ALEX P. MOWAT MB ChB FRCP DCH DObst RCOG
Consultant Paediatrician, Department of Child Health, King's College Hospital Medical School, Denmark Hill, London SE5 8RX

N. A. G. MOWAT MD ChB MRCP
Department of Medicine, University of Aberdeen

BENNETT E. ROTH MD
Department of Medicine, University of California, Los Angeles, California 90024, USA

DAVID R. SAUNDERS MD
Associate Professor of Medicine, University of Washington, Seattle, USA

E. A. SHAFFER MD
Department of Surgery and Division of Gastroenterology, McGill University and Montreal General Hospital, Montreal, Quebec

JOHN H. WALSH MD
Department of Medicine, University of California, Los Angeles, California 90024, USA

CONTENTS

Preface	v
Contributors	vii
1. Physiology of the Gastro-oesophageal Junction and Hiatus Hernia *William H. Lipshutz*	1
2. Fat Absorption *David R. Saunders George B. McDonald*	27
3. Hormone-secreting Tumours of the Gastrointestinal Tract *John H. Walsh Bennett E. Roth*	49
4. The Effects of Massive Small Bowel Resection *E. A. Shaffer, R. A. Brown J. W. Dutton*	73
5. Connective Tissue Disorders Affecting the Gastrointestinal Tract *A. M. Hoare C. F. Hawkins*	96
6. The Use and Abuse of Laxatives *John H. Cummings*	124
7. Alcohol and the Gastrointestinal Tract *N. A. G. Mowat P. W. Brunt*	150
8. Endoscopic Cannulation of the Papilla of Vater. Clinical and Research Developments *Peter B. Cotton*	178
9. Clinical Aspects of Bile Acid Metabolism *K. W. Heaton*	199
10. Shunts for Hepatic Disease *Ronald A. Malt*	231
11. Liver Disease in Infants and Children *Alex P. Mowat*	261
12. Cystic Fibrosis of the Pancreas *Charlotte M. Anderson*	297
Index	335

1
PHYSIOLOGY OF THE GASTRO-OESOPHAGEAL JUNCTION AND HIATUS HERNIA

William H. Lipshutz

This chapter reviews current understanding of oesophageal physiology and pathophysiology in an attempt to provide a rational basis for the diagnosis and treatment of common disorders of the oesophagus. A complete discussion of the importance of hiatus hernia in the production of gastro-oesophageal reflux, aided by a descriptive section of the anatomy of the gastro-oesophageal junction, will allow the reader to make his own decision about this problem. The lower oesophageal sphincter is discussed in detail and all current systems for the control of this area are included. Controversial issues and viewpoints are set forth so that the reader can be informed about the current controversy in this area. The medical and surgical treatment of gastro-oesophageal reflux is considered with a background of laboratory and human experimentation, so that the reader will have a sound physiological basis for the treatment of this disorder. Neuromuscular disorders of the oesophagus are discussed giving special attention to new drugs used in their treatment.

THE ANATOMICAL CONFIGURATION OF THE GASTRO-OESOPHAGEAL JUNCTION

There is general disagreement over the precise definition of the gastro-oesophageal junction and the surrounding anatomical structures which might contribute to the barrier preventing reflux (Jackson, 1922; Lerche, 1950; Sanchez, Kramer and Ingelfinger, 1953; Carey and Hollinshead, 1955; Fyke, Code and Schlegel, 1956; Lyons, Ellis and Olsen, 1956; Nauta, 1956; Atkinson et al, 1957; Botha, 1962; Code et al, 1958; Ingelfinger, 1958; Listerud and Harkins, 1958; Vantrappen et al, 1960; Edwards, 1967. The most frequently proposed definitions of the gastro-oesophageal junction are: (1) the junction of squamous and columnar epithelium; (2) the point at which the tubular oesophagus enters the dilated stomach; (3) the junction between the inner oesophageal muscle layer and the inner layer of gastric musculature, the oblique or sling fibres (Skinner, 1972).

The squamo-columnar junction represents the point at which peptic oesophagitis and stricture begin and it can be defined in normals by direct vision and oesophagoscopic biopsy. However, in diseased states its location is variable and carefully performed anatomic and histological studies by Lerche (1950) reveal that the distal end of the human oesophagus is lined by a columnar non-acid-secreting mucosa. Thus both therapeutic and diagnostic decisions based upon this definition of the gastro-oesophageal junction are subject to error.

The junction of the tubular oesophagus with the dilated stomach is easily visualised at necropsy, surgery, and by barium x-ray. However, this precise landmark is often difficult to define in patients with disease in this location which accounts for much of the disagreement over the presence and incidence of hiatus hernia. The junction between the inner layer of oesophageal muscle and the gastric sling fibers can be seen upon careful anatomic dissection, but in clinical practice this landmark is obscured in patients with hiatus hernia, oesophagitis and stricture of the oesophagus (Skinner, 1972).

Because of the difficulties encountered with the anatomic definition of the gastro-oesophagel junction recent studies employing physiological techniques have proposed that the lower oesophageal sphincter is the division between oesophagus and stomach. This definition of the junction albeit physiological and not anatomical allows a reproducible and clinically useful guide to study this area in both health and disease.

IMPORTANCE OF THE ANATOMICAL STRUCTURES SURROUNDING THE GASTRO-OESOPHAGEAL JUNCTION

Contraction of the diaphragmatic crura serving as a pinchcock on the oesophagus as it passes through the hiatus has been defined as a mechanism for the barrier to reflux (Jackson, 1922). However, this area is only appreciated during deep breathing, is not present during quiet respiration, and the surgical creation of a hiatus hernia in dogs with obliteration of this pinchcock mechanism fails to produce gastro-oesophageal reflux, oesophagitis or to diminish the high pressure zone in the lower end of the oesophagus (Hendrix, 1972).

The flap valve created by the oblique angle of entry of the oesophagus into the stomach is considered by some to be important in the control of gastro-oesophageal reflux (Barrett, 1954; Collis, Kelly and Wiley, 1954). It is claimed that this angle which is created by the diaphragmatic crura and the oblique muscle fibres of the cardia occludes the oesophageal lumen and thereby prevents reflux. The validity of this mechanism as a barrier to reflx can be questioned by the examination of patients who have hiatus hernia with loss of this angle and who have no evidence of reflux; and secondly by the many patients with a normal anatomical gastro-oesophageal junction and free reflux. Finally surgical elimination of this angle does not result in gastro-oesophageal reflux in animal models. (Hendrix, 1972).

The phreno-oesophageal membrane has also been thought to contribute to the barrier to reflux at the junction of oesophagus and stomach (Bombeck, Dillard and Nyhus, 1966). However, surgical experience with this structure indicates that it is not always present and when found is often of variable thickness. Animal studies with division of the membrane failed to produce alteration in sphincter pressure or any gastro-oesophageal reflux (Bremner, Schlegel and Ellis, 1970). Only those experiments in which the distal oesophagus or the oesophago-gastric junction or both was resected did functional incompetence of the sphincter mechanism develop (Ellis et al, 1967). These studies employed surgical techniques which obliterated the anatomical structures surrounding the gastro-oesophageal barrier but failed to produce gastro-oesophageal reflux, and they must cast serious doubt about the importance of these structures. Thus investigation began to focus upon the intrinsic lower oesophageal sphincter.

WHAT IS THE IMPORTANCE OF A CENTRAL SLIDING HIATUS HERNIA IN THE PRODUCTION OF GASTRO-OESOPHAGEAL REFLUX?

For many years the medical and lay community have been convinced that a central sliding hiatus hernia is a specific gastrointestinal disease. The most common symptoms ascribed to the hiatus hernia are those of gastro-oesophageal reflux; pyrosis, waterbrash, and the free reflux of gastric content into the mouth especially when supine or bending over after a hearty meal. Recently the claim that a hiatus hernia is the cause for gastro-oesophageal reflux has been challenged. Carefully controlled studies have shown that the presence of a hiatus hernia has little relation to the symptoms of reflux (Cohen and Harris, 1970; Cohen and Harris, 1971). Most studies now report that the symptoms of reflux are related to diminished lower oesophageal sphincter (LES) pressure irrespective of the presence or absence of a hiatus hernia (Wankling, Warrian and Lind, 1965; Winans and Harris, 1967; Pope, 1967; Haddad, 1970). The symptoms of reflux, and the endoscopic and histological changes of reflux correlate with diminished LES pressure and strength (Haddad, 1970; Ismail-Beigi, Horton and Pope, 1970). Asymptomatic patients with a large hiatus hernia have normal sphincter function under resting conditions and in response to increased intra-abdominal pressure. Conversely, patients with symptoms of gastro-oesophageal reflux and no demonstrable hiatus hernia have diminished LES pressure and strength (Cohen and Harris, 1970; Cohen and Harris, 1971). Recent evidence suggests therefore that the strength of the physiological LES is the major barrier to reflux of gastric content at the gastro-oesophageal junction and that the hiatus hernia itself is not responsible for either the symptoms or complications of any reflux of gastric contents into the gullet.

QUANTIFICATION OF THE BARRIER TO GASTRO-OESOPHAGEAL REFLUX: THE LOWER OESOPHAGEAL SPHINCTER

At the distal end of the human oesophagus is a zone of elevated pressure (2–5 cm in length) with a mean midrespiratory pressure (12–30 mmHg above gastric fundal pressure) that relaxes upon deglutition and oesophageal distension thereby permitting material to enter the stomach. In contrast to this tonically contracted sphincteric area the oesophageal body is relaxed under basal conditions and contracts in an orderly progressive peristaltic manner in response to swallowing or oesophageal distension (Fyke et al, 1956). This disparity between the body of the oesophagus and the high pressure zone at its distal end is evidence for a physiological sphincteric mechanism.

The major problem with the universal acceptance of the LES has been our inability to define it anatomically in man (Allison, 1951; Higgs, Kerr and Ellis, 1965). There is no discrete muscle mass at the distal end of the human oesophagus. However, physiological studies employing infused intraluminal catheters can consistently measure a zone of elevated pressure between oesophagus and stomach. Modernisation of the previous techniques of balloons and open tipped uninfused catheters with infused catheters and sensitive terminal transducers have made it possible to study accurately LES pressures and to differentiate normals from patients with gastro-oesophageal reflux (Winans and Harris, 1967; Pope, 1967; Haddad, 1970). Infused intraluminal manometry has been shown to measure pressures which correlate excellently with an objective measurement of sphincter strength (Cohen and Harris, 1970).

To further evaluate the LES high pressure zone divorced from the anatomical structures surrounding the LES studies were performed in vitro in a suitable animal model, the opossum. Circular smooth muscle strips obtained from the manometrically defined LES and the adjacent oesophagus and stomach were studied in baths of Krebs–Ringer solution. The isometric contraction in response to passive stretch and to active stimulation by neural and humoral agonists was evaluated. The results of these investigations revealed that the LES muscle responds to adrenergic and cholinergic agonists at a lower threshold dose. The muscle in this area develops a much greater peak active tension than does muscle from the adjacent oesophagus and stomach (Christensen, 1970; Lipshutz and Cohen, 1971). LES muscle response to gastrin I was marked by an exquisite sensitivity and greater peak tension than muscle from adjacent oesophagus and stomach (Lipshutz and Cohen, 1971). Mechanical characteristics of sphincteric smooth muscle also differed from adjacent oesophagus and stomach by showing a greater tension in response to passive stretch (Lipshutz and Cohen, 1971; Christensen, Freeman and Miller, 1973a; Christensen, Conklin and Freeman, 1973b).

Other in vitro studies on the LES muscle have shown that it has a specific response to electrical stimulation. Electrical stimulation applied during tonic contraction induced by cholinergic stimulation produces relaxation in the LES circular smooth muscle and contraction in adjacent oesophageal and gastric muscle (Christensen et al, 1973b; Tuch and Cohen, 1973). This data provides strong evidence that the specialised muscle comprising the distal end of the oesophagus contributes in a major way to the function of the LES in vivo. We now understand that part if not all of the LES is due to the neural and neurohumoral stimuli acting upon this specialised smooth muscle segment at the distal end of the oesophagus.

CONTROL OF THE LOWER OESOPHAGEAL SPHINCTER STRENGTH: ADAPTIVE RESPONSE TO INCREASED INTRA-ABDOMINAL PRESSURE

Oesophageal manometric studies performed with infused intraluminal catheters have shown that the LES pressure in normal subjects and is increased above intragastric pressure in response to stimuli which increase intra-abdominal pressure (Lind, Warrian and Wankling, 1966; Cohen and Harris, 1971). This increase in LES pressure above intragastric pressure is dependent upon the resting LES pressure. Asymptomatic subjects with or without a hiatus hernia who have normal resting LES pressures can generate a change in LES pressure which is approximately twice as great as the change in gastric pressure in response to increased intra-abdominal pressure produced by straight leg raising or inflation of an abdominal binder. The ratio of the change in LES pressure (ΔS) over the change in gastric pressure (ΔG) in patients with normal sphincters is 2. It is an adaptive mechanism of the sphincter to prevent the reflux of gastric content into the oesophagus during periods of increased intra-abdominal pressure. Patients with symptoms of gastro-oesophageal reflux who have diminished resting LES pressures also have abnormal LES responses to increased intra-abdominal pressure and markedly affected individuals will frequently develop gastric pressures that exceed LES pressure in response to straight leg raising. The $\Delta S/\Delta G$ ratio will be <1. This adaptive response of the LES can be obliterated by the intravenous injection of atropine sulphate (Lind, Crispin and McIver, 1968) and some reports indicate a diminished response following truncal vagotomy (Lind et al, 1969).

It is thought at present that this adaptive response of the LES to increased intra-abdominal pressure is a vago-vagal reflex with afferents arising in the gastric wall and efferents in the vagus nerve. However, Dodds et al (1975) employing similar methods in humans reported different results for they observed sphincter augmentation only in response to straight leg raising but not in response to inflation of an abdominal binder or during the Valsalva manoeuvre. In addition these investigators failed to show that atropine inhibits LES response to increased intra-abdominal pressure. Thus it will be evident that at present the mechanism of the sphincteric response to abdominal compression is not fully understood and further clinical experimentation is needed.

NEURAL CONTROL OF THE LOWER OESOPHAGEAL SPHINCTER

Division of the vagus nerves at the level of the gastro-oesophageal junction in dogs results in a significant decrease in resting LES pressure and in the sphincter response to abdominal compression allowing free reflux to occur (Lind et al, 1969). Transabdominal vagotomy in man (Blackman, Nasrullah and Thayer, 1971; Mazur et al, 1973; Mann and Hardcastle, 1968) and cervical vagotomy in the opossum (Christensen et al, 1973a; Rattan and Goyal, 1974) do not affect resting LES pressure. Electrical stimulation of the peripheral end of the transected cervical vagus nerve in the opossum produces sphincter relaxation, evidence for an inhibitory efferent pathway mediating sphincteric relaxation. Stimulation of the central end of the transected vagus results in sphincter contraction suggesting an afferent vagal pathway which mediates LES contraction (Rattan and Goyal, 1974). Pharmacological doses of the parasympathomimetic drug Urecholine (Bethanechol) produce significant increases in resting LES pressure in man (Roling, Farrell, Castell, 1972). This drug works directly on the muscle membrane and it is a congener of acetylcholine, the postganglionic cholinergic neural transmitter. Atropine, a muscarinic blocking drug reduces resting LES pressure (Lind et al, 1968) and diminishes the LES response to exogenous gastrin and Urecholine, endogenous gastrin release and to increased intra-abdominal pressure (Cohen and Lipshutz, 1970). Studies in vitro on LES circular smooth muscle indicate that acetylcholine produces a dose dependent increase in smooth muscle contraction (Christensen and Daniel, 1968; Lipshutz and Cohen, 1971). Although studies in vivo in animals and in vitro on LES smooth muscle indicate that cholinergic stimuli increase LES contractile response, the exact role of the cholinergic nervous system in the control of human LES function awaits further studies.

There is evidence that the adrenergic nervous system influences LES pressure. Alpha-adrenergic agonists contract LES circular smooth muscle in the cat and opossum (Christensen and Daniel, 1968; Lipshutz and Cohen, 1971). This contractile response is inhibited by specific alpha-adrenergic antagonists. Alpha-adrenergic stimulants produce an increase in LES pressure in the intact opossum that is inhibited by specific alpha-blocking drugs (DiMarino and Cohen, 1973). The alpha-adrenergic blocking drug phentolamine produced a mean reduction in resting LES pressure of 38.4 per cent in the anaesthetised opossum. Adrenergic denervation produced by 6-hydroxydopamine reduced basal LES pressure by 22.5 per cent in this animal model (DiMarino and Cohen, 1973). Beta-adrenergic agonists fail to contract

LES circular smooth muscle in vitro (Christensen, 1970; Lipshutz and Cohen, 1971) and diminish resting LES pressure in vivo. Only limited studies on the adrenergic control of human LES function have been reported and they confirm that beta-adrenergic agonists decrease human LES pressure (Zfass et al, 1970).

LOWER OESOPHAGEAL SPHINCTER RELAXATION

The ability of the tonically contracted high pressure zone at the distal end of the oesophagus to relax upon deglutition and oesophageal distension remained unexplained until recently. It has been shown that bilateral vagotomy in the opossum (Christensen et al, 1973b) truncal vagotomy in man (Blackman et al, 1971) and the vagolytic drug, atropine (Cohen and Lipshutz, 1970) do not effect relaxation of the LES. Alpha-adrenergic antagonists, adrenergic denervation, and beta-adrenergic stimulants do not affect sphincter relaxation (DiMarino and Cohen, 1973). These findings indicate that LES relaxation is mediated by neither adrenergic nor cholinergic stimuli. Studies in vitro on LES circular smooth muscles indicate that the inhibition produced by electrical stimulation of tonically contracted LES muscle is neurogenic (Tuch and Cohen, 1973). Inhibition in other areas of the gastrointestinal tract has been shown recently to be due to a specialised group of nerves that release purine compounds. Adenosine triphosphate or a related purine compound is the proposed chemical that is released from these purinergic nerve endings (Burnstock, 1972). Prostaglandin E_1 can cause relaxation of the LES in the opossum. The proposed mechanism for its action is the intracellular accumulation of cyclic AMP. Preliminary studies indicated that prostaglandin E_1-induced LES relaxation was not altered by neural antagonists, suggesting a direct action on the muscle. Isoproterenol and theophylline agents that work through increased cyclic AMP (isoproterenol increases synthesis and theophylline decreases degradation of cyclic AMP) mimic the action of prostaglandin E_1 on LES relaxation (Goyal and Rattan, 1973). The importance of the purinergic nervous system on LES relaxation in man awaits future investigation.

HORMONAL CONTROL OF THE LOWER OESOPHAGEAL SPHINCTER

Giles et al (1969) Castell and Harris (1970) reported that exogenous gastrin (hog or synthetic) and synthetic gastric pentapeptide (pentagastrin) increased LES pressure in man. It was shown subsequently in man that acidification of the gastric antrum decreases resting LES pressure and alkalinisation of the gastric antrum increases resting LES pressure. These observations were considered to indicate that there had been an alteration of endogenous gastrin release: acidification of the antrum decreasing gastrin release and alkalinisation of the antrum increasing gastrin release (Cohen and Lipshutz, 1971a). Further studies in man using exogenous intravenous synthetic gastrin I (Cohen and Lipshutz, 1971) and synthetic pentagastrin (pentapeptide amide) (Nebel and Castell, 1973) have reported full dose-response curves of LES pressure to these agonists.

Secretin was also shown to affect LES function in man. Low doses of exogenous intravenous pure natural secretin markedly inhibit the elevated LES pressure in man following stimulation by endogenous gastrin produced by antral alkalinisation (Cohen and Lipshutz, 1971a). However, only large pharmacological doses of secretin inhibited resting LES pressure in man. Secretin was also shown to competitively antagonise the action of gastrin on the LES in man. These studies indicate that exogenous gastrin, or the endogenous release of gastrin, increases LES pressure in man. Exogenous secretin or endogenously released secretin appears able to affect LES pressure by bringing the elevated gastrin stimulated sphincter pressure back to normal resting levels. These in vivo human studies were supported further by animal experiments both in vivo and in vitro. The potency of gastrin (molar concentration producing 50 per cent response) on LES circular smooth muscle in vitro was shown to be 10^7 times greater than the recognised neural transmitters acetylcholine and norephinephrine (Lipshutz and Cohen, 1971). Furthermore the action of gastrin on LES circular smooth muscle was specific for this area of the gastrointestinal tract.

Further evidence for the role of gastrin in the genesis of resting LES pressure came from studies on the opossum. Employing a gastrin-specific antiserum Lipshutz, Hughes and Cohen (1972) reported that the LES circular muscle response to gastrin in vitro could be antagonised specifically by the antiserum; and that the LES response to endogenous release and to exogenous administration of gastrin in vivo was diminished as was the resting LES pressure.

Recently, however, controversy has arisen regarding the physiological importance of gastrin in the control of LES function in man. The serum level of gastrin following intravenous and subcutaneous pulse doses of gastrin which increase human LES pressure, result in circulating gastrin levels far in excess of that found under physiologic conditions (Grossman, 1973). In addition recent reports fail to show a relationship between serum gastrin levels measured by radioimmunoassay and LES pressures during gastric acidification and alkalinisation (Hoke, et al, 1972; Rogers, Rothman and Arostegui, 1974). However, more recent studies have shown that both serum gastrin and LES pressure increase in the proper time relation following a protein meal in normal human subjects (Nebel and Castell, 1972; Farrell, Castell and McGuigan, 1974). In addition, continuous intravenous infusion of gastrin I at rates which produce serum levels similar to those following a protein meal produce submaximal increases in gastric acid output and significant increases in human LES pressure (Freeland et al, 1975).

This controversy over the physiological role of gastrin in the control of LES function in man is not resolved at present.

Other gastrointestinal hormones have been shown to alter LES function. Cholecystokinin and its synthetic octapeptide decrease resting LES pressure and competitively antagonise the sphincter response to gastrin (Resin et al,

Table 1.1 Factors causing an increase in lower oesophageal sphincter (LES) pressure

Drugs
1. Cholinergics (acetylcholine, urecholine, etc.)
2. Cholinesterase inhibitors (tensilon, physostigmine)
3. Metaclopramide (direct action)
4. Antacids (gastrin release?, local reflex?)
5. Adrenergic alpha stimulators

Hormones
Gastrin

Food
Protein

Surgery
1. Creation of a flap valve?
2. Reconstitution of LES?

Table 1.2 Factors causing a decrease in lower oesophageal sphincter (LES) pressure

Drugs
1. Anticholinergics
2. Beta-adrenergic stimulators
3. Prostaglandins E_1, E_2, A_2
4. Theophylline
5. Gastric acidification
6. Gastrin antiserum

Hormones
1. Secretin
2. Cholecystokinin
3. Glucagon

Foods
1. Chocolate (methylzanthines)
2. Coffee? (methylzanthines)
3. Fat (cholecystokinin release)
4. Smoking
5. Ethanol

1973; Sturdevant and Kun, 1974; Fisher, DiMarino and Cohen, 1974). Glucagon also decreases resting LES pressure and antagonises the LES response to gastrin (Jennewein et al, 1973; Jaffer et al, 1974). The full importance of these hormonal actions on the control of human LES function remains to be determined.

The agents that increase and decrease LES tone are shown in Tables 1.1

and 1.2 and a schematic representation for the current control of LES function is shown in Figure. 1.1.

CLINICAL EVALUATION AND MEDICAL TREATMENT OF GASTRO-OESOPHAGEAL REFLUX

The patient suffering from gastro-oesophageal reflux will usually experience retrosternal burning pain, travelling orad and accompanied by a sour or bitter regurgitation of gastric content into the mouth. The symptoms are usually made worse by bending over or reclining after a large meal (Winans and Harris, 1967; Edwards, 1973). Some patients complain of nocturnal cough and hoarseness due to aspiration of small amounts of gastric contents during sleep.

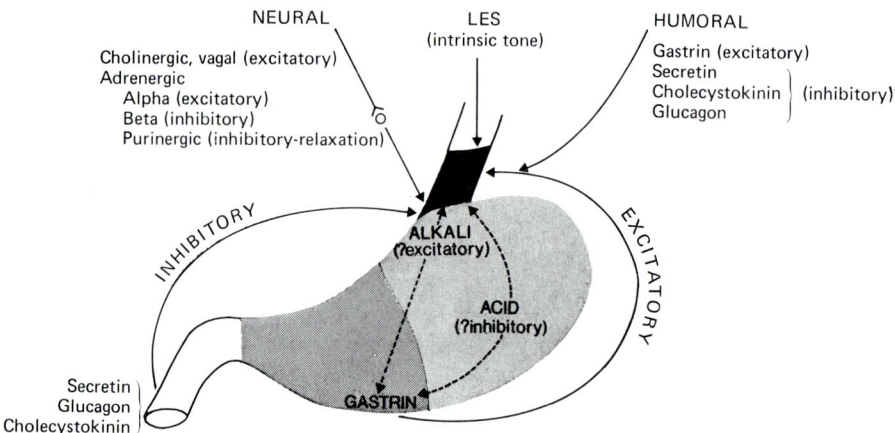

Figure 1.1 Control of the lower oesophageal sphincter (LES)

Pulmonary disease such as aspiration pneumonitis and lung abscess are recognised complications of severe reflux (Urschel and Paulson, 1967; Belsey, 1960). Following prolonged episodes of oesophageal inflammation, a stricture of the oesophagus can develop with consequent alterations of symptoms. Such patients usually complain of dysphagia for solids which can progress to involve liquids as well. Ultimately oropharyngeal secretions will not enter the stomach causing the patient to expectorate continuously. With the onset and progression of an oesophageal stricture patients loose weight, become anorexic and appear to be suffering from carcinoma of the oesophagus. During periods of acute oesophageal inflammation secondary to reflux the patient might complain of chest pain that is not unlike that of coronary artery disease (Bennett and Atkinson, 1966). The retrosternal tightness with radiation to the back and down the arms is usually due to associated oesophageal spasm secondary to the corrosive gastric content bathing the distal oesophagus.

The medical treatment and investigation of the patient suffering from gastro-oesophageal reflux depends upon the stage of the disease. The patient who experiences periodic heartburn can be managed easily by taking 15 to 30 ml of commercially available liquid antacids after meals and before bedtime and proper positional and dietary manipulation. These patients should be instructed to loose excess weight, to avoid bending, stooping and reclining after meals, and to sleep with the head of the bed elevated. This latter manoeuvre can be accomplished easily by placing 4 to 6 in. blocks under the feet of the head of the bed. The use of pillows or bolsters actually puts the patient at a disadvantage because of the increased intra-abdominal pressure which will be produced. The use of antacids in the treatment of gastro-oesophageal reflux serves two important purposes. Firstly, they neutralise the acid which has refluxed into the distal oesophagus; secondly antacids have been shown to increase LES pressure (Castell and Harris, 1970; Castell and Levine, 1971). The mechanism for this increase in LES pressure is not fully understood. It was thought that gastrin, released from the gastric antrum in response to the increased intragastric pH was responsible (Castell and Harris, 1970), but recent studies using a gastrin radioimmunoassay do not show measurable increases in serum gastrin following antacid therapy (Rogers et al, 1974; Higgs, Smith and Castell, 1974). Thus the exact mechanism for the increased LES pressure following antacid therapy has not been defined.

The next step in the medical treatment of pyrosis is to alert the patient about the various foods and drugs which may make the symptoms of reflux worse. Excessive fat in the diet is potentially harmful. Experimental studies in humans have shown that fat is capable of significantly decreasing LES pressure (Nebel and Castell, 1973). The proposed mechanism for this decrease in LES pressure is the endogenous release of cholecystokinin (CCK) produced by the presence of fat on the duodenal mucosa. CCK diminishes resting LES pressure and competitively inhibits the action of gastrin on the LES in man (Resin et al, 1973; Sturdevent and Kun, 1974). Other foods which might be harmful to the patient with reflux are chocolates and coffee. They contain methylxanthine which decreases LES pressure in man and in animal models (Nebel and Castell, 1972; Dennish and Castell, 1972). The proposed mechanism for the methylxanthine decrease in LES pressure is by the accumulation of cyclic AMP consequent upon the action of methylxanthine to inhibit the phosphodiestase enzyme system which metabolises cyclic AMP to 5'-AMP (Goyal and Rattan, 1973). Studies in humans have produced variable results. Earlier studies showed that coffee can inhibit human LES pressure (Dennish and Castell, 1972). A recent publication showed the reverse effect (Cohen and Booth, 1975) and indicated that coffee and decaffinated coffee increased human LES pressure.

Cigarette smoking also affects human LES pressure. Soon after the smoking of one or two cigarettes LES pressure falls precipitiously (Dennish and Castell, 1971). Anticholinergic drugs markedly diminish human LES pressure and can produce the symptoms of reflux in a patient with borderline LES function (Kantrowitz et al, 1960; Lind et al, 1968; Bettarello, Tuttle and Grossman, 1960). Ethanol has also been shown to diminish LES pressure in man (Hogan, Viegas De Andrade and Winship, 1972). Ulcerogenic drugs such as salicylates should be avoided.

The introduction of these dietary manipulations, the avoidance of potentially harmful food and drugs, and the liberal use of liquid antacids will render most patients asymptomatic within a few days.

The patient whose symptoms does not respond to this initial approach requires additional diagnostic and therapeutic procedures. Failure to respond to the initial therapeutic measures suggests either a mistaken diagnosis or a serious complication of gastro-oesophageal reflux. At this time barium x-ray, endoscopic and manometric studies might be in order. The use of the barium meal is not to look for the presence or absence of a hiatus hernia for it has been argued that a hernia by itself has little relation to the symptoms of reflux (Wankling et al, 1965; Cohen and Harris, 1971). The value of the barium study is to look for the reflux of barium from stomach to oesophagus, and to diagnose complication of reflux such as destroyed distal oesophageal mucosa, oesophageal ulceration and stricture. The observations of free gastro-oesophageal reflux, without procedures that increase intra-abdominal pressure, usually indicates a markedly incompetent LES. It is known, however, that the absence of reflux at the barium meal does in no way rule out the fact that reflux is occurring, since the x-ray is an insensitive method for the detection of gastro-oesophageal reflux (Pope, 1972). Another advantage to the barium upper gastrointestinal series is to look for other conditions which might produce symptoms of reflux such as peptic ulcer or neoplasm of oesophagus or stomach. Further refinement of radiographic techniques such as careful evaluation of swallowing by cine photography might detect reflux missed by the conventional barium studies and provide information about oesophageal peristalsis (Battle, Nyus and Bombeck, 1973). The use of abdominal compression with the patient lying in the Trendelenburg position will at times disclose reflux from stomach to oesophagus. The water siphonage test (Donner and Margulies, 1972) is probably too sensitive to detect reflux. LES relaxation during swallowing allows barium to move from stomach to oesophagus especially when the abdomen is manually compressed.

Upper gastrointestinal endoscopy with modern flexible fibreoptic instruments has provided a rapid and effective way of assessing the entire oesophagus, stomach, and duodenum with little patient discomfort (see Chapter 8). The oesophageal mucosa can be assessed directly for the presence of oesophagitis, ulceration and stricture (Akdamar et al, 1973). Oesophageal biopsy can be obtained under direct vision. Recent histological studies have shown that the pathological changes of reflux can be present even when the oesophageal mucosa appears normal under direct vision. (Ismail-Beigi et al, 1970).

Oesophageal manometry and pH reflux testing have been accepted universally as the most precise diagnostic methods available to assess oesophageal function. Previous techniques that employed balloons and uninfused catheters which over- or under-estimated true sphincter pressure, have now been replaced by infused catheters and sensitive terminal transducers (Winans and Harris, 1967; Pope, 1967; Haddad, 1970; Stef et al, 1974). LES pressure measured with infused catheters has been shown to be an accurate measurement of sphincter strength in vivo and in vitro (Pope, 1967; Cohen and Harris, 1970).

Recent studies indicate that conventional recording tubes, with three separate side orifices each at a different level, should be replaced by a tube having several recording apertures at the same radial level (Kaye and Showalter, 1971; Winans, 1972). These authors contend that the variation in human LES pressure between the conventional three recording orifices is due to the asymmetric way in which the oesophagus contracts. More than one orifice at each level arranged in a radial distribution would be able to detect the true pressure at each level and this problem of variability in sphincter pressure would be solved. The recent introduction of sensitive miniature transducers incorporated into recording tubes obviates the need for infusion pumps and external transducers and appears to measure the full range of oesophageal propulsive force (Stef et al, 1974; Hollis and Castell, 1972).

Most studies report that patients with symptoms of gastro-oesophageal reflux have diminished LES pressure. The normal mean LES pressure in most clinical laboratories is 15 mmHg (range 12–30 mmHg). Those patients with severe symptoms of gastro-oesophageal reflux have markedly diminished LES pressure (<5 mmHg) (Winans and Harris, 1967; Pope, 1967; Haddad, 1970; Cohen and Harris, 1971).

LES pressure, however, is an indirect method for the detection of gastro-oesophageal reflux. For this reason, procedures employing the instillation of 0.1 N-HCl have been devised. The first of these was the Bernstein acid perfusion test (Bernstein and Baker, 1958). This test should be performed in a double blind manner with the intra-oesophageal infusion of 0.1 N-HCl alternating with normal saline. If the symptoms of pyrosis and waterbrash are produced by HCl and not saline, and if the symptoms produced by HCl infusion mimic the patient's pain, then reflux is the proposed cause for the patient's symptoms. This test is best employed on patients who have chest pain of obscure aetiology. Some normal subjects will experience pyrosis during acid infusion and these can have normal LES function and no symptoms of gastro-oesophageal reflux. In addition a positive Bernstein test does not mean that the patient will have endoscopic or biopsy evidence of oesophagitis. Therefore, the acid infusion test gives information only about the sensitivity of the oesophagus to acid.

The acid reflux test (Tuttle and Grossman, 1958) employs a pH probe positioned 4 cm proximal to the manometrically defined LES. Following intragastric infusion of 0.1 N-HCl and the application of positive abdominal pressure, a drop in intra-oesophageal pH below 4 indicates a positive test. One variation of this test is to pull a pH probe from the stomach orad following gastric infusion of 0.1 N-HCl. The number of swallows required to raise the intra-oesophageal pH above 4 at a level 4 cm proximal to the LES is recorded. It should normally take 4 to 10 swallows to raise intra-oesophageal pH above 4 (Booth, Kemmer and Skinner, 1968).

The most recent attempt to provide a standardised easily performed test to detect gastro-oesophageal reflux employs radioactive scanning of the oesophagus following the ingestion of a radioactive test substance. This test obviates the need for nasogastric intubation and can be performed without patient discomfort. The authors' report that the radiation hazard is no greater than that following conventional liver or brain scanning (Fisher et al, 1975).

The multiplicity of diagnostic tests available to detect gastro-oesophageal reflux attests to the need for a simple, reliable, easily performed method for evaluating reflux.

The patient with symptomatic gastro-oesophageal reflux, proved by any one of the previously described tests, who does not respond to antacid, dietary and positional therapy, may benefit from additional pharmacotherapy. Bethanechol (urecholine), a postganglionic cholinergic drug, which works directly on the muscle membrane has been shown in a random double-blind study to reduce reflux symptoms and to lessen the need for antacid therapy. Bethanechol is beneficial for the patient with symptomatic reflux because it increases LES pressure and increases oesophageal propulsive force (Farrell, Roling and Castell, 1974). This drug also increases LES in man following vagotomy and antrectomy suggesting a further role in the treatment of bile reflux oesophagitis (Higgs and Castell, 1975). Metoclopramide employed orally or subcutaneously has also been shown to increase LES pressure and to accelerate the rate of emptying of acid infused into the oesophagus (Heitmann and Moller, 1970; Stanciu and Bennett, 1973; Dilawari and Misiewicz, 1973; McCallum et al, 1974). Controlled clinical trials with the use of placebo are needed to further assess the role of this drug.

Those patients whose symptoms do not respond to any of the above therapy or who develop a complication of reflux such as oesophageal ulceration, stricture or haemorrhage are candidates for surgical therapy.

SURGICAL TREATMENT OF GASTRO-OESOPHAGEAL REFLUX

In the early part of this century surgery enjoyed great popularity as the treatment of choice for hiatus hernia. Harrington (1928) reported the experience at the Mayo Clinic and was the first author to stimulate interest in surgery for hiatus hernia. His work covered all types of hiatus hernia and was concerned with the anatomical reconstruction of the hiatus. Allison (1951) clearly established that gastro-oesophageal reflux was the cause of symptoms in patients with hiatus hernia. He emphasised correction of the defect at the cardia as a proper mode of treatment for this disorder. Unfortunately the results of these operations for hiatus hernia were followed by an unacceptably high incidence of anatomical and clinical recurrence (Woodward, Thomas and McAlhany, 1971). It was soon appreciated that correction of the anatomical defect at the cardia was an unsatisfactory approach to the problem of reflux and surgical intervention for this disorder fell into disrepute.

Improved understanding of the physiology of the gastro-oesophageal region and the importance of the lower oesophageal sphincter enabled surgical treatment to play a new role in the management of this disorder. The creation of an intra-abdominal segment of oesophagus, first proposed by Collis et al (1954) and Boerema and Germs (1955) in addition to anatomical repair of the cardia produced better clinical and anatomical results in patients with reflux and hiatux hernia. The use of the stomach wrapped around the intra-abdominal segment of oesophagus was popularised in 1955 by Nissen in Switzerland and Belsey in England.

The present physiological data indicate quite conclusively that the LES is the major barrier to reflux at the gastro-oesophageal junction, and the newer methods of surgical treatment for reflux attempts to restore this barrier. Attention has drifted away from the mere anatomical correction of the patulous hiatus and is directed towards the establishment of a competent valve mechanism at the junction of oesophagus with stomach. We now recognise that patients can suffer from severe reflux and all its complications in the absence of a demonstrable hiatus hernia.

The three major operations in use today are: the Belsey Mark IV transthoracic repair (Skinner and Belsey, 1967), the Nissen transabdominal fundoplication (Nissen, 1961), and the Hill posterior gastropexy (Hill, 1967). The goals of these procedures are: reduction of the hernia if present, and calibration of the cardia; creation of an intra-abdominal segment of oesophagus exposed to positive intra-abdominal pressure; and suture of the stomach around the intra-abdominal oesophagus, which is then sutured to the pre-aortic fascia (Hill repair) or the under-surface of the diaphragm (Belsey repair). The Nissen fundoplication involves a 360° wrap of the stomach around the oesophagus whereas the Hill and Belsey repairs employ a wrap of 180°.

Many studies have appeared on the follow-up of patients who have undergone these operations and they have reported clinical, radiographic, endoscopic and manometric improvement. Csendes and Larrain (1972) reported that clinical and radiographic improvement after the Hill gastropexy was related to an increase in LES pressure from 3.5 mmHg before to 12.5 mmHg after operation. Moran, Pihl and Norton (1971) found an increase in LES pressure from 9.4 to 16.5 mmHg after the Nissen and Belsey repairs. Hill (1967) stated that 95 per cent of surgical repairs were followed by a return of resting LES pressures to normal levels. Other workers have also shown not only an increase in LES pressure postoperatively, but also a decrease in reflux by pH reflux testing (Pope, Eastwood and Eastwood, 1973; Moran et al, 1971; McAlhany, Thomas and Woodward, 1972).

The surgical treatment of choice for oesophageal stricture secondary to reflux oesophagitis (Collis, 1963; Thal, 1968) is still not agreed upon. Some authors advocate resection of the stricture with oesophagogastric anastomosis in the chest (Weaver, Large and Walt, 1970). This is a formidable operation with a high operative morbidity and mortality. Other authors feel that oesophageal resection with colon interposition is the treatment of choice (Belsey, 1965). Several recent reports (Larrain, Csendes and Pope, 1975; Hill et al, 1970) indicate that surgical correction of reflux by posterior gastropexy and cardiac calibration relieves dysphagia, corrects the reflux, and cures the strictures without dilitation.

Most surgical studies report good to excellent results in 85 to 90 per cent of patients (Woodward et al, 1971; Bave and Belsey, 1967; Skinner and Belsey, 1967; Hill, 1967). The more recent studies report not only clinical results, but also employ sophisticated manometric and reflux testing which indicate that clinical improvement is associated with manometric and radiographic improvement. Using the most sensitive technique available for showing reflux, pH reflux testing, it is possible to demonstrate that gastro-oesophageal reflux is diminished following operation (McAlhany et al, 1972; Pope et al, 1973; Moran et al, 1971).

In a recent study comparing the medical and surgical treatment of gastro-oesophageal reflux Behar et al (1975) found that 73 per cent of the surgical group (posterior gastropexy or anterior fundoplication) enjoyed good to excellent results as compared to 19 per cent of the medical group. Clinical improvement was positively correlated with normal acid infusion tests, normal oesophagoscopy and return of LES pressure to normal. The only problem with this study was that not enough antacid was given to the medical group, and Bethanechol and Metoclopramide, drugs which increase LES pressure and decrease gastroesophageal reflux, were not used.

The mechanism whereby surgery produces increased LES pressure is still unanswered. The postoperative increase in LES pressure is greater than that attributable by the sphincter pressure and intra-abdominal pressure (Behar et al, 1974). Resting LES pressure is not only normalised postoperatively but LES response to gastrin and tensilon is also improved (Lipshutz et al, 1974; Farrell, Higgs and Castell, 1974).

At present surgery appears to be indicated for the patient who has severe symptomatic gastro-oesophageal reflux and its complications and is unresponsive to intensive medical therapy. However, the surgical follow-up of these new procedures is still brief and the ultimate role for these new antereflux procedures awaits a longer period of follow-up. Ingelfinger (1971) expressed a note of pessimism when he stated 'A final possibility—one to be muttered sotto voce—is that the current popularity of Nissen, Belsey, Hill and cognate types of hernia repair will, like that of the Allison procedure, fade away, with a consequent depreciation of the ultimate position of the distal esophagus . . .'.

OTHER DISORDERS OF LOWER OESOPHAGEAL SPHINCTER FUNCTION

Achalasia

Achalasia is a neurological disorder of the oesophagus producing dysphagia for both liquids and solids, regurgitation of undigested food, pulmonary complications of aspiration, pneumonitis and lung abscess, odynophagia (painful swallowing) and retrosternal chest discomfort. Weight loss is mild, and bleeding from retentive oesophagitis or associated carcinoma of the oesophagus is rare (Roth and Stein, 1963; Cassella et al, 1964; Harris, 1969; Ellis and Olsen, 1969).

Radiographic evaluation will usually reveal a dilated gullet with an air fluid level, retained secretions, and a sharply tapered distal end producing the 'bird beak' or 'pen quill' sign (Code et al, 1958). Fluoroscopy reveals absence of oesophageal peristalsis and a hold-up of barium at the distal oesophagus which will open periodically to allow small amounts of barium to enter the stomach (Ellis and Olsen, 1969).

Oesophageal manometry reveals a triad of markedly elevated resting LES pressure, impaired LES relaxation upon swallowing and aperistalsis of the entire oesophagus (Cohen and Lipshutz, 1971b; Cohen, 1965; Kramer and Ingelfinger, 1949; Butin, 1953; Creamer, Olsen and Code, 1957). The subcutaneous injection (2–10 mg) of the parasympathomimetic drug methacholine (mecholyl) is followed by a rapid increase in intra-oesophageal pressure to more than 25 mmHg, intense chest and back pain, excessive salivation and ultimately regurgitation of the recording catheter (Kramer and Ingelfinger, 1951; Hightower, Olsen and Moersch, 1954). This response can be terminated quickly by the intravenous injection of atropine sulphate 0.4 to 1.0 mg. The oesophageal and LES hyperresponsiveness to mecholyl is an example of Cannon's law of denervation supersensitivity (Cannon and Rosenblueth, 1949). A positive mecholyl test is not specific for achalasia and has been reported in carcinoma of the cardia (Hawthorne, Frobese and Nemir, 1956) diffuse oesophageal spasm (Kramer et al, 1967) and Chagas' disease (Castro and Grossi, 1963).

Even though the radiographic, manometric and clinical findings may be highly suggestive of achalasia it is necessary, however, for thorough endoscopic evaluation to rule out gastric fundal carcinoma which can produce all of the features typical of achalasia (Herrara et al, 1970; Seaman, Wells and Flood, 1963; Kalodny et al, 1968).

The pathogenesis of achalasia is due to a denervation of the neural supply to the oesophagus. Careful histopathological study has shown a decrease in parasympathetic ganglion cells in the oesophageal wall (Lendrum, 1937; Misiewicz et al, 1969; Trounce et al, 1957), wallerian degeneration of the vagus nerve supplying the oesophagus and diminished number of cell bodies in the dorsal motor nucleus of the vagus (Cassella et al, 1964).

Physiological studies in patients with achalasia have shown that the oesophagus and LES are not only supersensitive to the postganglionic cholinergic drug methacoline, but also to gastrin (Cohen, Lipshutz and Hughes, 1971) and to a cholinesterase inhibitor edrophonium (tensilon) (Cohen, Fisher and Tuch, 1972). These data indicate that the genesis of achalasia is related to a site of neural denervation, proximal to the ganglion, and agrees with the histopathologic studies. Cohen et al (1971) have presented data showing that the LES hypertension in achalasia may be related to a supersensitivity of the LES to endogenous circulating gastrin.

The therapy of achalasia is aimed at a reduction of the elevated resting LES pressure. The absence of oesophageal peristalsis and the incomplete LES relaxation upon swallowing are unaffected by current therapy. The reduction in LES pressure produced by pneumatic dilatation (Vantrappen et al, 1971; Kurlander et al, 1963) or surgical myotomy (Heller, 1913; Ellis et al, 1967; Ellis, 1973) produces marked clinical improvement by decreasing the gradient between the oesophagus and stomach after a swallow.

Future treatment for this disorder may involve the use of specific drugs which decrease LES pressure and augment LES relaxation upon swallowing. The most promising candidate drugs are beta-adrenergic agonists (DiMarino and Cohen, 1975) and prostaglandins (Goyal, Mukhopadhyay and Rattan, 1974).

Incompetence of the Lower Oesophageal Sphincter

Gastro-oesophageal reflux and its complications are due to diminished LES pressure and strength. (Winans and Harris, 1967; Lipshutz et al, 1973; Farrell et al, 1974). Since there is no consistent anatomical explanation for this disorder investigation of other factors known to control LES pressure have been undertaken. Based upon the importance of endogenous gastrin in the control of resting LES pressure it was suggested that sphincter incompetence is the result of diminished endogenous gastrin release (Cohen and Harris, 1972). Lipshutz et al (1973) reported that the LES of reflux patients responded normally to cholinergic stimulation, to direct muscle stimulation, and to exogenous pentagastrin. These authors also reported that reflux patients differed from normals only in the LES response to endogenous gastrin release produced by intragastric infusion of alkali and glycine. In 1974 Lipshutz et al, reported that the diminished LES response in reflux patients to endogenous gastrin release produced by intragastric infusion of alkalinised glycine was due to a diminished release of endogenous gastrin. Farrell et al (1974) also reported that the integrated gastrin response following a protein meal was significantly less in reflux patients as compared to normals. These studies do suggest that there may be a deficiency of gastrin release in reflux patients. However, the failure to show a striking difference in serum gastrin levels under fasting conditions between reflux subjects and normals leaves unexplained the observed differences in resting LES pressure between these two groups. In addition the absolute LES pressure to drug and hormonal stimulation is significantly lower in reflux patients as compared to normals even though the percentage increase in pressure above basal is similar in the two groups (Farrell et al, 1974; Lipshutz et al, 1973). Sturdevant and Kun (1974) did not report a diminished gastrin release in reflux patients, and concluded that the LES muscle itself was the reason for sphincteric hypotension in reflux patients. Gastrin deficiency seems therefore to be only one factor responsible for LES incompetence in reflux patients, with the total defect being unknown at present.

Scleroderma

This systemic connective tissue disorder frequently involves the oesophagus as the earliest manifestation of visceral involvement (Treacy et al, 1963). Manometric studies reveal a very specific pattern of oesophageal involvement which separates this disease from the other connective tissue disorders. Diminished to absent LES pressure and weak to absent smooth muscle oesophageal peristalsis, with normal peristalsis in the skeletal muscle section of the upper one-third of the oesophagus, and normal upper oesophageal spincter and pharynx is virtually pathognomonic of this disease (Turner et al, 1973).

Physiological studies have shown normal LES response to methacholine which acts directly on the muscle membrane and impaired response to agents which work indirectly through cholinergic neurons (Cohen et al, 1972). These data reveal a primary cholinergic neuron dysfunction in this disease and are in good agreement with histological studies which report normal smooth muscle in areas of abnormal oesophageal motility (Treacy et al, 1963). The proposed explanation for this cholinergic neuron dysfunction in patients with scleroderma is the excessive sympathetic stimulation known to be present in this disorder and to be responsible for the vasospastic phenomena characteristic of this disease.

Decreased LES pressure and loss of distal oesophageal peristalsis account for the clinical problems of gastro-oesophageal reflux and its complications. Use of conventional antacids, bethanechol, and antireflux manoeuvres are the current treatments of choice. However controlled studies with drugs that interfere with sympathetic neural stimulation may offer a promising treatment for this disorder (see Chapter 5).

Diffuse Oesophageal Spasm

Oesophageal spasm can be a primary disorder or secondary to a variety of diseases. Primary oesophageal spasm is a motor disorder of the oesophagus presenting as a severe chest pain similar to angina pectoris associated with dysphagia for liquids and solids and severe odynophagia. Patients usually report most severe symptoms following the ingestion of liquids of extreme temperature, iced cold drinks or hot tea or coffee (Bennett and Hendrix, 1970; Fleshler, 1967; Respress et al, 1955). Radiographic studies reveal tertiary oesophageal contractions ranging from small ripples in the barium column to enormous contractions producing the 'corkscrew' or 'rosary bead' oesophagus (Roth and Fleshler, 1964; Stiennon, 1968; Ismay, 1952).

Oesophageal manometry reveals increased amplitude, non-peristaltic double and triple peaked contractions and spontaneous oesophageal contractions. One-third of the patients with spasm will have abnormal LES relaxation with or without elevated resting LES pressure.

Since the cause of this disorder is unknown the treatment remains unsatisfactory. Reassurance of the patient that coronary artery disease is not the cause of the symptoms and drugs aimed at counteracting the hypermotile oesophagus (anticholinergics and topical anaesthetics) have met with some clinical success. For those patients with marked dysphagia and odynophagia who have abnormalities of LES function, pneumatic dilatation may be helpful. More controlled trials with drugs shown to relax oesophageal and LES muscle are needed in this disorder.

REFERENCES

Akdamar, K., Maumus, L. T., Ichinose, H., Font, R. G. & Sparks, R. D. (1973) Clinical analysis of reflux esophagitis in symptomatic patients. *Gastrointestinal Endoscopy*, **19**, 172–173.

Allison, P. R. (1951) Reflux esophagitis, sliding hiatus hernia, and the anatomy of repair. *Surgery, Gynecology and Obstetrics*, **92**, 419–451.

Atkinson, M., Edwards, D. A. W., Honour, A. J. et al (1957) Comparison of cardiac and pyloric sphincters: a manometric study. *Lancet*, **2**, 918–922.

Barrett, N. R. (1954) Hiatus hernia—a review of some controversial points. *British Journal of Surgery*, **42**, 231.

Battle, W. A., Nyus, L. M. & Bombeck, C. T. (1973) Gastroesophageal reflux: diagnosis and treatment. *Annals of Surgery*, **177**, 560–565.

Bave, A. E. & Belsey, R. H. R. (1967) The treatment of sliding hiatus hernia and reflux esophagitis by the Mark IV technique. *Surgery*, **62**, 396–404.

Behar, J., Sheahan, D. G., Biancani, P., Spiro, H. M. & Storer, E. H. (1975) Medical and surgical management of reflux esophagitis. *New England Journal of Medicine*, **293**, 263–267.

Behar, J., Biancani, P., Spiro, H. M. et al (1974) Effect of an anterior fundoplication on lower esophageal sphincter competence. *Gastroenterology*, **67**, 209–215.

Belsey, R. H. R. (1960) The pulmonary complications of esophageal disease. *British Journal of Diseases of the Chest*, **54**, 342.

Belsey, R. H. R. (1965) Reconstruction of esophagus with left colon. *Journal of Thoracic and Cardiovascular Surgery*, **49**, 33.

THE GASTRO-OESOPHAGEAL JUNCTION AND HIATUS HERNIA 21

Bennett, J. R. & Atkinson, M. (1966) The differentiation between oesophageal and cardiac pain. *Lancet*, **2**, 1123.
Bennett, J. R. & Hendrix, T. R. (1970) Diffuse esophageal spasm: a disorder with more than one cause. *Gastroenterology*, **59**, 273–279.
Bernstein, L. M. & Baker, L. A. (1958) A clinical test for esophagitis. *Gastroenterology*, **34**, 760–781.
Bettarello, A., Tuttle, S. G. & Grossman, M. I. (1960) Effect of autonomic drugs on gastroesophageal reflux. *Gastroenterology*, **39**, 340–346.
Blackman, A. H., Nasrullah, M. & Thayer, W. R. (1971) Transabdominal vagectomy and lower esophageal function. *Archives of Surgery*, **102**, 6–8.
Boerema, I. & Germs, R. (1955) Fixation of the lesser curvature of the stomach to the anterior abdominal wall after reposition of the hernia through the esophageal hiatus. *Archivum Chirurgicum Neerlandicum*, **7**, 351.
Bombeck, C. T., Dillard, D. H. & Nyhys, L. M. (1966) Muscular anatomy of the gastroesophageal junction and role of the phrenoesophageal ligament, autopsy study of sphincter mechanism. *Annals of Surgery*, **164**, 643.
Booth, D. J., Kemmer, W. T. & Skinner, D. B. (1968) Acid clearing from the distal esophagus. *Archives of Surgery*, **96**, 731.
Botha, G. S. M., Ed. (1962) *The Gastroesophageal Junction*. Boston: Little Brown.
Bremner, C. G., Schlegel, J. F. & Ellis, H. F. Jr (1970) Studies of the gastroesophageal sphincter mechanism: the role of the phrenoesophageal membrane. *Surgery*, **67**, 735–740.
Burnstock, G. (1972) Purinergic nerves. *Pharmacological Reviews*, **24**, 509–581.
Butin, J. W. (1953) A study of esophageal pressures in normal persons and patients with cardiospasm. *Gastroenterology*, **23**, 278–286.
Cannon, W. (1939) A law of denervation (Abstract). *American Journal of Medical Sciences*, **198**, 739.
Cannon, W. B. & Rosenblueth, A. (1949) *The Supersensitivity of Denervated Structures. A Law of Denervation*. New York: Macmillan.
Carey, J. M. & Hollinshead, W. H. (1955) An anatomic study of the esophageal hiatus. *Surgery, Gynecology and Obstetrics*, **100**, 196–200.
Cassella, R. R., Brown, A. L., Sayre, G. P. & Ellis, F. H. (1964) Achalasia of the esophagus: pathologic and etiologic considerations. *Annals of Surgery*, **160**, 474–487.
Castell, D. O. & Harris, L. D. (1970) Hormonal control of gastroesophageal sphincter strength. *New England Journal of Medicine*, **282**, 886–889.
Castell, D. O. & Levine, S. M. (1971) Lower esophageal sphincter response to gastric alkalinisation. A new mechanism for treatment of heartburn with antacids. *Annals of Internal Medicine*, **74**, 223–227.
Castro, L. de P. & Grossi, C. A. (1963) O teste do mecolil no diagnostico de aperistalsis do esofago. *Review Goiana Medicine*, **9**, 3–19.
Christensen, J. (1970) Pharmacologic identification of the lower esophageal sphincter. *Journal of Clinical Investigation*, **49**, 681–691.
Christensen, J., Freeman, B. W. & Miller, J. K. (1973a) Some physiological characteristics of the esophagogastric junction in the opossum. *Gastroenterology*, **64**, 1119–1125.
Christensen, J., Conklin, J. L. & Freeman, B. W. (1973b) Physiologic specialisation at esophagogastric junction in three species. *American Journal of Physiology*, **225**, 1265–1270.
Christensen, J. & Daniel, E. E. (1968) Effects of some autonomic drugs on circular esophageal smooth muscle. *Journal of Pharmacology and Experimental Therapeutics*, **159**, 243–249.
Code, C. F., Creamer, B., Schlegel, J. F., Olsen, A. M., Donoghue, F. E. & Andersen, H. A. (1958) *An Atlas of Esophageal Motility in Health and Diseases*. Springfield: Thomas.
Cohen, B. R. (1965) Cardiospasm in achalasia: demonstration of an abnormally elevated esophagogastric sphincter pressure with partial relaxation on swallowing (Abstract). *Gastroenterology*, **48**, 864.
Cohen, S. & Booth, G. H. Jr (1975) Gastric acid secretion and LES pressure in response to coffee and caffeine. *New England Journal of Medicine*, **293**, 897–900.
Cohen, B. R. & Guelrad, M. (1971) Cardiospasm in achalasia: demonstration of supersensitivity of the lower esophageal sphincter (Abstract). *Gastroenterology*, **60**, 769.
Cohen, S. & Harris, L. D. (1970) Lower esophageal sphincter pressure as an index of lower esophageal sphincter strength. *Gastroenterology*, **58**, 157–162.

Cohen, S. & Harris, L. D. (1971) Does hiatus hernia affect competence of the gastroesophageal sphincter? *New England Journal of Medicine*, **284**, 1053–1056.

Cohen, S. & Lipshutz, W. H. (1970) Anticholinergic therapy: a triple threat to lower esophageal sphincter competence (Abstract). *Annals of Internal Medicine*, **72**, 792.

Cohen, S. & Lipshutz, W. H. (1971a) Hormonal regulation of human lower esophageal sphincter strength: interaction of gastrin and secretin. *Journal of Clinical Investigation*, **50**, 449–454.

Cohen, S. & Lipshutz, W. H. (1971b) Lower esophageal sphincter dysfunction in achalasia. *Gastroenterology*, **61**, 814–819.

Cohen, S., Lipshutz, W. H. & Hughes, W. (1971) Role of gastrin supersensitivity in the pathogenesis of lower esophageal sphincter hypertension in achalasia. *Journal of Clinical Investigation*, **50**, 1241–1247.

Cohen, S., Fisher, R. S. & Tuch, A. (1972) The site of denervation in achalasia. *Gut*, **13**, 556–559.

Cohen, S. & Harris, L. D. (1972) The lower esophageal sphincter. *Gastroenterology*, **63**, 1066–1073.

Cohen, S., Fisher, R. S., Lipshutz, W. H. et al (1972) The pathogenesis of esophageal dysfunction in scleroderma and Raynaud's disease. *Journal of Clinical Investigation*, **51**, 2663–2668.

Collis, J. L., Kelly, T. D. & Wiley, A. N. (1954) Anatomy of the crura of the diaphragm and the surgery of hiatus hernia. *Thorax*, **9**, 175.

Collis, J. L. (1963) Gastroplasty. *Thoraxchirurgie*, **11**, 57.

Creamer, B., Olsen, A. M. & Code, C. F. (1957) The esophageal sphincters in achalasia of the cardia (cardiospasm). *Gastroenterology*, **33**, 293–301.

Crispin, J. S., McIver, D. K. & Lind, J. F. (1967) Manometric study of the effect of vagotomy on the gastroesophageal sphincter. *Candian Journal of Surgery*, **10**, 299–303.

Csendes, A. & Larrain, A. (1972) Effect of posterior gastropexy on gastroesophageal sphincter pressure and symptomatic reflux in patients with hiatal hernia. *Gastroenterology*, **63**, 19–24.

Dennish, G. W. & Castell, D. O. (1972) Caffeine and the lower esophageal sphincter. *American Journal of Digestive Disease*, **17**, 993–996.

Dennish, G. W. & Castell, D. O. (1971) Inhibitory effect of smoking on the lower esophageal sphincter. *New England Journal of Medicine*, **284**, 1136–1137.

Dilawari, J. B. & Misiewicz, J. J. (1973). Action of oral metaclopramide on the gastroesophageal junction in man. *Gut*, **14**, 380–382.

DiMarino, A. J. & Cohen, S. (1973) The adrenergic control of lower esophageal sphincter function. *Journal of Clinical Investigation*, **52**, 2264–2271.

DiMarino, A. J. & Cohen, S. (1975) Adrenergic control of lower esophageal sphincter function: response to beta$_2$-adrenergic agonists. *Proceedings of the Society for Experimental Biology and Medicine*, **148**, 1265–1269.

Dodds, W. J., Hogan, W. J., Stef, J. J., Arndorfer, R. C. & Laydon, S. B. (1975) Effect of increased intra-abdominal pressure on lower esophageal sphincter pressure. *American Journal of Digestive Disease*, **20**, 298–308.

Donner, M. W. & Margulies, S. I. (1972) Radiographic examination. In *Gastroesophageal Reflux and Hiatus Hernia*. Ed. Skinner, D. B., Ch. 6. Boston: Little Brown.

Earlam, R. J. & Ellis, F. H. Jr (1967) Repair of experimental hiatus hernia in dogs. *Archives of Surgery*, **95**, 585–594.

Edwards, D. A. W. (1967) Sphincter mechanisms in the gastrointestinal tract. *American Journal of Digestive Disease*, **12**, 267–276.

Edwards, D. A. W. (1973) Symposium on gastroesophageal reflux and its complications. *Gut*, **14**, 233–253.

Ellis, F. H. Jr, Kiser, J. C., Schlegel, J. F., Earlam, R. J., McVey, J. L. & Olsen, A. M. (1967) Esophagomyotomy for esophageal achalasia: experimental, clinical and manometric aspects. *Annals of Surgery*, **166**, 640–656.

Ellis, F. H. Jr (1973) Esophagomyotomy for esophageal achalasia. *Surgical Clinics of North America*, **53**, 319–324.

Ellis, F. H. Jr & Olsen, A. M. (1969) *Achalasia of the Esophagus*, p. 221. Philadelphia: W. B. Saunders Co.

Farrell, R. L., Castell, D. O. & McGuigan, J. E. (1974) Measurements and comparisons of the lower esophageal sphincter pressures and serum gastrin levels in patients with gastro-oesophageal reflux. *Gastroenterology*, **67**, 415–422.

Farrell, R. L., Roling, G. T. & Castell, D. O. (1974) Cholinergic therapy of chronic heartburn. A controlled trial. *Annals of Internal Medicine*, **80**, 573–576.

Farrell, R. L., Higgs, R. H. & Castell, D. O. (1974) Dynamics of the lower esophageal high pressure zone before and after belsey fundoplasty (Abstract). *Gastroenterology*, **66**, 690.

Fisher, R. S., DiMarino, A. J. & Cohen, S. (1974) Mechanism of cholecystokinin induced inhibition of lower esophageal sphincter pressure (Abstract). *Clinical Research*, **22**, 358.

Fisher, R. S., Roberts, G. S., Lobis, I. F. & Malmud, L. S. (1975) Use of gastroesophageal scintiscan to evaluate anti-reflux maneuvers. *Gastroenterology*, **68**, 893.

Fleshler, B. (1967) Diffuse esophageal spasm. *Gastroenterology*, **52**, 559–564.

Freeland, G. R., Higgs, R. H., Castell, D. O. & McGuigan J. E. (1975) Lower esophageal sphincter and gastric acid responses to intravenous infusions of synthetic human gastrin heptadecapeptide I (Abstract). *Gastroenterology*, **68**, 700.

Fyke, R. E., Code, C. F. & Schlegel, J. F. (1956) The gastroesophageal sphincter in healthy human beings. *Gastroenterologia*, **86**, 135–150.

Giles, G. R., Mason, M. C., Humphries, C. & Clark, C. G. (1969) Action of gastrin on the lower esophageal sphincter in man. *Gut*, **10**, 730–734.

Goyal, R. K. & Rattan, S. (1973) Mechanism of the lower esophageal sphincter relaxation. Action of prostaglandin E_1 and theophylline. *Journal of Clinical Investigation*, **52**, 337–341.

Goyal, R. K., Mukhopadhyay, A. & Rattan, S. (1974) Effect of prostaglandin E_2 on the lower esophageal sphincter in normal subjects and patients with achalasia (Abstract). *Clinical Research*, **22**, 358.

Grossman, M. I. (1973) What is physiological? (Abstract). *Gastroenterology*, **65**, 994.

Haddad, J. K. (1970) Relation of gastroesophageal reflux to yield sphincter pressures. *Gastroenterology*, **58**, 175–184.

Harrington, S. W. (1928) Diaphragmatic hernia. *Archives of Surgery*, **16**, 386.

Harris, L. D. (1969) Dysphagia. *Advances in Internal Medicine*, **15**, 203–219.

Hawthorne, H. R., Frobese, A. S. & Nemir, P. (1956) The surgical management of achalasia of the esophagus. *Annals of Surgery*, **144**, 653–663.

Heitmann, P. & Moller, N. (1970) The effect of metaclopramide on the gastroesophageal junctional zone and the distal esophagus in man. *Scandinavian Journal of Gastroenterology*, **5**, 621–625.

Heller, E. (1913) Extramuköse Cardiaplastik beim Chronischen Cardiospasmus mit dilatation des Oesophagus. *Mitteilungen aus den Grenzgebieten der Medizin und Chirurgie*, **27**, 141–149.

Hendrix, T. R. (1972) Function of the gastroesophageal segment. In *Gastroesophageal Reflux and Hiatus Hernia*, ed. Skinner, D. B., Belsey, R. H., Hendrix, T. R. & Zuidema, G. D., Ch. 2. Boston: Little Brown.

Herrara, A. F., Colon, J., Valdes-Dapena, A. & Roth, J. L. A. (1970) Achalasia or carcinoma? The significance of the mecholyl test. *American Journal of Digestive Disease*, **15**, 1073–1081.

Hiebert, C. A. & Belsey, R. H. R. (1961) Incompentency of the gastric cardia without radiologic evidence of hiatus hernia. *Journal of Thoracic and Cardiovascular Surgery*, **42**, 352.

Higgs, B., Kerr, F. W. L. & Ellis, F. H. Jr (1965) A study of the anatomy of the human esophagus with special reference to the gastroesophageal sphincter. *Journal of Surgical Research*, **5**, 503–507.

Higgs, R. H., Smith, R. D. & Castell, D. O. (1974) Gastric alkalinisation: effect on lower esophageal sphincter pressure and serum gastrin. *New England Journal of Medicine*, **291**, 486–490.

Higgs, R. H. & Castell, D. O. (1975) Cholinergic stimulation of the lower esophageal sphincter in patients with vagotomy and antrectomy. *American Journal of Digestive Disease*, **20**, 190–195.

Hightower, N. C., Olsen, A. M. & Moersch, H. J. (1954) A Comparison of the effects of acetyl-beta-methyl-choline chloride (Mecholyl) on esophageal intraluminal pressure in normal persons and patients with cardiospasm. *Gastroenterology*, **26**, 592–600.

Hill, L. D. (1967) An effective operation for hiatal hernia: an eight year appraisal. *Annals of Surgery*, **166**, 681–692.
Hill, L. D., Gelfand, M. & Bauermeister, O. (1970) Simplified management of reflux esophagitis with stricture. *Annals of Surgery*, **172**, 628–646.
Hogan, W. J., Viegas De Andrade, S. R. & Winship, D. H. (1972) Ethanol induced acute esophageal motor dysfunction. *Journal Applied Physiology*, **36**, 755–760.
Hoke, S. E., Reid, D. P., Hogan, W. J., Kalkhoff, R. K. & Arndorfer, R. C. (1972) Effect of glucagon on esophageal motor function (Abstract). *Clinical Research*, **20**, 732.
Hollis, J. B. & Castell, D. O. (1972) Amplitude of esophageal peristalsis as determined by rapid infusion. *Gastroenterology*, **63**, 417–422.
Ingelfinger, F. J. (1958) Esophageal motility. *Physiology Review*, **38**, 533–584.
Ingelfinger, F. J. (1971) The sphincter that is a Sphinx. *New England Journal of Medicine*, **285**, 1095–1096.
Ismail-Beigi, F., Horton, P. F. & Pope, C. E. II (1970) Histological consequences of gastroesophageal reflux in man. *Gastroenterology*, **58**, 163–174.
Ismay, G. (1952) Painful spasm of the oesophagus ('corkscrew' oesophagus). *British Medical Journal*, **2**, 697–703.
Jackson, C. (1922) Diaphragmatic pinchock in so-called 'cardiospasm'. *Laryngoscope*, **32**, 199–242.
Jaffer, S. S., Makhlouf, G. M., Schorr, B. A. & Zfass, A. M. (1974) Nature and kinetics of inhibition of lower esophageal sphincter pressure by glucagon. *Gastroenterology*, **67**, 42–46.
Jennewein, H. M., Waldeck, F., Siewert, R., Weiser, F. & Thimm, R. (1973) The interaction of glucagon and pentagastrin on the lower esophageal sphincter in man and dog. *Gut*, **14**, 861–864.
Kalodny, M., Schrader, Z. R., Rubin, W., Hochman, R. & Sleisenger, M. H. (1968) Esophageal achalasia probably due to gastric carcinoma. *Annals of Internal Medicine*, **69**, 569–573.
Kantrowitz, P. A., Siegel, C. I., Strong, M. J. et al (1970) Response of the human esophagus to d-tubocuraine and atropine. *Gut*, **11**, 47.
Kaye, M. D. & Showalter, J. P. (1971) Manometric configuration of the lower esophageal sphincter in normal human subjects. *Gastroenterology*, **61**, 213–223.
Kramer, P. & Ingelfinger, F. J. (1949) Motility of the human esophagus in control subjects and in patients with esophageal disorders. *American Journal of Medicine*, **7**, 168–174.
Kramer, P. & Ingelfinger, F. J. (1951) Esophageal sensitivity to mecholyl in cardiospasm. *Gastroenterology*, **19**, 242–251.
Kramer, P., Fleshler, B., McNally, E. & Harris, L. D. (1967) Oesophageal sensitivity to mecholyl in symptomatic diffuse spasm. *Gut*, **8**, 120–127.
Kurlander, D. J., Raskin, H. F., Kirsner, J. B. & Palmer, W. L. (1963) Therapeutic value of the pneumatic dilator in achalasia of the esophagus. *Gastroenterology*, **45**, 604–613.
Larrain, A., Csendes, A. & Pope, C. E. II (1975) Surgical correction of reflux. An effective therapy for esophageal strictures. *Gastroenterology*, **69**, 578–583.
Lendrum, F. C. (1937) Anatomic features of the cardiac orifice of the stomach. *Archives of Internal Medicine*, **59**, 474–480.
Lerche, W, (1950) The Esophagus and *Pharynx in Action*. Springfield, Ill.: Charles C. Thomas.
Lind, J. F., Warrian, W. G. & Wankling, W. J. (1966) Responses of the gastroesophageal junction to increases in abdominal pressure. *Candian Journal of Surgery*, **91**, 32–40.
Lind, J. F., Crispin, J. S. & McIver, D. K. (1968) The effect of atropine on the gastroesophageal sphincter. *Candian Journal of Physiology and Pharmacology*, **46**, 233–238.
Lind, J. F., Cotton, D. J., Blanchard, R., Crippin, J. S. & Dimopolos, G. E. (1969) Effect of thoracic displacement and vagotomy on the canine gastroesophageal junctional zone. *Gastroenterology*, **56**, 1078–1085.
Linsman, J. (1965) Gastroesophageal reflux elicited while drinking water (water siphonage test): its correlation with pyrosis. *Medical Journal of Roentgenology, Radium Therapeutics, Nuclear Medicine*, **94**, 325–332.
Lipshutz, W. H. & Cohen, S. (1971) Physiological determinants of lower esophageal sphincter function. *Gastroenterology*, **61**, 16–24.
Lipshutz, W. H., Hughes, W. & Cohen, S. (1972) The genesis of lower esophageal sphincter pressure: its identification through the use of gastrin antiserum. *Journal of Clinical Investigation*, **51**, 522–529.

Lipshutz, W. H., Eckert, R. J., Gaskins, R. D., Blanton, D. E. & Lukash, W. M. (1974) Normal lower esophageal sphincter function after surgical treatment of gastroesophageal reflux. *New England Journal of Medicine*, **291**, 1107–1110.

Lipshutz, W. H., Gaskins, R. D., Lukash, W. M. & Sode, J. (1973) Pathogenesis of lower esophageal sphincter incompetence. *New England Journal of Medicine*, **289**, 182–184.

Lipshutz, W. H., Gaskins, R. D., Lukash, W. M., & Sode, J. (1974) Hypogastrinemia in patients with lower esophageal sphincter incompetence. *Gastroenterology*, **67**, 423–427.

Listerud, M. & Harkins, H. (1958) Anatomy of the esophageal hiatus. *AMA Arch. Surg.*, **76**, 835–842.

Lyons, W. S., Ellis, F. H. & Olsen, A. M. (1956) The gastroesophageal sphincter in healthy human beings. *Gastroenterologia*, **86**, 135–150.

McAlhany, J. C., Thomas, H. F. & Woodward, E. R. (1972) Gastroesophageal reflux after operative procedures for sliding hiatal hernia. *American Journal of Surgery*, **123**, 657–662.

McCallum, R., Kline, M., Curry, N. & Sturdevant, R. (1974) Comparative effects of metaclopramide and urecholine on lower esophageal sphincter pressure in reflux patients (Abstract). *Gastroenterology*, **66**, 742.

Mann, C. V. & Hardcastle, J. D. (1968) The effect of vagotomy on the human gastroesophageal sphincter. *Gut*, **9**, 688–695.

Mazur, J. M., Skinner, D. B., Jones, E. L. & Zuidema, G. D. (1973) Effect of transabdominal vagotomy on the human gastroesophageal high pressure zone. *Surgery*, **73**, 818–822.

Misiewicz, J. J., Waller, S. L., Anthony, P. P. & Gummer, J. W. P. (1969) Achalasia of the cardia: pharmacology and histopathology of isolated cardiac sphincteric muscle from patients with and without achalasia. *Quarterly Journal of Medicine*, **38**, 17–30.

Moran, J. M., Pihl, C. O. & Norton, R. A. (1971) The hiatal hernia–reflux complex: current approaches to correction and evaluation of results. *American Journal of Surgery*, **121**, 404–411.

Nauta, J. (1956) The closing mechanism between the esophagus and the stomach. *Gastroenterologia*, **86**, 219–222.

Nebel, O. T. & Castell, D. O. (1973) Kinetics of fat inhibition of the lower esophageal sphincter. *Journal of Applied Physiology*, **35**, 6–8.

Nebel, O. T. & Castell, D. O. (1972) Lower esophageal sphincter pressure changes after food ingestion. *Gastroenterology*, **63**, 778–783.

Nissen, R. (1961) Gastropexy and 'fundoplication' in surgical treatment of hiatal hernia. *American Journal of Digestive Disease*, **6**, 954.

Pearson, J. B. & Gray, J. G. (1967) Esophageal hiatus hernia: long-term results of the conventional thoracic operation. *British Journal of Surgery*, **54**, 530–533.

Pope, C. E. II (1967) A dynamic test of sphincter strength: its application to the lower esophageal sphincter. *Gastroenterology*, **52**, 779–786.

Pope, C. E. II (1972) Recognition and management of gastroesophageal reflux. *Viewpoints in Digestive Disease*, **4**, 1–4.

Pope, C. E. II, Eastwood, L. F. & Eastwood, I. R. (1973) Objective results of anti-reflux surgery. *Clinical Research*, **21**, 208A.

Rattan, S. & Goyal, R. K. (1974) Neural control of the lower esophageal sphincter. *Journal of Clinical Investigation*, **54**, 899–906.

Resin, H., Stern, D. H., Sturdevant, R. A. et al (1973) Effect of the C-terminal octapeptide of cholescystokinin on lower esophageal sphincter pressure in man. *Gastroenterology*, **64**, 946–949.

Respress, J. C., Ingelfinger, F. J., Hendrix, T. R. & Kramer, P. (1955) The effect of cold on motor mechanism of the human esophagus. *Clinical Research Proceedings*, **3**, 130.

Rogers, A. I., Rothman, S. L. & Arostegui, M. (1974) Lower esophageal sphincter responsiveness to postprandial antacids. *Journal Clinical Research*, **22**, 23.

Roling, G. T., Farrell, R. L. & Castell, D. O. (1972) Cholinergic response of the lower esophageal sphincter. *American Journal of Physiology*, **222**, 967–972.

Roth, H. P. & Fleshler, B. (1964) Diffuse esophageal spasm. Clinical, radiological and manometric observations. *Annals of Internal Medicine*, **61**, 914–922.

Roth, J. L. A. & Stein, G. N. (1963) *Achalasia (Cardiospasm)* in *Gastroenterology* ed. by Bockus, H. L. Vol. 1, pp. 145–168. Philadelphia and London: W. B. Saunders Co.

Sanchez, G. C., Kramer, P. & Ingelfinger, F. J. (1953) Motor mechanisms of the esophagus, particularly of its distal portion. *Gastroenterology*, **25**, 321–332.

Seaman, W. B., Wells, J. & Flood, C. A. (1963) Diagnostic problems of esophageal cancer. *American Journal of Roentgenology, Radium Therapy and Nuclear Medicine*, **90**, 778–791.

Sicular, A., Cohen, B., Zimmerman, A. & Kark, A. E. (1967) The significance of an intraabdominal segment of canine esophagus as a competent antereflux mechanism. *Surgery*, **61**, 784–790.

Skinner, D. B. (1972) *Anatomy in gastroesophageal Reflux and Hiatus Hernia*, ed. Skinner, D. B., Belsey, R. H. R., Hendrix, T. R. & Zuidema, G. D., Ch. 1. Boston: Little Brown.

Skinner, D. B. & Belsey, R. H. R. (1967) Surgical management of esophageal reflux and hiatus hernia. *Journal of Thoracic and Cardiovascular Surgery*, **53**, 33.

Soergel, K. H., Zboralske, F. F. & Amberg, J. R. (1964) Presbyesophagus: esophageal motility in nonagenarians. *Journal of Clinical Investigation*, **43**, 1472.

Stanciu, C. & Bennett, J. R. (1973) Metaclopramide in gastroesophageal reflux. *Gut*, **14**, 275–279.

Stef, J. J., Dodds, W. J. & Hogan, W. J. (1974) Intraluminal esophageal manometry: component analysis of systems used to record intraluminal pressure. In *Proceedings of Fourth International Symposium on Gastrointestinal Motility*, ed. Daniel, E. E. pp. 337–346. Vancouver: Mitchell Press.

Stiennon, O. A. (1968) On the cause of tertiary contractions and related disturbances of the esophagus. *American Journal of Roentgenology, Radium Therapy, and Nuclear Medicine*, **104**, 617–624.

Sturdevant, R. & Kun, T. (1974) Interaction of pentagastrin and the octapeptide of cholecystokinin on the human lower esophageal sphincter. *Gut*, **15**, 700–702.

Sturdevant, R. & Kun, T. (1974) Gastrin and gastroesophageal sphinter incompetence. In *Proceedings of the Fourth International Symposium on Gastrointestinal Motility*, ed. Daniell, E. E., pp. 125–130. Vancouver: Mitchell Press.

Thal, A. P. (1968) A unified approach to surgical problems of the esophagogastric junction. *Annals of Surgery*, **168**, 542.

Treacy, W. L., Baggenstoss, A. H., Slocumb, C. H. & Code, C. F. (1963) Scleroderma of the esophagus, a correlation of histologic and physiological findings. *Annals of Internal Medicine*, **59**, 351–356.

Trounce, J. R., Deuchar, D. C., Kauntze, R. & Thomas, G. A. (1957) Studies in achalasia of the cardia. *Quarterly Journal of Medicine*, **26**, 433–456.

Tuch, A. & Cohen, S. (1973) Lower esophageal sphincter relaxation: studies on the neurogenic inhibitory mechanism. *Journal of Clinical Investigation*, **52**, 14–20.

Turner, R., Lipshutz, W. H., Miller, W., Rittenberg, G., Schumaker, H. R. & Cohen, S. (1973) Esophageal dysfunction in collagen disease. *American Journal of the Medical Sciences*, **265**, 191–199.

Tuttle, S. G. & Grossman, M. I. (1958) Detection of gastroesophageal reflux by simultaneous measurement of intraluminal pressures and pH. *Proceedings of the Society of Experimental Biology and Medicine*, **98**, 225.

Urschel, H. C. Jr & Paulson, D. L. (1967) Gastroesophageal reflux and hiatal hernia: complications and therapy. *Journal of Thoracic and Cardiovascular Surgery*, **53**, 21–32.

Vantrappen, G., Texter, E. C., Barborka, C. F. & Vandenbroucke, J. (1960) The closing mechanism at the gastroesophageal junction. *American Journal of Medicine*, **28**, 564–577.

Vantrappen, G., Hellemans, J., Deloof, W., Valembois, P. & Vandenbroucke, J. (1971) Treatment of achalasia with pneumatic dilatations. *Gut*, **12**, 268–275.

Wankling, W. J., Warrian, W. G. & Lind, J. F. (1965) The gastroesophageal sphincter in hiatus hernia. *Canadian Journal of Surgery*, **8**, 61–67.

Weaver, A. W., Large, A. M. & Walt, A. J. (1970) Surgical management of severe reflux esophagitis. Eight to seventeen year follow-up study. *American Journal of Surgery*, **119**, 15.

Winans, C. S. & Harris, L. D. (1967) Quantitation of lower esophageal sphincter competence. *Gastroenterology*, **52**, 773–778.

Winans, C. S. (1972) Manometric asymmetry of the lower esophageal high pressure zone (Abstract). *Gastroenterology*, **62**, 830.

Woodward, E. D., Thomas, H. F. & McAlhany, J. C. (1971) Comparison of crural repair and nissen fundoplication in the treatment of esophageal hernia with peptic esophagitis. *Annals of Surgery*, **171**, 782–789.

Zfass, A. M., Prince, R., Allen, F. N. et al (1970) Inhibitory beta-adrenergic receptors in the human distal esophagus. *American Journal of Digestive Disease*, **15**, 303–310.

2
FAT ABSORPTION

David R. Saunders   George B. McDonald

We wish to present the practising gastroenterologist with an overview of fat absorption which will place advances in physiology into clinical perspective. A large volume of new information about fat absorption has been distilled into several reviews (Hofmann and Mekhjian, 1973; Borgström, 1974; Ockner and Isselbacher, 1974; Gangl and Ockner, 1975), and into an excellent, didactic approach (Hofmann, 1974).

DEFINITION OF THE PROBLEM

To understand how fat is absorbed we must fathom how a water-insoluble substance is transported through the watery contents of the intestine, through the surface lipid membrane of intestinal absorptive cells, and finally through the absorptive cells into the aqueous lymph. Triglycerides of long-chain fatty acids (9 kcal/g) constitute 40 per cent of many Westerners' caloric intake. Cholesterol, lecithins, and fat-soluble vitamins are other nutritionally important lipids whose fate in the intestine must be pondered.

FAECAL FAT

Origin of Faecal Fat

Once it was believed that almost all of the fat in normal faeces was of endogenous origin. The coefficient of absorption of radioactive oleic acid was better than 98 per cent (Blomstrand, 1955) and the composition of faecal fatty acids bore little resemblance to dietary fat (Webb, James and Kellock, 1963). The issue has been clarified by studying patients with ileostomies, who excrete about 0.5 g of fat daily when fasting, and about 3 g of fat daily when ingesting 50 g of corn oil (Wiggins et al, 1969). A minor portion of fat in normal faeces is of endogenous origin, therefore, and the remainder is of dietary origin which is modified by colonic bacteria.

Research for this chapter was supported by Research Grant NIAMDD AM16059 from the National Institute of Health, United States of America.

Measurement of Faecal Fat

The most commonly used technique in the clinical laboratory for measuring faecal fat involves hydrolysing the triglycerides in homogenised faeces and titrating the lipid-soluble fatty acids. The aptness of the dietary fatty intake (Annegers, 1949), vagaries of faecal flow (Weijers, Drion and Van de Kamer, 1960) and possible errors in the laboratory (Bliss, Small and Donaldson, 1971) often demote the usual quantitative fat balance to a qualitative status. The Van de Kamer technique is inappropriate when patients are ingesting medium-chain triglycerides, because the resulting fatty acids are incompletely extracted (Van de Kamer, 1953).

The capacity of the normal human small intestine to absorb fat is truly prodigious: one of Dr Kasper's subjects absorbed 98 per cent of the 639 g of his daily corn and olive oil (Kasper, 1970). The ability to absorb fat reaches adult efficiency at about one year of age (Weijers et al, 1960), coincident with adequate bile acid production (Watkins, 1974). Thereafter, about 95 per cent of normal dietary fat is absorbed so that there is a rough direct correlation between dietary intake and fat excretion (Kasper, 1970). Annegers (1949) analysed the relationship between faecal fat and dietary intake in patients with malabsorption: the coefficient of fat absorption was 54 per cent in patients who lacked bile and was 32 per cent in patients who lacked pancreatic juice. Increasing the dietary intake of fat in a patient with suspected malabsorption may dramatically increase the amount of fat in the stools (Walker et al, 1973).

DIAGNOSIS OF MALABSORPTION

A physician can make a confident diagnosis of malabsorption if his patient is losing weight yet is eating adequately and is passing bulky, putty-like stools which contain many sudanophilic droplets. Oily droplets in the toilet water usually signify pancreatic insufficiency, or insufficient time for triglyceride to be hydrolysed in the small intestine. Floating stools are not a reliable indicator of steatorrhoea; flotation depends on faecal gas content and not on content of buoyant fat (Levitt and Duane, 1972). Mild malabsorption may be difficult to prove without a carefully undertaken faecal fat balance. Several screening tests for malabsorption may be helpful, but each has its problems. A serum carotene of less than 20 μg/100 ml accurately predicts steatorrhoea, but higher values have little predictive value (Onstad and Zieve, 1972). D-Xylose is a poorly metabolised pentose whose absorption depends upon a normal small intestinal mucosa; the D-xylose absorption test errs 30 per cent of the time, however (Sladen and Kumar, 1973; Krawitt and Beeken, 1975). Low serum folate appears to be a reliable screening test of coeliac disease, especially in children (Weir and Hourihane, 1974). Rarely the effects of iron or calcium deficiency may direct attention to underlying intestinal disease.

Defects in ileal function may be screened by measuring the urinary excretion of radioactivity after feeding ^{57}Co-vitamin B_{12} plus intrinsic factor, or the pulmonary excretion of radioactivity after feeding ^{14}C-glycine-glycocholate. In the latter test, the unabsorbed bile salt is deconjugated by colonic bacteria, the glycine is metabolised, and $^{14}CO_2$ is expelled in the breath (Hepner, 1974; Newman, 1974). Both tests will be affected by excessive population of the small intestine by bacteria, or by too rapid transit through the small intestine (see also Chapter 9).

Examining a 24-hr specimen of stool is as reasonable a screening test as any other. A pasty, greyish, glistening, rancid stool which contains many sudanophilic droplets, and which weighs more than 200 g/day should be adequate evidence for malabsorption (Raffensperger et al, 1967).

ROLE OF THE STOMACH IN FAT ABSORPTION

It is believed that relatively little digestion of fat occurs in the stomach although there are lipases in gastric juice and in pharyngeal secretions (Hamosh et al, 1975). The churning action of the antrum may aid in emulsifying ingested fat, but the main contribution of the stomach to fat absorption is in metering its contents into the duodenum so that the absorptive capacity of the upper small intestine is not overwhelmed. Normally food remains in the stomach about 4 h after eating a solid meal (Malagelada, Go and Summerskill, 1975). The rate of gastric emptying is regulated via duodenal receptors excited by tonicity, acidity, fat and amino acids. Fatty acids seem to be the most potent of these inhibitors of gastric emptying (Cooke, 1975). Two of three normal subjects in whom we injected 25 g of ^{131}I triolein rapidly intraduodenally excreted an excessive amount of ^{131}I in their faeces subsequently, as did both of the subjects given a 50 g dose. All subjects had a low amount of faecal ^{131}I after ingesting the triolein. Gastric resection or antral denervation may be expected to reduce the efficiency of fat absorption.

THE LUMINAL PHASE OF FAT ABSORPTION

Most molecules of dietary lipid have a hydrophobic, carbon skeleton on which is engrafted hydrophilic, polar groups. The balance between these moieties determines how the molecule reacts in aqueous solutions of bile salts (Carey and Small, 1972). Some molecules, such as sterol esters, behave as nonpolar compounds, that is, they cannot dissolve within water. Slightly polar triglycerides of long-chain fatty acids are also insoluble in water and they are virtually unabsorbable. After digestion, however, the free sterol, the free fatty acids (FFA) and monoglycerides are more polar; these molecules can now be transported through luminal water to the intestinal absorptive cells. What steps are involved in this process?

Mixing and Emulsification

The kneading action of the gastric antrum and the segmental contractions of the small intestine should help to emulsify fat. Bile salts and phospholipids would stabilise the emulsion. There are no data, however, on emulsification in the human upper intestinal tract and on whether a possible defect in emulsification is important in the pathogenesis of steatorrhoea in disorders of small intestinal motility such as intestinal pseudo-obstruction (Maldonado et al, 1970).

Release of Cholecystokinin-Pancreozymin (CCK–PZ)

Fatty acids and amino acids in the proximal small intestine evoke release of CCK–PZ from cells in the crypts of Lieberkühn. CCK–PZ elicits contraction of the gall bladder, and discharge of zymogen granules into pancreatic acini. The process of releasing CCK–PZ is self-perpetuating as long as digestion of fat and protein continues in the intestinal lumen. High concentrations of bile salts may serve as the inhibitory arc of an autoregulating system (Malagelada et al, 1973).

Hydrolysis by Pancreatic Enzymes

Lipase is secreted by the pancreas in an active form, and in great excess. Even patients who have had 95 per cent of their pancreas excised can absorb 80 per cent of their dietary fat (Kalser, Leite and Warren, 1968). A coenzyme, colipase, is present in pancreatic juice. The physicochemical association between lipase and colipase appears to facilitate interaction of lipase with triglyceride substrate and to protect lipase against inactivation (Borgström and Erlanson, 1971). Lipase attacks the outside ester linkages of triglyceride molecules at the surface of emulsion droplets. The hydrolytic products, 2-monoglyceride and FFA, form mixed micelles with bile salts, and leave the reaction site.

The pancreas also secretes a non-specific esterase which hydrolyses sterol esters. Bile salts seem to be necessary and specific for this reaction (Hyun, Treadwell and Vahouny, 1972). There is a pancreatic phospholipase which is secreted as a proenzyme to be activated in the intestinal lumen by trypsin. This enzyme hydrolyses the fatty acid ester linkage at the 2-position of lecithins forming lysolecithins and FFA (De Haas et al, 1968). Lysolecithins are water soluble and their detergent properties may assist solubilisation of lipids in intestinal contents.

Formation of Bile Salt Micelles

The two bile salts synthesised in the human liver are cholic acid (3,7,12-trihydroxycholanic acid) and chenodeoxycholic acid (3,7-dihydroxycholanic acid), which are conjugated with taurine or glycine. Conjugates of deoxycholic acid (3,12-dihydroxycholanic acid) are also present in human bile; deoxycholate is formed from cholic acid by the action of a bacterial dehydroxylase in the lumen of the ileum and colon. Bile salts possess a hydrophobic, steroidal skeleton and several hydrophilic groups. They are amphiphiles which are highly soluble in water at pH levels above their pK_a, that is, when they are completely ionised. Conjugated bile salts have pK_as of less than 4.5 so that they exist as anions at the pH of about 6 in the proximal small intestine when unconjugated bile salts with higher pK_as may precipitate.

After an overnight fast, most of the total body pool of bile acids, amounting to 2.5 to 4.5 g, is concentrated in the gallbladder ready to be propelled into the intestine. High concentrations of bile salts are achieved in the upper small intestine during the hours needed for digestion of a meal. Little absorption of bile occurs in the jejunum, where most nutrients are absorbed; active absorption of both conjugated and unconjugated bile salts occurs in the ileum. Portal blood delivers these bile salts to the liver, where they are virtually completely extracted and secreted into the bile (see also Chapter 9).

Can these aspects of bile salt physiology be measured in man? The amount of circulating bile salts per day is the product of the pool size and the number of enterohepatic circulations. The pool size is readily measured by using isotopic bile salts, since the biologic half-life of bile salts is two to three days (Tyor, Garbutt and Lack, 1971). The number of enterohepatic circulations can be determined, but duodenal contents must be aspirated continuously (Brunner et al, 1974). The effective pool size is about 8 g bile salts per meal because of the very efficient enterohepatic circulation.

Why is it important to have high concentrations of conjugated bile salts in the intestine during digestion? Below a concentration of about 2 mmol, bile salts merely dissolve in intestinal water. At a certain concentration, the bile salt molecules form aggregates, called micelles; and above this concentration all additional bile salts are maintained in these aggregates. The concentration of unaggregated bile salt molecules becomes constant, but the molecules flit rapidly in and out of the aggregates.

Lipids which have some interaction with water such as fatty acids, lecithins, and monoglycerides can form multimolecular aggregates with bile salts and these are then called mixed micelles. These mixed micelles, in turn, can solubilise lipids which have virtually no interaction with water, such as fat-soluble vitamins.

What is the importance of bile salt micelles? The surface of the intestinal absorptive cells is covered by a relatively unstirred layer of water through which molecules must pass (Wilson, Sallee and Dietschy, 1971). This unstirred layer may be as thick as 1 mm in the human small intestine (Gray, 1975). Diffusion through the unstirred layer depends on the size of a molecule and its solubility. Bile salt micelles may seem cumbersome compared with smaller molecules of monoglyceride, but water-insoluble monoglyceride can only cross the diffusion barrier in quantity when transported by micellar carriers.

INVESTIGATING THE LUMINAL PHASE OF FAT ABSORPTION

Fat digestion and solubilisation can be assessed by feeding a standard test meal and by sampling intestinal contents from the proximal jejunum. The output of pancreatic enzymes and bile salts can be quantified (Brunner et al, 1974), but often only the concentrations of these substances are measured (Lundh, 1958).

Whether digestion of dietary triglyceride is normal can be assessed by comparing the amount of FFA with the amount of unhydrolysed fatty acid; whether the products of digestion are normally solubilised can be judged by quantifying the lipids which are dissolved in the aqueous phase of intestinal contents. Pursuing the answer to the latter question involves removing the oily droplets of intestinal contents by either centrifugation (Go et al, 1970) or ultrafiltration (Porter and Saunders, 1971). All these techniques are somewhat problematic (Saunders, 1972), but they have yielded important physioloigcal information (Hofmann and Borgström, 1964): the aqueous micellar phase of normal human jejunal contents contains bile salt, monoglyceride, and fatty acid, but virtually no triglyceride or diglyceride.

How the composition of intestinal contents is affected by several disease states is recorded in Table 2.1. The fatty acid content of the micellar phase is especially impoverished in patients with external biliary fistulae. Some lipolysis occurs in intestinal contents of patients with chronic alcoholic pancreatitis; micellar FFA is one-fifth of normal concentration, yet it is fifty-fold higher than in bile salt deficiency. The composition of intestinal contents may be nearly normal in some patients with small intestinal stasis despite excessive dilution of the test meal. These data, however, do not indicate whether fatty acids are being absorbed from the proximal small intestine; such information could be decided directly by measuring fatty acid absorption from intestinal contents under steady state conditions (Northfield and Hofmann, 1975), or indirectly, by examining the intestinal absorptive cells histologically (Rubin, 1966). To understand the interrelationships between intestinal contents and absorptive cells it is necessary to consider the mucosal phase of fat absorption.

THE MUCOSAL PHASE OF FAT ABSORPTION

Uptake of Lipids

There are three anatomic adaptations of the small intestine which account for its remarkable surface area. First, there are circular mucosal folds. Second, there are innumerable, 1 mm-long villi covering the circular folds which multiply the absorptive area about eight times. Third, there are microvilli of about 1 μm in length covering the luminal surface of the absorptive cells. The microvilli increase the absorptive surface area a further 14 to 24-fold so that the total area becomes 200 to 500 m^2 (Davenport, 1971). Almost half of the total absorptive surface area is present in the first quarter of the human small intestine because its circular mucosal folds are more prominent, its villi are longer, and its population of mucus-secreting goblet cells is less than in the ileum.

Ingested food and trophic hormones influence the small intestinal mucosa. When animals are fed parenterally the intestinal weight decreases (Johnson et al, 1975) unless pentagastrin is given (Johnson et al, 1975). When the human intestine is resected, the remaining mucosa can undergo hyperplasia by increasing the number of epithelial cells per unit length of villus (Porus, 1965). And in rats, the ileum can adapt to compensate for the loss of proximal small intestine (Weser, 1971); pancreatic secretions in the intestinal lumen seem to mediate this hyperplastic change (Altmann, 1972).

Covering the surface of the microvilli is a layer of negatively charged mucopolysaccharides called the glycocalyx. How this layer interacts with the adjacent water layer or with the products of fat digestion is unknown. It is believed that lipids are absorbed as molecules from those which are dispersed in aqueous solution adjacent to the microvillus membrane. Uptake is independent of bile salts for lipids with finite solubility in water, such as short-chain or as unsaturated long-chain fatty acids. Bile salts, on the other hand, are obligatory for the absorption of cholesterol and fat-soluble vitamins, as discussed above.

The intact mixed micelle does not enter the intestinal absorptive cell (Wilson and Dietschy, 1972) and conjugated bile salts remain within the lumen where they can continue to solubilise lipid. Monoglyceride and FFA are passively absorbed; their absorption continues even when cellular enzymes are numbed by cold (Strauss, 1966). Absorption of FFA into the surface microvillous membrane of absorptive cells can be regarded as a partitioning between luminal water and lipid membrane. This partitioning of FFA into the membrane may be enhanced by a fatty acid binding protein in the cytosol of absorptive cells which transports FFA from the microvillous membrane to the endoplasmic reticulum (Ockner and Manning, 1974).

Intracellular Fates of Absorbed Lipid

The liberated fatty acids and monoglycerides are resynthesised into triglyceride within the intestinal absorptive cells. One benefit of this resynthesis is to lower the concentration of FFA within the absorptive cell so that diffusion of FFA into the absorptive cells is favoured. There are two biochemical pathways by which triglycerides can be synthesised within intestinal absorptive cells. The major, monoglyceride, pathway has been shown to predominate in man (Kayden, Senior and Mattson, 1967). This pathway involves activation of the long-chain fatty acids with coenzyme A, formation of 1,2-diglyceride from absorbed 2-monoglyceride and fatty acid-CoA, and, finally, condensation of another fatty acid-CoA with the diglyceride. The component enzymes of this pathway are purified simultaneously when the biochemist conjures with intestinal microsomes—an observation which suggests that the enzymes exist as a complex. This complex has been called triglyceride synthetase (Rao and Johnston, 1966). Similarly, hamster intestinal microsomes can resynthesise lecithin from absorbed lysolecithin and fatty acid (Mansbach, 1973).

The other minor route for triglyceride synthesis is the α-glycerophosphate pathway in which glycerophosphate from the glycolytic cycle or from absorbed glycerol reacts with two molecules of fatty acid-CoA. The phosphate ester is then cleaved so that the diglyceride can react with another molecule of fatty acid-CoA to form triglyceride or perhaps with a molecule of phosphoryl choline to form lecithin.

What factors may influence triglyceride synthesis? Fatty acids whose hydrocarbon chain is less than 12 carbons are less readily activated to acetyl-CoA derivatives (Brindley and Hübscher, 1966). Medium and shorter chain fatty acids are not transported predominantely as chylomicron triglyceride but as FFA in portal venous blood (Bloom, Chaikoff and Reinhardt, 1951). An increased availability of long-chain fatty acid substrate is associated with an increase in the specific activities of components of triglyceride synthetase (Singh et al, 1972). It is not surprising that there have been difficulties in trying to prove that bile salts have intracellular effects on intestinal mucosa because their stimulation of triglyceride synthesis (Dawson and Isselbacher, 1960) may be due to their increasing the availability of fatty acid substrate.

Formation of Intestinal Lipid Particles

The intestinal absorptive cell must now solve the problem of transporting the reconstituted triglyceride in a form which is compatible with water. The solution is to envelop the triglyceride with a hydrophilic coating so that the resulting particles can be dispersed in water without coalescing.

The intestinal absorptive cells manufacture a spectrum of lipid particles. After a fatty meal, chylomicrons—particles of more than 100 nm (1000 Å)—appear in intestinal absorptive cells, intestinal lymphatics and peripheral blood. They have a hydrophobic core of triglyceride and cholesterol ester surrounded by a hydrophilic coating of protein, phospholipid, and free cholesterol (Zilversmit, 1968).

Smaller intestinal lipid particles are present in fasting human jejunal absorptive cells (Tytgat, Rubin and Saunders, 1971). They have the same size distribution as plasma very low density lipoproteins (VLDL). These intestinal particles are reduced in number in patients with a biliary fistula (Porter et al, 1971), and are absent in patients who lack β-lipoprotein (Tytgat et al, 1971). These observations suggest that endogenous lipids such as those from bile are transported from small intestinal absorptive cells as VLDL-like particles.

The relationship between intestinal chylomicron-like particles and VLDL-like particles is poorly understood. The 'lumpers' argue that these particles are part of a continuous spectrum. In their view, chylomicrons are VLDL particles whose triglyceride component is expanded during fat absorption. The 'splitters' point to differences in apoprotein composition which indicate that chylomicrons and VLDL are distinct classes of lipoproteins (Glickman and Kirsch, 1974). Resolution of the argument is complicated by plasma

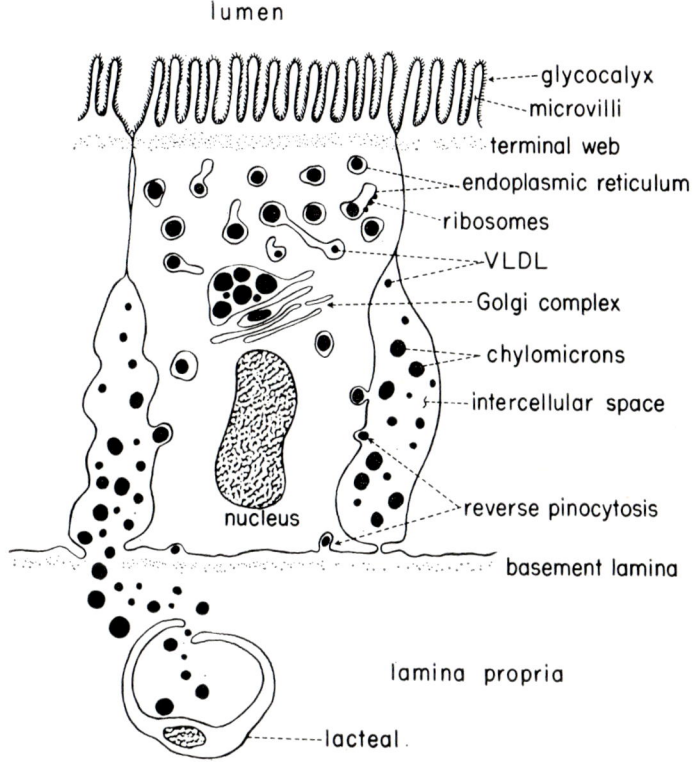

Figure 2.1 An electron microscopist's view of a jejunal absorptive cell during a fatty meal. The microvilli of the brush border face the lumen. The nucleus is located basally

proteins contaminating intestinal lipid particles during fat absorption (Wollin and Jaques, 1973), and by the structure of absorbed fatty acids influencing the size of intestinal lipid particles (Ockner and Jones, 1970).

How these lipid particles reach intestinal lymphatics is outlined in Figure 2.1. During the fasting state, only osmiophilic droplets of less than 0.1 μm diameter, the very low density lipoprotein particles (VLDL), are seen within the absorptive cells, the intercellular spaces, the lamina propria and the lacteals.

After a fatty meal, a variety of sizes of lipid particles from less than 100 to 750 nm in diameter is present in the same places where VLDL particles were seen during the fasting state. The only difference is that the larger postprandial lipid particles, or chylomicrons, predominate. Passive non-ionic diffusion of fatty acid and monoglyceride molecules through the glycocalyx, microvillous plasma membrane and terminal web is invisible. When lipid appears within profiles of the endoplasmic reticulum, it is as resynthesised triglyceride. The lipid particles are then transported via the interconnecting tubules of the endoplasmic reticulum to a specialised area above the nucleus, the cisternae of the Golgi complex. Here the particles are delayed temporarily while they may receive envelopes of phospholipid and protein before finding their way to the lateral and basal plasma membrane. The lipoprotein particles are extruded predominantly into the intercellular space by reverse pinocytosis. From the intercellular space the lipoprotein particles move through gaps in the basement lamina into the extracellular spaces of the lamina propria. After a relatively long journey through the lamina propria they enter lacteals. In contrast, radioautographic studies show that medium-chain fatty acids, which are transported as FFA in portal venous blood, do not frequent the Golgi complex or the lacteals (Carlier and Bezard, 1975).

The importance of intestinal lipid particles may reach beyond their role in transporting endogenous and exogenous lipid from absorptive cells. Possibly the manufacture of these particles may be at fault in some hyperlipemic states such as those induced by ethanol (Mistilis and Ockner, 1972) or by carbohydrate (Den Besten et al, 1973).

INVESTIGATING THE MUCOSAL PHASE OF FAT ABSORPTION

There is no simple method for studying human duodenojejunal mucosa. A peroral biopsy of the fasting proximal small intestine usually suffices for the investigation of a patient with steatorrhoea who then improves with a gluten-free diet. A thorough review of small intestinal biopsy was published recently (Perera, Weinstein and Rubin, 1975). Occasionally, electron microscopy of postprandial mucosa may reveal abnormalities which help to explain the pathogenesis of puzzling streatorrhoea (Ament et al, 1972).

An indirect method of assessing mucosal function would be to measure the amount of triglyceride absorbed by the time a meal reached a point just beyond the duodenojejunal junction. Because all the jejunal contents cannot be removed through a narrow peroral tube, reference to a non-absorbable marker has been advocated. The fraction of triglyceride absorbed could be calculated from the ratios of marker to triglyceride in the meal and in a sample of jejunal contents. Markers of the watery phase of a meal, however, tend to separate from triglyceride in the stomach (Wiggins and Dawson, 1961). Markers in the oily phase may also separate from triglyceride in the stomach (Saunders,

O'Brien and Smith, 1972), and should tend to separate in the intestine as triglyceride is digested and its products move into the aqueous phase of intestinal contents. Marker techniques in the small intestine should be regarded with suspicion. However, fatty markers may prove to be of value when fat absorption is assessed by faecal analysis (Hoving et al, 1975).

SUMMARY OF DIGESTION AND ABSORPTION OF TRIGLYCERIDE

The process of fat absorption can be thought of as as a series of way-stations in order to dramatise possible derailments. Normal gastric emptying ensures that dietary triglyceride is mixed well with bile and pancreatic juice. Triglyceride digestion involves hydrolysis to more hydrophilic monoglyceride and fatty acid, and solubilisation of these products in luminal water with bile salts. Aided by the churning action of the small intestine, solubilised fatty acid and monoglyceride can penetrate the poorly stirred layer adjacent to the microvillous membrane. They diffuse passively into the absorptive cells where they are resynthesised to triglyceride. To render the triglyceride compatible with water, chylomicrons are formed, and are delivered into the intercellular spaces and, from there, into intestinal lymphatics.

This process is so efficient in normal man that about 80 per cent of ingested triglyceride seems to be absorbed in the proximal half of the small intestine (Borgström, Dahlquist and Lundh, 1962).

ABNORMALITIES THAT AFFECT THE LUMINAL PHASE PREDOMINANTLY

Abnormal Gastric Emptying

Gastric emptying is deranged after vagotomy and pyloroplasty (Cooke, 1975). A mild steatorrhoea ensues; usually the coefficient of fat absorption is higher than 85 per cent (Edwards et al, 1974). More serious disturbances occur after gastric resection when intestinal continuity is restored by gastrojejunostomy. The main part of a meal may be well down into the jejunum before pancreatic enzymes are secreted so that there is poor mixing (Lundh, 1958). Gastric surgery could result in catastrophic malabsorption if it were added to underlying disorders which have diminished the absorptive surface of the small intestine, for example coeliac disease or intestinal resection.

Deficient Release of CCK–PZ

Effective levels of CCK–PZ could be abnormally low in disease which affect the proximal small intestinal mucosa. In coeliac disease, defects in the output of bile salts, and of pancreatic lipase have been identified after meals, but not after intravenous CCK-PZ (DiMagno, Go and Summerskill, 1972). Whether such defects contribute to steatorrhoea in this disease is difficult to assess because pancreatic enzymes seem to be secreted in superabundance.

Bile Salt Deficiency

Bile salts are not obligatory for the absorption of dietary fatty acids. Munk (1890) was the first to show that animals with bile fistulae continue to absorb more than 50 per cent of their dietary fat. Luminal digestion of triglyceride seems to be normal, at least as revealed by the normal concentration of free fatty acids in jejunal contents (Knoebel and Ryan, 1963; Porter et al, 1971), but the free fatty acid resides almost entirely in the oily phase of intestinal contents (Table 2.1). Depressed rates of fatty acid absorption in the proximal

Table 2.1 Duodenojejunal contents after a fatty meal[a]

	Unseparated phases					Aqueous phase	
	pH	Phenol red (μmol)	Trypsin (μg/ml)	Lipolysis (%)	FFA (mmol)	Bile salts (mmol)	FFA (mmol)
Normal (12)	6 ± 0.5	90 ± 12	630 ± 160	34 ± 7	17 ± 4	9 ± 2	10 ± 3
Bile fistula (4)	6 ± 0.7	80 ± 16	530 ± 80	31 ± 10	10 ± 4	0.8 ± 0.2	0.04 ± 0.01
Chronic alcoholic pancreatitis (4)	6 ± 0.6	90 ± 8	<5	11 ± 8	4 ± 2	9 ± 2	2 ± 1
Intestinal stasis syndrome (1)	6.0	48	260	47.4	14.8	4.4	8.2

[a] The aqueous phase of intestinal contents was obtained by filtration (Porter and Saunders, 1971). The test meal contained phenol red, 160 μmol. The values are means ± s.d.

small intestine (Kern and Borgström, 1965) leads to an increased delivery of fatty acid to the ileum (Knoebel and Ryan, 1963).

Borgström (1953) showed that absorbed palmitic acid was transported from the bile-deficient rat intestine presumably by the portal vein because only one-quarter of the absorbed radioactivity was recovered in intestinal lymph. Some absorbed long-chain fatty acids seem to be transported from the bile-deficient, human small intestine via the portal vein (Blomstrand, Carlberger and Forsgren, 1969), although some appear to utilise the chylomicron-lymphatic pathway (Porter et al, 1971).

Why might chylomicron formation be impaired in bile-deficient animals? One factor might be a depression of those microsomal enzymes which re-synthesise triglyceride (Rodgers, Tandon and O'Brien, 1973). Another factor may be the loss of 4 to 8 g of biliary lecithin per day (Arnesjö et al, 1969) which would ordinarily contribute to chylomicron synthesis (O'Doherty, Kakis and Kuksis, 1973). Under these circumstances, it is not surprising that some sparingly soluble long-chain fatty acids might be swept away in portal venous blood which flows some 500 times faster than intestinal lymph and which constitutes the major route of transport for absorbed freely soluble short-chain fatty acids.

The loss of the absorptive surface of the ileum through resection, by-pass, or disease greatly worsens the steatorrhoea which results from simply interrupting the enterohepatic circulation of bile salts. If one can extrapolate from experiments with monkeys (Small, Dowling and Redinger, 1972), loss of the active transport system for bile salts in the human ileum constitutes an interruption of the enterohepatic circulation of 50 per cent. Increased hepatic synthesis of bile salts cannot compensate for the deficit and, consequently, the size of the bile salt pool falls. Patients who have a functioning gall bladder will store bile salts during their usual overnight fasts. At the time of breakfast there will be a normal complement of bile salts in the proximal small intestine. However, about half the bile salts produced at breakfast may be lost into the stools. Bile salt concentrations will retrogress during the subsequent meals of the day (Van Deest, et al, 1968) (see also Chapter 9).

Certain drugs may decrease the concentration of soluble bile salts in intestinal contents. The cationic amino groups of neomycin bind and precipitate bile salt, as well as fatty acid anions (Thompson et al, 1971). Neomycin also adversely affects the small intestinal mucosa (Dobbins, Herrero and Mansbach, 1968). Cholestyramine, an anionic exchange resin, can bind bile salts and increase their faecal excretion (Hofmann and Poley, 1969).

Insufficiency of Pancreatic Enzymes

Steatorrhoea does not ensue until pancreatic enzyme output is reduced by 90 per cent (DiMagno, Go and Summerskill, 1973). Theoretically, in pancreatic insufficiency triglyceride hydrolysis should be markedly impaired. Some long-chain fatty acids may be liberated by the action of pharyngeal and gastric lipases and of residual amounts of pancreatic lipase. Any liberated long-chain fatty acids should dissolve readily in luminal water because bile salts are present. In fact, in our patients with chronic alcoholic pancreatitis hydrolysis was one-third of normal, and solubilised fatty acid was one-fifth of normal (Table 2.1). In spite of a seemingly adequate concentration of solubilised fatty acid, fifty-fold that of bile fistula subjects, no evidence of fat absorption by jejunal mucosa was uncovered by the electron microscope. Lipid particles were not present in the apical cytoplasm of absorptive cells at villous tips; chylomicrons did not appear in the intercellular spaces. These electron-microscopic abnormalities could be reversed by adding pancreatic enzymes to the test meal, or by feeding a predigested fatty meal whose enzymes were inactivated (Shimoda et al, 1974). Patients with untreated pancreatic insufficiency absorb a third of their dietary fat despite their electron-microscopic abnormalities. Perhaps the pathogenesis of the steatorrhoea is more complex than mere depression of triglyceride hydrolysis;

perhaps there are other abnormalities in the intestinal lumen. The oily phase of intestinal contents will be expanded by unhydrolysed triglyceride and will conceal FFA and fat-soluble vitamins. The aqueous phase of intestinal contents may be abnormal. Lecithins depress the rate of fatty acid absorption in vitro (Rampone, 1973). When lecithin hydrolysis is impaired a relative excess of lecithins and bile salts may retard fatty acid absorption by favouring partitioning of fatty acids into the aqueous phase rather than into the lipid membrane. The mucosal phase may be abnormal because the rate of entry of FFA into absorptive cells is slow. In pancreatic insufficiency FFA may leave absorptive cells as monomers in portal blood or as triglyceride in very small lipid particles which cannot be visualised by electron microscopy.

Pancreatic lipase may be ineffective in acidic intestinal contents of patients with gastrinomas and gastric acid hypersecretion because it is inactivated below a pH of 3. Other defects in fat absorption occur in these patients. Dihydroxy-bile salts are precipitated because the luminal pH is less than their pK_a; trihydroxy-bile salts are diluted (Go et al, 1970). The duodenojejunal mucosa is injured, presumably due to acid and pepsin (Shimoda, Saunders and Rubin, 1968).

Stagnation of Jejunal Contents with Bacterial Overgrowth

The interior of the small intestinal cylinder is a physiological dead space because absorption occurs from peripheral intestinal contents immediately adjacent to the microvillous membrane. Much of the fluid in dilated, aperistaltic jejunal loops may be unstirred, and may be regarded as being in an expanded dead space. Test meals, bile salts, and pancreatic enzymes may be diluted excessively in the duodenum of such patients (Table 2.1). Bacteria can grow exuberantly in the fluid-filled intestinal loops, they can interfere with the absorption of vitamin B_{12}, and deconjugate and dehydroxylate bile salts. Deconjugated bile salts can be absorbed by passive diffusion which reduces the concentration of bile salts in the micellar phase. Metabolites such as deoxycholic acid may contribute to the extensive mucosal damage which can be seen in this disease (Ament et al, 1972; Shimoda, O'Brien and Saunders, 1974).

ABNORMALITIES IN THE MUCOSAL PHASE OF FAT ABSORPTION

The Coeliac Disease Lesion

The small intestine seems to respond to injury in a characteristic fashion. Villous architecture is deranged in almost all mucosal diseases. A great deal of absorptive surface is lost especially if microvilli are also injured. The severity of the small intestinal mucosal injury is inversely related to the distance from the pylorus if the noxious agent enters from the stomach. Fortunately for logic, the severity of malabsorption appears to correlate directly with the length of small intestine that is injured (Perera et al, 1975). The most common cause of the coeliac disease lesion in North America is related to the ingestion of gluten. Diagnosis requires a characteristic proximal small intestinal biopsy and a clinical response to a gluten-free diet.

Deficiency of Apo-β-lipoprotein

Abetalipoproteinaemia is a rare disorder in which the number of investigators far exceeds the number of patients. Nevertheless, the disease represents an important natural experiment because it shows that, without apo-β-lipoprotein, chylomicrons are not formed after a fatty meal. Dietary fatty acids appear to enter absorptive cells of the proximal small intestine but triglycerides accumulate in the cells (Ways et al, 1967). These patients, however, absorb more than 80 per cent of their dietary fatty acids which suggest that fatty acids must be leaving from the mucosa by an alternate pathway such as the portal venous route. The concept that inhibited protein synthesis impairs fat absorption was confirmed recently (Glickman, Kirsch and Isselbacher, 1972). Rats poisoned with cycloheximide transported less infused fatty acid in their intestinal lymph and their lymph chlomicrons were abnormally large.

Obstruction of the Intestinal Lymphatics

This may be a congenital or acquired disease in which dilated intestinal lymphatics filled with chylomicrons are present even in the fasting state. In addition to the block in chylomicron transport some of the dilated lymphatics may rupture and spill their contents into the intestinal lumen or into the peritoneal cavity. The health of such patients can be improved by substituting medium-chain for long-chain triglycerides. The medium-chain fatty acids leave the small intestine via the portal venous pathway.

SOME CONSEQUENCES OF FAT MALABSORPTION

Watery Diarrhoea

Diarrhoea is a common but not invariable symptom of those diseases which cause fat malabsorption. In some of them inefficiency of salt and water absorption is inherent; for example, the jejunum in untreated coeliac disease secretes water (Fordtran et al, 1967; Kumar et al, 1974). But even when the small intestine and colon are structurally sound watery diarrhoea may accompany steatorrhoea.

The original concept of 'fatty acid diarrhoea' supposed that intestinal bacteria transformed long-chain fatty acids into castor-oil-like hydroxy fatty acids (James, Webb and Kellock, 1961; Kim and Spritz, 1968; Soong et al,

1972), but faecal hydroxy fatty acid concentrations do not correlate well with stool water content in patients with steatorrhoea (Bliss, Small and Donaldson, 1973; Wiggins, Cummings and Pearson, 1974). However, excessive luminal fatty acids will themselves inhibit the absorption of salt and water by the human small bowel and colon (Ammon and Phillips, 1973; Ammon, Thomas and Phillips, 1974). Perhaps both mechanisms conspire to add a watery component to steatorrhoea.

Several manipulations may reduce diarrhoea in patients with fat malabsorption. Obviously the underlying disease should be treated. Another manipulation is to lower the dietary fat content, which will lower faecal fat excretion and watery diarrhoea (Andersson, Isaksson and Sjögren, 1974). In patients who need the fatty calories, substitution of medium-chain triglyceride will lower stool water output (Bochenek, Rodgers and Balint, 1970; Hofmann and Poley, 1972). Finally, the use of oral fluids with a composition similar to that used in cholera may prevent dehydration in patients with excessive diarrhoea, because glucose continues to enhance water absorption in the presence of fatty acid-induced fluid secretion (Brown and Ammon, 1974).

Decreased Calcium and Magnesium Absorption

Divalent ion absorption is decreased in steatorrhoea particularly because long-chain fatty acids bind calcium and magnesium. As the amount of fatty acid in the stool increases, the amount of insoluble fatty acid salts of calcium and magnesium increases (Bliss, Small and Donaldson, 1972). Any disorder causing steatorrhoea may lead to calcium malabsorption (Agnew and Holdsworth, 1971). Further decreases in calcium absorption occur when there is bile salt deficiency or severe mucosal damage which would impair the absorption of vitamin D.

It may be important to give calcium and magnesium supplements without food, since absorption of radioactive calcium is normal in patients with steatorrhoea when calcium is given in the fasting state (Agnew, Kehayoglou and Holdsworth, 1969).

Oxalic Acid Absorption

Oxalic acid, a constituent of many foods, is poorly absorbed from the normal intestine. Absorption of oxalate is abnormally high in patients with a variety of intestinal disorders, such as ileal resection (Chadwick, Modha and Dowling, 1973; Stauffer, Humphreys and Weir, 1973; Earnest et al, 1974); regional enteritis (Smith, Fromm and Hofmann, 1972; Dowling, Rose and Sutor, 1971); small bowel bypass operations (Dickstein and Frame, 1973; Fikri and Casella, 1975); pancreatic insufficiency (Stauffer, Steward and Bertrand, 1974); and coeliac disease (Smith et al, 1972; McDonald, Earnest and Admirand, 1975). Fat malabsorption is common to these conditions and there is a good correlation between intestinal absorption of dietary oxalate and the quantity of faecal fat. This association has been noted in patients with ileal resection (Earnest et al, 1974) and with coeliac disease (McDonald et al, 1975).

The colon may be the site of this excessive oxalate absorption, for ileostomy patients with fat malabsorption do not develop hyperoxaluria on high-oxalate diets (Earnest et al, 1974). Studies of regional differences in oxalate absorption in rat intestine also support the concept that increased oxalate absorption occurs primarily in the colon when there is steatorrhoea (Saunders, Sillery and McDonald 1975).

These observations may be relevant to the pathogenesis of oxalate renal stones in patients with small bowel disease.

REFERENCES

Agnew, J. E. & Holdsworth, C. D. (1971) The effect of fat on calcium absorption from a mixed meal in normal subjects, patients with malabsorption disease, and patients with a partial gastrectomy. *Gut*, **12**, 973.
Agnew, J. E., Kehayoglou, A. K. & Holdsworth, C. D. (1969) Comparison of three isotopic methods for the study of calcium absorption. *Gut*, **10**, 590.
Altmann, G. G. (1972) Influence of starvation and refeeding on mucosal size and epithelial renewal in the rat small intestine. *American Journal of Anatomy*, **133**, 391.
Ament, M. E., Shimoda, S. S., Saunders, D. R. & Rubin, C. E. (1972) Pathogenesis of steatorrhea in three cases of small intestinal stasis syndrome. *Gastroenterology*, **63**, 728.
Ammon, H. V. & Phillips, S. F. (1973) Inhibition of colonic water and electrolyte absorption by fatty acids in man. *Gastroenterology*, **65**, 744.
Ammon, H. V., Thomas, P. J. & Phillips, S. F. (1974) Effects of oleic acid and ricinoleic acid on net jejunal water and electrolyte movement. Perfusion studies in man. *Journal of Clinical Investigation*, **53**, 374.
Andersson, H., Isaksson, B. & Sjögren, B. (1974) Fat-reduced diet in the symptomatic treatment of small bowel disease. *Gut*, **15**, 351.
Annegers, J. H. (1949) Fecal excretion of nutrients in impaired absorption. *Northwestern University Quarterly Bulletin*, **23**, 202.
Arnesjö, B., Nilsson, A., Barrowman, J. & Borgström, B. (1969) Intestinal digestion and absorption of cholesterol and lecithin in the human. *Scandinavian Journal of Gastroenterology*, **4**, 653.
Bliss, C. M., Small, D. M. & Donaldson, R. M. (1971) The use of sonication to eliminate sampling and storage errors in stool fat determinations. *Clinical Research*, **19**, 387.
Bliss, C. M., Small, D. M. & Donaldson, R. M. (1972) The excretion of calcium and magnesium fatty acid soaps in steatorrhea (Abstract). *Gastroenterology*, **62**, 724.
Bliss, C. M., Small, D. M. & Donaldson, R. M. (1973) Water phase fatty acid excretion in diarrhea (Abstract). *Gastroenterology*, **64**, 701.
Blomstrand, R. (1955) A study on the intestinal absorption of fat in normal adults and in non-tropical sprue with carbon-labelled oleic acid and palmitic acid. *Acta medica scandinavica*, **152**, 129.
Blomstrand, R., Carlberger, G. & Forsgren, L. (1969) Intestinal absorption and metabolism of ^{14}C-labelled fatty acids in the absence of bile in man. *Acta chirurgica scandinavica*, **135**, 329.
Bloom, B., Chaikoff, I. L. & Reinhardt, W. O. (1951) Intestinal lymph as pathway for transport of absorbed fatty acids of different chain lengths. *American Journal of Physiology*, **166**, 451.
Bochenek, W., Rodgers, J. B. & Balint, J. A. (1970) Effects of changes in dietary lipids on intestinal fluid loss in the short-bowel syndrome. *Annals of Internal Medicine*, **72**, 205.

Borgström, B. (1953) The effect of bile diversion on fat absorption in the rat. *Acta physiologica scandinavica*, **28**, 279.
Borgström, B. (1974) Bile salts—their physiological functions in the gastrointestinal tract. *Acta medica scandinavica*. **196**, 1.
Borgström, B. & Erlanson, C. (1971) Pancreatic juice co-lipase: physiological importance. *Biochimica et biophysica acta*, **242**, 509.
Borgström, B., Dahlquist, A. & Lundh, G. (1962) On the site of absorption of fat from the human small intestine. *Gut*, **3**, 315.
Brindley, D. N. & Hübscher, G. (1966) The effect of chain length on the activation and subsequent incorporation into glycerides by the small intestinal mucosa. *Biochimica et biophysica acta*, **125**, 92.
Brown, D. B. & Ammon, H. V. (1974) Continuing glucose enchanced water absorption during fluid secretion induced by glycodeoxycholic acid (GDC) and oleic acid (OA) in man (Abstract). *Clinical Research*, **22**, 601A.
Brunner, H., Northfield, T. C., Hofmann, A. F., Go, V. L. W. & Summerskill, W. H. J. (1974) Gastric emptying and secretion of bile acids, cholesterol, and pancreatic enzymes during digestion. *Mayo Clinic Proceedings*, **49**, 851.
Carey, M. C. & Small, D. M. (1972) Micelle formation by bile salts. *Archives of Internal Medicine*, **130**, 506.
Carlier, H. & Bezard, J. (1975) Electron microscope autoradiographic study of intestinal absorption of decanoic and octanoic acids in the rat. *Journal of Cell Biology*, **65**, 383.
Chadwick, V. S., Modha, K. & Dowling, R. H. (1973) Mechanism of hyperoxaluria in patients with ileal dysfunction. *New England Journal of Medicine*, **289**, 172.
Cooke, A. R. (1975) Control of gastric emptying and motility. *Gastroenterology*, **68**, 804.
Davenport, H. W. (1971) *Physiology of the Digestive Tract*, 3rd edn, p. 171. Chicago: Year Book Medical Publishers.
Dawson, A. M. & Isselbacher, K. J. (1960) Studies in lipid metabolism in the small intestine with observations on the role of bile salts. *Journal of Clinical Investigation*, **39**, 730.
Den Besten, L., Reyna, R. H., Connor, W. E. & Stegink, L. D. (1973) The different effects on the serum lipids and fecal steroids of high carbohydrate diets given orally or intravenously. *Journal of Clinical Investigation*, **52**, 1384.
De Haas, G. H., Postema, N. M., Nieuwen Huizen, W. & Van Deenven, L. L. M. (1968) Purification and properties of an anionic zymogen of phospholipase A from porcine pancreas. *Biochimica et biophysica acta*, **159**, 118.
Dickstein, S. S. & Frame, B. (1973) Urinary tract calculi after intestinal shunt operations for the treatment of obesity. *Surgery, Gynecology and Obstetrics*, **136**, 257.
DiMagno, E. P., Go, V. L. W. & Summerskill, W. H. J. (1972) Impaired cholecystokinin–pancreozymin secretion, intraluminal dilution, and maldigestion of fat in sprue. *Gastroenterology*, **63**, 25.
DiMagno, E. P., Go, V. L. W. & Summerskill, W. H. J. (1973) Relations between pancreatic enzyme outputs and malabsorption in severe pancreatic insufficiency. *New England Journal of Medicine*, **288**, 813.
Dobbins, W. O. III, Herrero, B. A. & Mansbach, C. M. (1968) Morphological alterations associated with neomycin induced malabsorption. *American Journal of Medical Science*, **255**, 63.
Dowling, R. H., Rose, G. A. & Sutor, D. J. (1971) Hyperoxaluria and renal calculi in ileal disease. *Lancet*, **1**, 1103.
Earnest, D. L., Johnson, G., Williams, H. E. & Admirand, W. H. (1974) Hyperoxaluria in patients with ileal resection: an abnormality in dietary oxalate absorption. *Gastroenterology*, **66**, 1114.
Edwards, J. P., Lyndon, P. J., Smith, R. B. & Johnston, D. (1974) Faecal fat excretion after truncal, selective, and highly selective vagotomy for duodenal ulcer. *Gut*, **15**, 521.
Fikri, E. & Casella, R. R. (1975) Hyperoxaluria and urinary tract calculi after jejunoileal bypass. *American Journal of Surgery*, **129**, 334.
Fordtran, J. S., Recton, F. C., Locklear, T. W. & Ewton, M. R. (1967) Water and solute movement in the small intestine of patients with sprue. *Journal of Clinical Investigation*, **46**, 287.
Gangl, A. & Ockner, R. K. (1975) Intestinal metabolism of lipids and lipoproteins. *Gastroenterology*, **68**, 167.

Glickman, R. M. & Kirsch, K. (1974) The apoproteins of various size classes of human chylous fluid lipoproteins. *Biochimica et biophysica acta*, **371**, 255.

Glickman, R. M., Kirsch, K. & Isselbacher, K. J. (1972) Fat absorption during inhibition of protein synthesis: studies of lymph chylomicrons. *Journal of Clinical Investigation*, **51**, 356.

Go, V. L. W., Poley, J. R., Hofmann, A. F. & Summerskill, W. H. J. (1970) Disturbances in fat digestion induced by acidic jejunal pH due to gastric hypersecretion in man. *Gastroenterology*, **58**, 638.

Gray, G. M. (1975) Carbohydrate digestion and absorption. Role of the small intestine. *New England Journal of Medicine*, **292**, 1225.

Hamosh, M., Klaeveman, H. L., Wolf, R. O. & Scow, R. O. (1975) Pharyngeal lipase and digestion of dietary triglyceride in man. *Journal of Clinical Investigation*, **55**, 908.

Hepner, G. W. (1974) Breath analysis: gastroenterological applications. *Gastroenterology*, **67**, 1250.

Hofmann, A. F. (1974) Lipid digestion and absorption, Unit V, Undergraduate Teaching Project, American Gastroenterological Association. Distributed by Milner Fenwick, Baltimore, Md.

Hofmann, A. F. & Borgström, B. (1964) The intraluminal phase of fat digestion in man: the lipid content of the micellar and oil phases of intestinal content during fat digestion and absorption. *Journal of Clinical Investigation*, **43**, 247.

Hofmann, A. F. & Mekhjian, H. S. (1973) Bile acids and the intestinal absorption of fat and electrolytes in health and disease. In *The Bile Acids*, Vol. II, pp. 103-152. New York: Plenum Press.

Hofmann, A. F. & Poley, J. R. (1969) Cholestyramine treatment of diarrhea associated with ileal resection. *New England Journal of Medicine*, **281**, 397.

Hofmann, A. F. & Poley, J. R. (1972) Role of bile acid malabsorption in pathogenesis of diarrhea and steatorrhea in patients with ileal resection. I. Response to cholestyramine or replacement of dietary long-chain triglyceride by medium-chain triglyceride. *Gastroenterology*, **62**, 918.

Hoving, J., Valkema, A. J., Wilson, H. M. P. & Woldring, M. D. (1975) Properties of glycerol-^{75}Se-triether: a lipid-soluble marker for the estimation of intestinal fat absorption. *Journal of Laboratory and Clinical Medicine*, **86**, 286.

Hyun, J., Treadwell, C. R. & Vahouny, G. V. (1972) Pancreatic juice cholesterol esterase. Studies on molecular weight and bile salt induced polymerisation. *Archives of Biochemistry and Biophysics*, **153**, 233.

James, A. T., Webb, J. & Kellock, T. D. (1961) The occurrence of unusual fatty acids in faecal lipids from human beings with normal and abnormal fat absorption. *Biochemical Journal*, **78**, 333.

Johnson, L. R., Copeland, E. M., Dudrick, S. J., Lichtenberger, L. M. & Castro, G. A. (1975) Structural and hormonal alterations in the gastrointestinal tract of parenterally fed rats. *Gastroenterology*, **68**, 1177.

Johnson, L. R., Lichtenberger, L. M., Copeland, E. M., Dudrick, S. J. & Castro, G. A. (1975) Action of gastrin on gastrointestinal structure and function. *Gastroenterology*, **68**, 1184.

Kalser, M. H., Leite, C. A. & Warren, W. D. (1968) Fat assimilation after massive distal pancreatectomy. *New England Journal of Medicine*, **279**, 570.

Kasper, H. (1970) Fecal fat excretion, diarrhea and subjective complaints with highly dosed oral fat intake. *Digestion*, **3**, 321.

Kayden, H. J., Senior, J. R. & Mattson, F. H. (1967) The monoglyceride pathway of fat absorption in man. *Journal of Clinical Investigation*, **46**, 1695.

Kern, F. & Borgström, B. (1965) The effect of a conjugated bile on oleic acid absorption in the rat. *Gastroenterology*, **49**, 623.

Kim, Y. S. & Spritz, N. (1968) Hydroxy acid excretion in steatorrhea of pancreatic and nonpancreatic origin. *New England Journal of Medicine*, **279**, 1424.

Knoebel, L. K. & Ryan, J. M. (1963) Digestion and absorption of fat in normal and bile-deficient dogs. *American Journal of Physiology*, **204**, 509.

Krawitt, E. L. & Beeken, W. L. (1975) Limitations of the usefulness of the D-xylose absorption test. *American Journal of Clinical Pathology*, **63**, 261.

Kumar, P. J., Silk, D. B. A., Rousseau, B., Pagaltsos, A. S., Clark, M. L., Dawson, A. M. & Marks, R. (1974) Assessment of jejunal function in patients with dermatitis herpetiformis and adult coeliac disease using a perfusion technique. *Scandinavian Journal of Gastroeneterology*, **9**, 793.
Levitt, M. D. & Duane, W. C. (1972) Floating stools—flatus versus fat. *New England Journal of Medicine*, **286**, 973.
Lundh, G. (1958) Intestinal digestion and absorption after gastrectomy. *Acta chirurgica scandinavica*, Suppl. 231.
Malagelada, J. R., Go, V. L. W. & Summerskill, W. H. J. (1975) Gastric functions in response to solid and homogenised meals. *Clinical Research*, **23**, 387.
Malagelada, J. R., Go, V. L. W., DiMagno, E. P. & Summerskill, W. H. J. (1973) Interactions between intraluminal bile acids and digestive products on pancreatic and gall bladder function. *Journal of Clinical Investigation*, **52**, 2160.
Maldonado, J. E., Gregg, J. A., Green, P. A. & Brown, A. L. (1970) Chronic idiopathic intestinal pseudo-obstruction. *American Journal of Medicine*, **49**, 203.
Mansbach, C. M. II (1973) Complex lipid synthesis in hamster intestine. *Biochimica biophysica acta*, **296**, 386.
Mansbach, C. M. (1975) Effect of fat feeding on complex lipid synthesis in hamster intestine. *Gastroenterology*, **68**, 708.
Mistilis, S. P. & Ockner, R. K. (1972) Effects of ethanol on endogenous lipid and lipoprotein metabolism in small intestine. *Journal of Laboratory and Clinical Medicine*, **80**, 34.
Munk, I. (1890) Uber die resorption von fetten und festen fettsäuren nach ausschluss der galle vom darmkanel. *Virchows Archiv Pathologie und Anatomie*, **122**, 302.
McDonald, G. B., Earnest, D. L. & Admirand, W. H. (1975) Hyperoxaluria correlates with steatorrhea in patients with celiac sprue (Abstract). *Gastroenterology*, **68**, 949.
Newman, A. (1974) Progress report. Breath analysis tests in gastroenterology. *Gut*, **15**, 308.
Northfield, T. C. & Hofmann, A. F. (1975) Biliary lipid output during three meals and an overnight fast. *Gut*, **16**, 1.
Ockner, R. K. & Isselbacher (1974) Recent concepts of intestinal fat absorption. *Review of Physiology, Biochemistry, and Pharmacology*, **71**, 107.
Ockner, R. K. & Jones, A. L. (1970) An electron microscopic and functional study of very low density lipoproteins in intestinal lymph. *Journal of Lipid Research*, **11**, 284.
Ockner, R. K. & Manning, J. (1974) Fatty acid binding protein in small intestine: identification, isolation, and evidence for its role in cellular fatty acid transport. *Journal of Clinical Investigation*, **54**, 326.
O'Doherty, P. J. A., Kakis, G. & Kuksis, A. (1973) Role of luminal lecithin in intestinal fat absorption. *Lipids*, **8**, 249.
Onstad, G. R. & Zieve, L. (1972) Carotene absorption. A screening test for steatorrhea. *Journal of the American Medical Association*, **221**, 677.
Perera, D. R., Weinstein, W. M. & Rubin, C. E. (1975) Small intestinal biopsy. *Human Pathology*, **6**, 157.
Porter, H. P. & Saunders, D. R. (1971) Isolation of the aqueous phase of human intestinal contents during the digestion of a fatty meal. *Gastroenterology*, **60**, 997.
Porter, H. P., Saunders, D. R., Tytgat, G., Brunser, O. & Rubin, C. E. (1971) Fat absorption in bile fistula man, a morphological and biochemical study. *Gastroenterology*, **60**, 1008.
Porus, R. L. (1965) Epithelial hyperplasia following massive small bowel resection in man. *Gastroenterology*, **48**, 753.
Raffensperger, E. C., D'Agostino, F., Manfredo, H., Ramirez, M., Brooks, F. P. & O'Neill, F. (1967) Fecal fat excretion: an analysis of four years' experience. *Archives of Internal Medicine*, **119**, 573.
Rampone, A. J. (1973) Studies on micellar fatty acid uptake by rat intestine in vitro with reference to the role of bile. *Journal of Physiology*, **229**, 495.
Rao, G. A. & Johnston, J. M. (1966) Purification and properties of triglyceride synthetase from the intestinal mucosa. *Biochimica et biophysica acta*, **125**, 465.
Rodgers, J. B., Tandon, R. & O'Brien, R. J. (1973) Activities of lipid resterifying enzymes in jejunal microsomes of bile fistula rats—attempts to correlate enzyme activities with microsomal phospholipid content. *Biochimica biophysica acta*, **326**, 345.
Rubin, C. E. (1966) Electron microscopic studies of triglyceride absorption in man. *Gastroenterology*, **50**, 65.

Saunders, D. R. (1972) Testing fat absorption in the human proximal small intestine: the state of the art. *Gastroenterology*, **63**, 186.

Saunders, D. R., O'Brien, T. K. & Smith, K. (1972) Disappointment with triethers as markers for measuring triglyceride absorption in man. *Gut*, **13**, 867.

Saunders, D. R., Sillery, J. & McDonald, G. B. (1975) Regional differences in oxalate absorption by rat intestine: evidence for excessive absorption by the colon in steatorrhoea. *Gut*, **16**, 543.

Shimoda, S. S., O'Brien, T. K. & Saunders, D. R. (1974) Fat absorption after infusing bile salts into the human small intestine. *Gastroenterology*, **67**, 7.

Shimoda, S. S., Saunders, D. R. & Rubin, C. E. (1968). The Zollinger-Ellison syndrome with steatorrhea. The mechanisms of fat and vitamin B_{12} malabsorption. *Gastroenterology*, **55**, 705.

Shimoda, S. S., Saunders, D. R., Schuffler, M. D. & Leinbach, G. L. (1974) Electron microscopy of small intestinal mucosa in pancreatic insufficiency. *Gastroenterology*, **67**, 19.

Singh, A., Balint, J. A., Edmonds, R. H. & Rodgers, J. B. (1972) Adaptive changes of the rat small intestine in response to a high fat diet. *Biochimica biophysica Aeta* **260**, 708.

Sladen, G. E. & Kumar, P. J. (1973) Is the xylose test still a worthwile investigation? *British Medical Journal*, **3**, 223.

Small, D. M., Dowling, R. H. & Redinger, R. N. (1972) The enterohepatic circulation of bile salts. *Archives of Internal Medicine*, **130**, 552.

Smith, L. H., Fromm, H. & Hofmann, A. F. (1972) Acquired hyperoxaluria, nephrolithiasis and intestinal disease. *New England Journal of Medicine*, **286**, 1371.

Soong, C. S., Thompson, J. B., Poley, J. R. & Hess, D. R. (1972) Hydroxy fatty acids in human diarrhea. *Gastroenterology*, **63**, 748.

Stauffer, J. Q., Humphreys, M. H. & Weir, G. J. (1973) Acquired hyperoxaluria with regional enteritis after ileal resection: role of dietary oxalate. *Annals of Internal Medicine*, **79**, 383.

Stauffer, J. Q., Stewart, R. J. & Bertrand, G. (1974) Acquired hyperoxaluria: relationship to dietary calcium content and severity of steatorrhea (Abstract). *Gastroenterology*, **66**, 783.

Strauss, E. W. (1966) Electron microscopic study of intestinal fat absorption in vitro from mixed micelles containing linolenic acid, monolein, and bile salt. *Journal of Lipid Research*, **7**, 307.

Thompson, G. R., Barrowman, J., Gutierrez, L. & Dowling, R. H. (1971) Action of neomycin on the intraluminal phase of lipid absorption. *Journal of Clinical Investigation*, **50**, 319.

Tyor, M. P., Garbutt, J. T. & Lack, L. (1971) Metabolism and transport of bile salts in the intestine. *American Journal of Medicine*, **51**, 614.

Tytgat, G. N., Rubin, C. E. & Saunders, D. R. (1971) Synthesis and transport of lipoprotein particles by intestinal absorptive cells in man. *Journal of Clinical Investigation*, **50**, 2065.

Van Deest, B. W., Fordtran, J. S., Morawski, S. G. & Wilson, J. D. (1968) Bile salt and micellar fat concentration in proximal small bowel contents of ileectomy patients. *Journal of Clinical Investigation*, **47**, 1314.

Van de Kamer, J. H. (1953) Quantitative determination of the saturated and unsaturated higher fatty acids in fecal fat. *Scandinavian Journal of Clinical and Laboratory Investigation*, **5**, 30.

Walker, B. E., Kelleher, J., Davies, T., Smith, C. L. & Losowsky, M. S. (1973) Influence of dietary fat on fecal fat. *Gastroenterology*, **64**, 233.

Watkins, J. B. (1974) Bile acid metabolism and fat absorption in newborn infants. *Pediatric Clinics of North America*, **21**, 501.

Ways, P. O., Parmentier, C. M., Kayden, H. J., Jones, J. W., Saunders, D. R. & Rubin, C.E. (1967) Studies on the absorptive detect for triglyceride in abetalipoproteinemia. *Journal of Clinical Investigation*, **46**, 35.

Webb, J. P., James, A. T. & Kellock, T. D. (1963) The influence of diet on the quality of fecal fat in patients with and without steatorrhea. *Gut*, **4**, 37.

Weijers, H. A., Drion, E. F. & Van de Kamer, J. H. (1960) Analysis and interpretation of the fat absorption coefficient. *Acta paediatrica*, **49**, 615.

Weir, D. G. & Hourihane, D. O'B. (1974) Coeliac disease during the teenage period: the value of serial serum folate estimations. *Gut*, **15**, 450.

Weser, E. (1971) Intestinal adaption to small bowel resection. *American Journal of Clinical Nutrition*, **24**, 133.

Wiggins, H. S. & Dawson, A. M. (1961) An evaluation of unabsorbable markers in the study of fat absorption. *Gut*, **2**, 373.
Wiggins, H. S., Cummings, J. H. & Pearson, J. R. (1974) Hydroxystearic acid and diarrhoea following ileal resection. *Gut*, **15**, 392.
Wiggins, H. S., Howell, K. E., Kellock, T. D. & Stadler, J. (1969) The origin of fecal fat. *Gut*, **10**, 400.
Wilson, F. A. & Dietschy, J. M. (1972) Characterisation of bile acid absorption across the unstirred water layer and brush order of the rat jejunum. *Journal of Clinical Investigation*, **51**, 3015.
Wilson, F. A., Sallee, V. L. & Dietschy, J. M. (1971) Unstirred water layers in intestine: rate determinant of fatty acid absorption from micellar solutions. *Science*, **174**, 2031.
Wollin, A. & Jaques, L. B. (1973) Plasma protein escape from the intestinal circulation to the lymphatics during fat absorption. *Proceedings of the Society for Experimental Biology and Medicine*, **142**, 1114.
Zilversmit, D. B. (1968) The surface coat of chylomicrons: lipid chemistry. *Journal of Lipid Research*, **9**, 180.

3
HORMONE-SECRETING TUMOURS OF THE GASTROINTESTINAL TRACT

John H. Walsh   Bennett E. Roth

During the past decade, knowledge of hormone-secreting tumours of the digestive tract has increased markedly, due in large part to the widespread application of radioimmunoassay (RIA) techniques for measurement of circulating hormones. These techniques were pioneered by Yalow and Berson (1960) for measurement of circulating insulin. These workers demonstrated that circulating insulin concentrations in patients with insulinoma were physiologically inappropriate even when the values fell within the 'normal' range (Yalow and Berson, 1965). Similar observations have been made by use of RIA in a variety of other hormone-secreting tumours.

The most important example of hormone hypersecretion affecting gastrointestinal function is the Zollinger-Ellison syndrome caused by a gastrin-secreting tumour or gastrinoma (Isenberg, Walsh and Grossman, 1973). In this condition increased serum gastrin concentrations are inappropriate because of concurrent gastric acid hypersecretion, whereas elevated serum gastrin is appropriate in patients with achlorhydria. Several types of endocrine tumours are capable of producing diarrhoea. The best-known example is the carcinoid syndrome which usually is caused by carcinoid tumours metastatic to the liver. These tumours produce serotonin and can be identified by the presence of abnormal amounts of the metabolite 5-hydroxyindole acetic acid (5-HIAA) in the urine. There is recent evidence that many of the manifestations of the carcinoid syndrome may be caused by tumour products other than serotonin such as prostaglandins and vasoactive peptides.

Another diarrhoeal syndrome caused by an endocrine tumour is uncommon but dramatic in its clinical presentation. This condition is called pancreatic cholera, Verner-Morrison syndrome, or watery diarrhoea, hypokalaemia, achlorhydria (WDHA) syndrome. The peptide responsible for the severe water diarrhoea in this condition only recently has been isolated (Said and Mutt, 1970). It is known as vasoactive intestinal peptide, or VIP, and has been demonstrated in high concentrations in plasma and tumours of patients with pancreatic cholera (Bloom, Polak and Pearse, 1973). Glucagon-secreting tumours recently have been described as a cause of diabetes, an unusual skin rash (necrolytic migratory erythema) and sometimes diarrhoea (Mallinson

---

The authors of this chapter are supported by grants AM 17294 and AM 17328 of the National Institutes of Health.

et al, 1974). Specific measurement of hormones has facilitated precise diagnosis in all of these conditions. In this chapter we will consider the pathophysiology, endocrine pathology, diagnosis, and management of hormone-producing tumours which are manifest clinically by peptic ulcer disease or diarrhoea.

CELLULAR ORIGINS AND PATHOLOGY

Endocrine tumours which produce the carcinoid, Zollinger–Ellison, and pancreatic cholera syndromes are difficult to tell apart by ordinary light microscopy (Fig. 3.1). The similar morphological appearances of these tumours are a reflection of their common embryological origin from the neural crest (Pearse, 1975). Hormone-producing cells of the pancreatic islets, stomach, and intestine as well as calcitonin-producing cells of the thyroid gland are included in the peripheral neuroendocrine division of the APUD series (*A*mine content and/or *A*mine *P*recursor *U*ptake and *D*ecarboxylation) of cells. Tumours arising from these cells have been called 'apudomas', with the following biological and pathological definitions (Pearse, 1975):

Biologically an apudoma is a tumour, derived from an APUD cell and thus neuro-ectodermal in quality, which is secreting either its normal peptide hormone (or variants thereof), or one or more of the hormones, prohormones, or carrier peptides of the APUD cell series or, additionally or solely, one or more of the amine hormones associated with the series. Pathologically an apudoma is an 'endocrine' tumour possessing the A–P–U–D and associated cytochemical qualities of its presumptive precursor cell, characterised ultrastructurally by the presence of specific storage granules of endocrine type containing a peptide component with or without catechol- or indolalkylamine. The peptide may or may not be identifiable by immunocytochemistry, and the amine may or may not be identifiable by cytofluorometry.

APUD cells may be identified by lead haematoxylin or silver stains, by identification of intracellular esterases, by identification of formalin-induced fluorescence after incubation with L-dopa or L-5-hydroxytryptophan, by specific immunocytochemistry, or by ultrastructural demonstration of specific granules such as B granules in an insulinoma.

Gastrinomas most often arise in the pancreas, but the cell of origin is not certain. Granules contained in gastrinoma cells sometimes resemble G-cell granules found in antral G-cells, but often are atypical (Fig. 3.2). Creutzfeldt et al (1973) have pointed out that gastrinomas and insulinomas both commonly contain small granules which do not have an ultrastructural appearance typical of any of the granules found in normal gut endocrine cells. VIP-secreting tumours have not yet been studied extensively by electron microscopy. The carcinoid syndrome is produced in a small proportion of patients with all histological types of carcinoid tumours, usually only after hepatic metastasis. Many of these tumours produce peptide hormones as well as serotonin (Pearse, Polak, and Heath, 1974). Carcinoid tumours may produce gastrin, insulin, calcitonin, ACTH or VIP and may produce more than one peptide hormone.

HORMONE-SECRETING TUMOURS 51

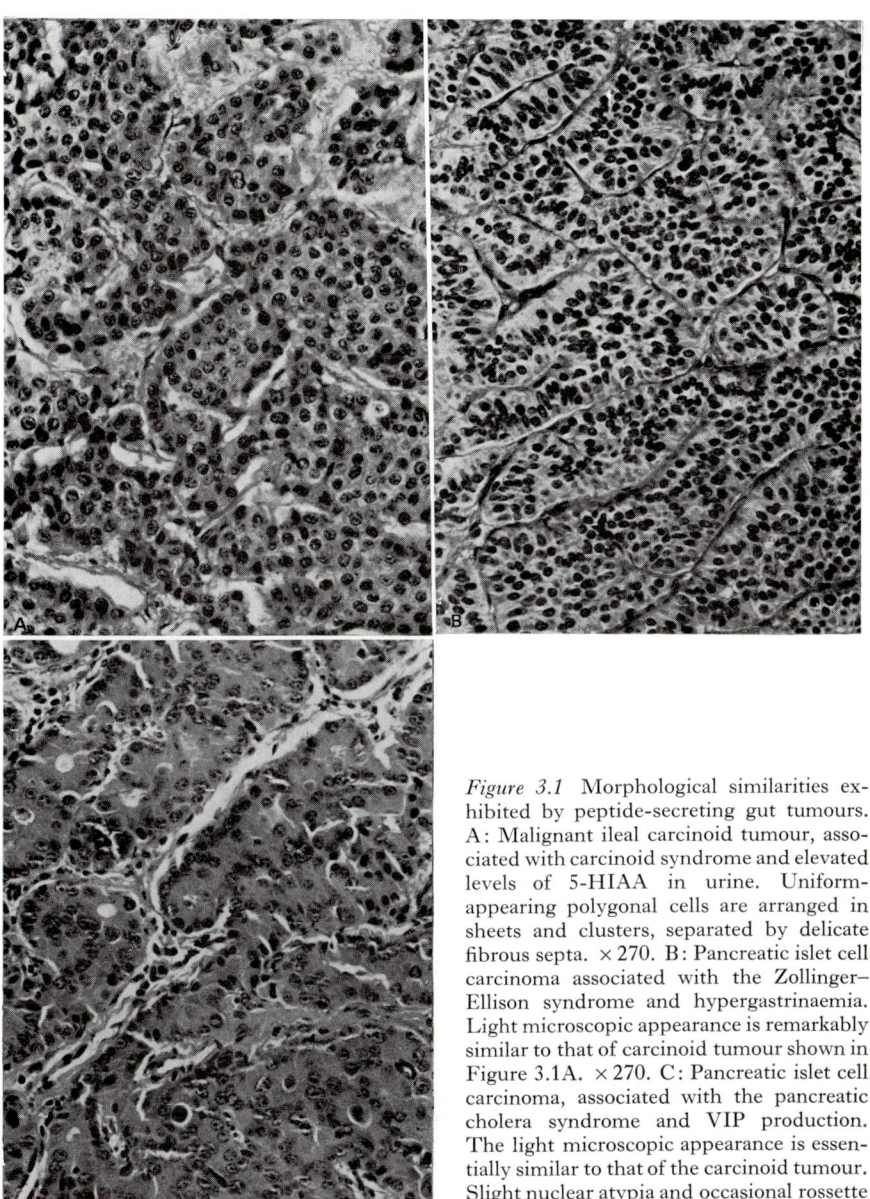

Figure 3.1 Morphological similarities exhibited by peptide-secreting gut tumours. A: Malignant ileal carcinoid tumour, associated with carcinoid syndrome and elevated levels of 5-HIAA in urine. Uniform-appearing polygonal cells are arranged in sheets and clusters, separated by delicate fibrous septa. × 270. B: Pancreatic islet cell carcinoma associated with the Zollinger–Ellison syndrome and hypergastrinaemia. Light microscopic appearance is remarkably similar to that of carcinoid tumour shown in Figure 3.1A. × 270. C: Pancreatic islet cell carcinoma, associated with the pancreatic cholera syndrome and VIP production. The light microscopic appearance is essentially similar to that of the carcinoid tumour. Slight nuclear atypia and occasional rossette formation can be noted here. × 270.

(Courtesy Dr Juan Lechago)

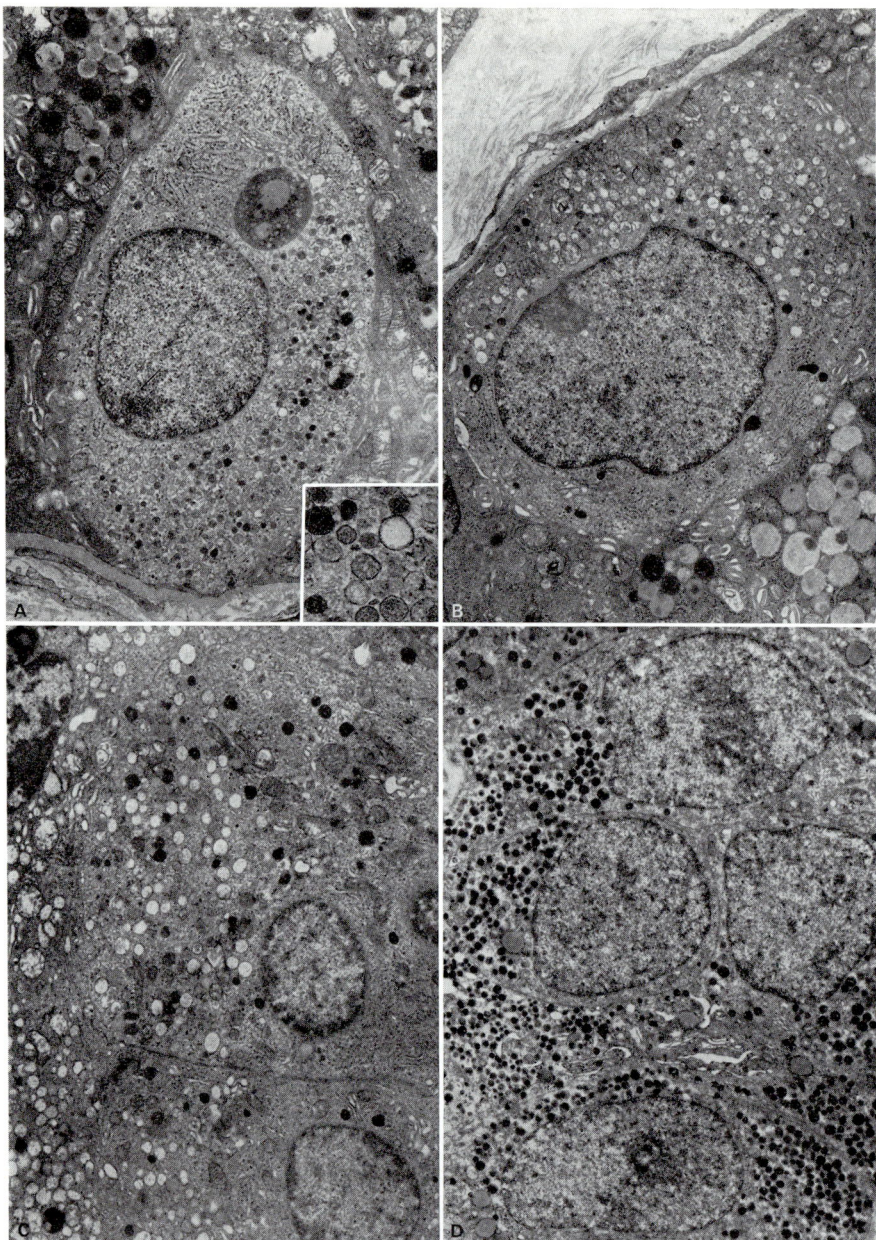

Figure 3.2 Electron micrographs. A: Human gastrin-producing cell shown in a resting state with numerous cytoplasmic granules accumulating towards the pole resting on the basal lamina. × 6500. *Inset:* Detail of gastrin cell secretory granules. These measure between 120 and 250 nm and their density varies from dark to almost empty vacuoles. × 21 000. B: An activated gastrin cell in a patient with achlorhydria. Most of the basally located secretory granules are of the pale vacuolated variety. × 6500. C: Another gastrinoma with cells containing scattered pale vacuolated secretory granules which resemble closely those of the activated antral gastrin cell. × 6500. D: A gastrinoma showing several cells which contain numerous secretory granules. These are uncharacteristically small with dark somewhat heterogeneous cores. × 6500. (Courtesy Dr Juan Lechago.)

The most reliable method for specific identification of peptide hormones contained within endocrine tumours is extraction of the tumours and measurement of hormone content by radioimmunoassay. Immunocytochemical techniques also may produce positive reactions, but may give negative results when granule content is low and are at least two orders of magnitude less sensitive for hormone detection than radioimmunoassay.

More than one apudoma may occur in a single patient, either in familial genetic dominant or non-familial pattern. The most common associations are pancreatic islet, parathyroid, and pituitary (Multiple Endocrine Adenoma syndrome, MEA-I) and parathyroid, adrenal medulla, and medullary thyroid (MEA-II).

ZOLLINGER–ELLISON (GASTRINOMA) SYNDROME

More than two decades have passed since Zollinger and Ellison (1955) described two patients with fulminant peptic ulcer disease associated with non-beta-cell tumours of the pancreatic islet cells. Peptic ulcer disease in this condition results from massive gastric acid hypersecretion which is stimulated by gastrin released from these tumours. The gastrin is indistinguishable from antral gastrin (Grossman, Tracy and Gregory, 1961) and the tumours have been called gastrinomas (Grossman, 1972). Markedly elevated serum gastrin concentrations often are measured by RIA in patients with gastrinoma (McGuigan and Trudeau, 1968), but an increasing number of gastrinoma patients are being identified with only modest elevations in serum gastrin. In these patients, provocative tests with agents such as calcium and secretin combined with radioimmunoassay often clarify the diagnosis. It has been suggested that the Zollinger–Ellison syndrome may be mimicked by primary hyperplasia of antral gastrin cells leading to hypergastrinaemia (Polak, Stagg and Pearse, 1972), but well-documented cases of this condition have been difficult to identify. Many other patients have markedly increased rates of basal acid secretion associated with peptic ulcer disease but with normal serum gastrin concentrations. The cause of their hypersecretion remains unexplained. Gastrinomas often are associated with hyperparathyroidism due to tumours or hyperplasia of the parathyroid glands. This association may explain the high incidence of peptic ulcer which has been reported in patients with hyperparathyroidism.

Clinical Manifestations

The clinical presentation of Zollinger–Ellison syndrome often is not remarkably different from that of ordinary duodenal ulcer disease. No strong clustering according to age or sex has been identified. The familial form, often associated with other apudomas, accounts for only a small minority of patients with the disease. The most frequent symptoms are epigastric pain, diarrhoea, haematemesis and/or melaena, and vomiting. Of these, only diarrhoea is relatively uncommon in untreated patients with ordinary ulcer disease, and this symptom is common after treatment with magnesium-containing antacids.

There are several clues which should lead to an increased suspicion of the presence of gastrinoma (Isenberg et al, 1973). Recurrent ulcer after vagotomy or gastric resection for treatment of peptic ulcer unfortunately remains the first clue all too often. Recurrence with bleeding or perforation in the early postoperative period is especially likely in patients with gastrinoma. A history of pancreatic, parathyroid, or pituitary endocrine tumours in the ulcer patient or his close relatives makes evaluation for gastrinoma mandatory. The radiolocial appearance of the upper gastrointestinal tract may suggest the diagnosis. Ulcers in the distal duodenum or jejunum are almost diagnostic but occur only in a minority of patients with gastrinoma. Usually the ulcer is located in the duodenal bulb and a number of patients have had no demonstrable ulcer. The gastric folds usually are large, due to mucosal hyperplasia, the barium meal usually becomes diluted by the large volume of gastric contents, and the proximal small intestine frequently has a dilated lumen with an abnormal mucosal pattern. This constellation of findings is suggestive but not diagnostic of gastrinoma and may be found in other patients with gastric acid hypersecretion. More specific diagnosis is provided by the combination of basal gastric acid hypersecretion and increased serum gastrin concentration.

Diagnosis

Acid secretion studies

In patients with gastrinoma, basal acid secretion rates usually are greater than those found in patients with ordinary duodenal ulcer. In the unoperated patient, failure to find basal acid output (BAO) greater than 5 mmol/h essentially excludes the diagnosis. In patients with previous gastric operations acid secretion studies may be unreliable, due to reflux of intestinal contents into the stomach, and the presence of recurrent ulcer may be taken as sufficient evidence for excessive acid secretion. Maximal acid output after histamine or pentagastrin stimulation (MAO) also is increased in many patients with gastrinoma but proportionately less than BAO. There are several acid secretory findings which are highly suggestive of the presence of a gastrinoma (Isenberg et al, 1973). These include overnight 12 h acid secretion >100 mmol, BAO >10 to 15 mmol/h, BAO/MAO ratio >0.6, ratio of basal to maximal acid concentration (BAC/MAC) >0.6 in the unoperated patient or BAO >5 mmol/h in a patient with previous gastric surgery. Acid studies taken alone may yield false positive and false negative results and should always be analysed together with other clinical and laboratory data including serum gastrin concentration.

A considerable proportion of patients with basal acid hypersecretion have no gastrin-secreting tumour, have normal serum gastrin concentration, and can be considered to have idiopathic acid hypersecretion. In our own experience (unpublished observations), nearly half of all patients with gastrinoma failed to meet the standard criteria for acid hypersecretion. One-fourth had BAO less than 10 mmol/h, half had BAO/MAO ratio less than 0.6, and one-fifth had BAO/MAO less than 0.4. Lower rates of acid secretion are especially common after successful parathyroid resection for treatment of hyperparathyroidism in patients who have an associated gastrinoma.

Table 3.1 Amino acid sequences of chemically characterised human gastrins

Human big gastrin (HG-34). Molecular weight 3839

1   2   3   4   5   6   7   8   9   10 11 12 13 14 15 16 17 18
Pyro–Leu–Gly–Pro–Gln–Gly–His–Pro–Ser–Leu–Val–Ala–Asp–Pro–Ser–Lys–Lys–Gln–

19 20 21 22 23 24 25 26 27 28 29 30 31 32 33 34
Gly–Pro–Trp–Leu–Glu–Glu–Glu–Glu–Glu–Ala–Tyr–Gly–Trp–Met–Asp–Phe–NH$_2$
                                            |
                                            R

Human heptadecapeptide (little) gastrin (HG–17). Molecular weight 2098

1   2   3   4   5   6   7   8   9   10 11 12 13 14 15 16 17
Pyro–Gly–Pro–Trp–Leu–Glu–Glu–Glu–Glu–Glu–Ala–Tyr–Gly–Trp–Met–Asp–Phe–NH$_2$
                                        |
                                        R

Human minigastrin (HG–14). Molecular weight 1851

1   2   3   4   5   6   7   8   9   10 11 12 13 14
Trp–Leu–Glu–Glu–Glu–Glu–Glu–Ala–Tyr–Gly–Trp–Met–Asp–Phe–NH$_2$
                            |
                            R

Pyro = pyroglutamyl   Gastrin I, R = H   Gastrin II, R = SO$_3$H

Serum gastrin measurements

STRUCTURE AND BIOLOGICAL ACTIVITY OF GASTRIN

The major biologically active forms of gastrin found in serum and tissues are known as 'big gastrin' (G-34 I and II) and heptadecapeptide or 'little gastrin' (G-17-I and II). The subscripts I and II refer to the absence or presence of a sulphate radical on the tyrosine side chain, but this substitution does not appear to alter biological activity or metabolism (Walsh and Grossman, 1975). Another molecular form, identified occasionally in serum, is 'minigastrin'. Very recently 'minigastrin' has been found to contain 14 amino acids (Harris, unpublished observations) rather than 13, so the trivial name for this peptide should be G-14. G-17 and G-14 are carboxy-terminal fragments of G-34 (Table 3.1). Two other forms of gastrin immunoreactivity have been identified by radioimmunoassay, both with larger apparent molecular weight than G-34. These are 'big-big gastrin' (Yallow and Wu, 1973) and 'Component I' (Rehfeld, Stadil and Vikelsoe, 1974).

Gastrin is stored in specialised endocrine cells (G-cells) located in the mucosa of the gastric antrum. In man, the duodenum also contains a considerable amount of gastrin and small amounts can be extracted from more distal portions of the small intestine. Antral gastrin is released when antral mucosa is exposed to protein digestion products and this release is inhibited by intragastric acidification (Walsh, Richardson and Fordtran, 1975). Gastrin release is not inhibited in man by vagotomy or by administration of atropine. Antral gastrin release in response to food is inhibited by intravenous infusion of secretin in contrast to stimulation of gastrin release from gastrinoma tissue during secretin infusion in most patients with Zollinger–Ellison syndrome.

The major physiological target of gastrin is the acid-secreting mucosa of the stomach. Doses of gastrin which increase serum gastrin to an extent similar to increases produced by a protein meal are sufficient to cause approximately half-maximal gastric acid secretion (Walsh et al, 1976). Another possible physiological action of gastrin is its trophic effect on the stomach, small intestine and pancreas. Johnson (1975) has reported that atrophy of of these organs in the rat during starvation can be prevented by doses of pentagastrin which are submaximal for stimulation of acid secretion. Gastrin also may play a physiological role in maintenance of the pressure of the lower oesophageal sphincter and in stimulation of pancreatic secretion, but these effects have not been definitely established as physiological. Large doses of gastrin produce pharmacological effects on water and electrolyte secretion and absorption, enzyme secretion, and smooth muscle function throughout the gastrointestinal tract but only in doses outside the physiological range.

G-17 is cleared from the circulation more rapidly than G-34; the half lives in man are approximately 6 and 40 min, respectively (Walsh et al, 1976). The difference in clearance rates probably accounts for the observation that G-34 is the most abundant active from of gastrin in the circulation although G-17 is the most abundant form in gastrin-secreting tissues. The kidney is one of the organs responsible for removal of gastrin from the circulation, but the rapid turnover of G-17 cannot be explained entirely by renal extraction and other organs such as small intestine also contribute to gastrin removal. The liver does not appear to remove significant amounts of G-17 or G-34 from the circulation although it is capable of removing small gastrin fragments quite efficiently.

RADIOIMMUNOASSAY OF GASTRIN

Gastrin radioimmunoassay methods now are sufficiently sensitive and specific to permit the measurement of immunoreactive gastrin under physiological conditions. Bioassay methods have been used successfully to identify markedly increased gastrin concentrations in serum of some patients with gastrinoma but are at least 1000 times less sensitive than RIA. Antibodies used routinely for gastrin RIA are specific for the carboxyterminal biologically active portion of the gastrin molecule. Immunoreactive gastrin concentrations measured with these antibodies do not distinguish among the various gastrin components (big-big gastrin, Component-I, G-34, G-17 and G-14). The most abundant forms of gastrin measured in normal subjects are big-big gastrin and G-34, whereas G-34, G-17, and Component-I predominate in hypergastrinaemic subjects (Rehfeld et al, 1974). Most gastrin antibodies have similar reactivity with sulphated and non-sulphated forms of G-17 and G-34 so that total gastrin concentration measured in hypergastrinaemic subjects is a reasonable reflection of total molar abundance of gastrin components. More accurate measurement of individual components can be achieved by fractionation of serum on gel filtration columns and RIA of individual fractions. This type of analysis could be important clinically to identify patients with relatively low total immunoreactive gastrin who secreted only the highly active G-17 molecule. However, most hypergastrinaemic patients, including those with gastrinoma, have more G-34 than G-17 in the circulation (Dockray, Walsh and Passaro, 1975). Antibodies with unusual specificity patterns have been used to identify circulating fragments of G-17 in gastrinoma patients (Dockray and Walsh, 1975).

Serum gastrin concentrations usually are expressed in units of pg/ml, representing immunoreactive gastrin in terms of a G-17-I standard. Actual values obtained for fasting gastrin in normal subjects average between 30 and 120 pg/ml in various laboratories (Blair et al, 1975). This four-fold difference among laboratories must be kept in mind when interpreting gastrin values. Assay conditions, standard solutions used, and patterns of antibody specificity all contribute to these differences. Peak mean increments in serum gastrin after a protein meal have varied between 50 and 200 pg/ml in various laboratories, and various types of protein appear to produce equivalent responses (Blair et al, 1975). Interpretation of serum gastrin concentrations thus must be done with knowledge of normal values obtained in the laboratory which performs the tests.

SERUM GASTRIN IN GASTRINOMA PATIENTS

When serum gastrin concentration is elevated more than 10 times higher than values found in normal or ordinary duodenal ulcer subjects in a patient with basal acid hypersecretion, the diagnosis of gastrinoma is highly probable. The differential diagnosis is limited. Primary antral G-cell hyperplasia (Polak et al, 1972) must be a very rare condition since no patients with this syndrome have been found among several groups which have studied large numbers of patients with gastrinoma. Hypergastrinaemia also occurs in patients with renal failure or with intestinal resection, but most of these patients have low acid secretion. Hypergastrinaemia may be quite marked in achlorhydric patients with atrophic gastritis but they have none of the clinical features of Zollinger–Ellison syndrome. In patients with previous gastric resection and gastrojejunostomy, isolated retained antrum must be considered, but few well-documented cases with markedly increased serum gastrin have been reported. Gastric outlet obstruction may lead to modest increases in serum gastrin associated with high rates of acid secretion. Some controversy exists about the aetiology of hypergastrinaemia and gastric hypersecretion in patients with hyperparathyroidism, especially in those patients whose values return to normal after parathyroidectomy. We feel that most, if not all, of these patients have occult gastrinomas which are responsive to changes in serum calcium concentration. Evidence in support of this view is offered by persistence of abnormal serum gastrin responses to calcium (Trudeau and McGuigan, 1969) and to secretin (Isenberg et al, 1972) after parathyroidectomy and by re-emergence of hypergastrinaemia and clinical manifestations of the Zollinger–Ellison syndrome in many patients without evidence for recurrent hyperparathyroidism.

As the use of radioimmunoassay has increased, more patients have been identified with less overt manifestations of gastrinoma and with serum gastrin concentrations only moderately increased over normal. In our own experience with documented or probable gastrinoma patients, 12 of 28 had fasting gastrin concentrations less than 300 pg/ml. Thompson et al (1975) studied 280 patients with potential Zollinger–Ellison syndrome and considered the diagnosis proved or probable in 45 patients of whom 10 had at least one serum gastrin value less than 250 pg/ml. They were unable to identify any patient with antral G-cell hyperplasia. Creutzfeldt et al (1975) reported serum gastrin concentrations less than 300 pg/ml in 3 of 17 patients with proved gastrinoma. Ivey and Hansky (1975) reported a patient in whom serum gastrin concentrations were normal when measured with an antibody which did not detect sulphated forms of gastrin but abnormal when measured with another antibody with broad reactivity, emphasising the importance of antibody selection in identifying hypergastrinaemic patients.

Stimulation tests provide additional diagnostic information in patients with suspected gastrinoma and borderline gastrin values. The two most useful tests are calcium infusion and secretin infusion. In our series of 12 gastrinoma patients with basal gastrin less than 300 pg/ml, 11 demonstrated greater than 100 per cent increase in serum gastrin either during the first 10 min after rapid intravenous injection of secretin (1 u/kg) or during intravenous infusion of calcium gluconate (15 mg Ca^{2+}/kg over 3 h). Other subjects with duodenal ulcer had minimal responses to these stimulants. Creutzfeldt et al (1975) found that secretin produced more than 100 per cent increase over basal gastrin in 6 of 9 patients with gastrinoma, while calcium infusion produced more than 100 per cent increase in each of 8 patients. Thompson et al (1975) obtained a similar incidence of 100 per cent or greater responses to secretin infusion (10 of 11) and calcium infusion (9 of 9) in gastrinoma patients. Both groups found glucagon to be less effective than secretin in stimulating tumour gastrin release. Both also found that a protein meal produced significant increases in gastrin in several gastrinoma patients and that a positive response to food therefore was not a reliable criterion by which to distinguish patients with gastrinoma from those with G-cell hyperplasia.

Treatment

Total gastrectomy remains the treatment of choice for patients with symptomatic gastrinoma (Isenberg et al, 1973). Addition of partial pancreatic resection to the procedure does not improve survival rates. The great majority of gastrinomas are multifocal or metastatic at the time of operation (Creutzfeldt et al, 1975) and cannot be resected. Pancreatic resection only adds to postoperative nutritional problems encountered in these patients after gastrectomy. Resection of gastrinomas which arise in the duodenal wall has been successful in some hands (Oberhelman and Nelsen, 1964) but does not apply to the majority of patients. Fox et al (1974) reported median survival of 5.5 years in gastrinoma patients with total gastrectomy compared with 1.2 years for patients with lesser procedures. Metastatic tumour was responsible for death in 17 per cent of patients in the former and 30 per cent of patients in the latter group. Earlier reports concerning use of chemotherapy in patients with metastatic gastrinoma have been discouraging, but Stadil et al (1976) have obtained good results with intra-arterial perfusion of streptozotocin into the coeliac or superior mesenteric artery in two patients with extensive hepatic metastases.

Under certain circumstances total gastrectomy may be postponed and other forms of therapy used initially. Patients with associated hyperparathyroidism may achieve prolonged clinical remissions after successful parathyroidectomy. In other patients with relatively mild symptoms of peptic ulcer or diarrhoea the diagnosis may be made fortuitously and treatment with antacids and anticholinergic agents may be successful on a temporary basis. The histamine H-2 receptor blocking agents metiamide and cimetidine are powerful inhibitors of gastrin-stimulated acid secretion. These agents have been used successfully in patients in whom operation was refused or technically impossible and to induce clinical remission of symptoms, prevent steatorrhoea and allow weight gain prior to elective surgery (Richardson and Walsh, 1976). In the future, cimetidine probably will be used extensively in place of metiamide which produces agranulocytosis in some patients.

CARCINOID SYNDROME

Carcinoid tumours were among the first apudomas to be described (Lubarsch, 1888), but the carcinoid syndrome and its association with serotonin were not recognised until 1953 (Hajdu, Winawer and Myers, 1974). Carcinoid tumours may arise in a variety of sites and have varied histological appearances and secretory products (Table 3.2). They are found with greatest frequency in the appendix followed by the jejuno-ileum, colon and rectum, lung, stomach, pancreas, ovary and duodenum. Carcinoid syndrome is produced by less than 10 per cent of all carcinoid tumours, usually occurs only after distant metastasis, and is most common with tumours arising in the jejuno-ileum and ovary and least common with appendiceal and rectal carcinoids. As with gastrinoma, malignancy is difficult to evaluate by histological appearance of the tumour cells. Superficially invasive tumours rarely metastasise while 85 per cent of deeply invasive carcinoids do so. Tumour cells can be stained by the same silver impregnation techniques used to identify the enterochromaffin cells of the small intestine (Soga and Tazawa, 1971).

Table 3.2 Carcinoid tumours

Embryological origin		Organs involved	Secretory products	Clinical expression
Foregut		Bronchus	5-HTP	Flush and other
Argentaffin	(−)	Stomach	Histamine	symptoms may be
Argyrophil	(+)	Pancreas	5-HT	provoked by eating
		Gallbladder		
Midgut		Jejunum	5-HT	Classical malignant
Argentaffin	(+)	Ileum	Bradykinin	carcinoid syndrome
Argyrophil	(+)	Appendix	? Prostaglandins	
		Ovary		
Hindgut		Colon	Rarely 5-HT	Rarely produce
Argentaffin	(−)	Rectum		carcinoid syndrome
Argyrophil	(−)			

Clinical Manifestations

General

Carcinoids of the appendix most often are asymptomatic and are discovered only at the time of appendectomy or at autopsy. Rarely they may be the cause of appendicitis or may metastasise and produce the carcinoid syndrome. Other intestinal carcinoid tumours also may be asymptomatic or they may present with local symptoms which resemble those produced by other gastrointestinal tumours including obstruction, pain, and bleeding. They metastasise first to regional lymph nodes and then to liver and bone. Bronchial carcinoids often produce dyspnoea or haematemesis when they are symptomatic.

Carcinoid syndrome

The carcinoid syndrome is produced when secretory products of the carcinoid tumour enter the circulation in excessive amounts. The principal manifestations are flushing, diarrhoea, and wheezing. Other problems encountered less often include cardiac lesions, oedema, retroperitoneal fibrosis, Peyronie's disease, and symptoms due to production of other hormones such as ACTH or gastrin.

FLUSHING

Four different types of flushing have been described in various forms of the carcinoid syndrome:

1. Short-lived diffuse erythaematous flush affecting the face, neck, and upper chest lasting less than 10 min.
2. Violaceous flush with similar distribution but longer duration and with eventual production of a permanent cyanotic flush, facial telangectasia, watery eyes, and conjunctival suffusion.
3. Prolonged flushes lasting two to three days and sometimes involving the entire body associated with watery eyes, enlarged salivary glands and face, and hypotension. These are most common with bronchial carcinoids.
4. Bright red patchy flushing, probably due to excessive histamine production, found in patients with gastric carcinoids.

Type 3 flushing may be caused by bradykinin alone while types 1 and 2 are thought to be produced by a combination of bradykinin and serotonin.

DIARRHOEA

The diarrhoea of the carcinoid syndrome may occur without any of the other symptoms. It is usually periodic and not associated with marked increases in faecal water and electrolyte excretion. Intestinal hypermotility is a prominent feature of the syndrome and is manifest by cramping abdominal pains and increased bowel sounds. In addition to hyperactive bowel sounds, examination of the abdomen usually reveals a distinctly enlarged nodular liver.

OTHER SYMPTOMS AND SIGNS

Wheezing occurs in about 25 per cent of patients with the syndrome and usually accompanies flushing attacks. Oedema may occur during carcinoid attacks only or may be chronic when congestive heart failure develops as a consequence of carcinoid heart disease. High output failure with valvular lesions involving the tricuspid and pulmonic valves is the most common form of heart disease. Lesions of the mitral and aortic valves are less common, are usually accompanied by right-sided involvement, and are found most often with bronchial carcinoids (Carpena et al, 1973). Pericardial effusion has been reported rarely. Skin lesions resembling those found in pellagra have been described and appear to result from nicotinamide deficiency produced when dietary tryptophan is diverted to serotonin production (Grahame-Smith, 1968).

Overt carcinoid syndrome usually is found only when humoral mediators of the syndrome are able to escape inactivation by the liver. Most patients with the syndrome have extensive hepatic metastases. The major exceptions to this rule are tumours whose venous drainage passes directly into the systemic circulation such as bronchial and ovarian carcinoids. The earliest manifestations of the syndrome are episodic attacks which may be brought on by alcohol, eating, emotional stress, exercise, or straining at stool. Attacks also may be induced pharmacologically by infusions of norepinephrine or calcium.

Diagnosis

Measurement of serotonin metabolites

Serotonin is one of the major products of carcinoid tumours and appears to be responsible for many of the clinical manifestations of the carcinoid syndrome. Serotonin (5-hydroxytryptamine, 5-HT) is a product of dietary L-tryptophan resulting from 5-hydroxylation to 5-hydroxytryptophan (5-HTP) followed by decarboxylation to 5-HT. Some of the 5-HT is metabolised within the tumour to 5-hydroxyindolacetaldehyde by monamine oxidase and subsequently to 5-hydroxyindoleacetic acid (5-HIAA) by aldehyde dehydrogenase. The remainder is released into the circulation where it is partially bound to platelets. Circulating 5-HT is metabolised to 5-HIAA by enzymes in the liver, lung, and other organs. Some tumours of foregut origin release 5-HTP into the circulation which is converted to 5-HT and eventually to 5-HIAA in other organs. Free circulating 5-HT probably mediates diarrhoea and intestinal hypermotility found in patients with the carcinoid syndrome (Sjoerdsma et al, 1957). The role played by serotonin in carcinoid flush, bronchoconstriction, oedema, and valvular heart lesions is not clear, but there is good evidence that other humoral agents are involved in their pathogenesis.

The most useful test for diagnosis of carcinoid syndrome is quantitative measurement of urinary excretion of 5-HIAA over a 24 h period. Urinary excretion of more than 25 mg 5-HIAA/24 h is abnormal and patients with the syndrome usually excrete considerably greater amounts than this, ranging up to 1000 mg. Care must be taken to prevent false-positive elevations resulting from ingestion of certain foods and drugs. Foods rich in serotonin, including bananas, tomatoes, avocadoes, red plums, walnuts, and eggplant, should be discontinued. Drugs which may result in false elevations include reserpine, mephanesin carbonate, phenothiazine compounds, glyceryl guaiacolate, and mandelamine (Pedersen et al, 1970). Direct measurement of circulating serotonin by radioimmunoassay now is possible (Kellum and Jaffe, 1975) and may further simplify the diagnosis. Free urinary 5-HT also can be measured. Excretion of more than 1 to 2 mg/24 h indicates release of 5-HTP into the circulation by a tumour originating in the foregut, most often the stomach. Provocative testing with epinephrine and norepinephrine to reproduce flushing attacks has been generally discontinued because of severe side effects. However, a stimulation test with direct measurement of blood serotonin during calcium infusion has been described recently (Kaplan, Jaffe and Peskin, 1972).

Measurement of other tumour products

Carcinoid tumours also synthesise the enzyme kallikrein which acts on circulating kinogen to release a decapeptide, lysyl-bradykinin, which is converted to bradykinin. These two kinin peptides are potent vasodilators and their infusion intravenously produces flushing similar to that seen in carcinoid attacks. Oates, Pettinger and Doctor (1966) demonstrated increased concentration of bradykinin in hepatic venous blood draining carcinoid metastases. Kallikrein has been identified in carcinoid tumours from patients with flushing. Other effects of bradykinin which may contribute to the carcinoid syndrome include hypotension, salivation, lacrimation, oedema, and increased cardiac output. Bradykinin-like peptides probably play a major role in the typical carcinoid attack.

Certain gastric and bronchial carcinoids secrete histamine. This substance may account for gastric hypersecretion in occasional cases. However, the incidence of peptic ulcer is not increased in patients with the carcinoid syndrome. When gastric hypersecretion is identified in a patient with carcinoid tumour, secretion of gastrin by the tumour also should be evaluated. Prostaglandins, calcitonin, and epinephrine also have been identified in carcinoid tumours, but the role of these substances in production of the carcinoid syndrome has not been defined.

Treatment

Surgical

Primary tumour resection, when possible, is the preferred treatment for all carcinoid tumours. Unfortunately this is not possible in most patients with the carcinoid syndrome because of the presence of distant metastases. However, resection of a major fraction of functioning tumour mass may produce significant palliation of symptoms. Severe bronchospasm and hypotension may be produced in patients with carcinoid syndrome when the tumour is manipulated or during induction of anaesthesia. Pretreatment with serotonin antagonists may be helpful in prevention of such problems.

Small carcinoid tumours without evidence of tissue invasion may be treated by local resection. More extensive resection is required when there is invasion into the bowel wall. In the presence of lymphatic or distant metastasis, chemotherapy may be added to or substituted for local resection. The five year survival for patients with benign carcinoids approaches 100 per cent but is only 40 per cent for malignant rectal carcinoids (Orloff, 1971). Palliation of carcinoid symptoms has been reported with a combination of resection and radiation therapy of metastatic lesions (Reed et al, 1963).

Medical

Agents which have been used in attempts to antagonise the effects of humoral agents responsible for carcinoid symptoms have been listed by Kowlessar (1973). Parachlorophenylalanine is an inhibitor of serotonin synthesis which is most effective against nausea, vomiting, and diarrhoea but may produce altered central nervous system function. Methysergide maleate (Sansert) and cyproheptidine (Periactin) are peripheral antagonists of serotonin. They have been used for control of diarrhoea, flushing, and asthmatic attacks, but are most effective for control of diarrhoea. A variety of other drugs have been used in an attempt to control flushing. Corticosteroids have been dramatically effective in a small number of patients and probably prevent release of kallekrein from certain tumours. Phenoxybenzamine also may alleviate flushing by preventing kallekrein release. Antihistamines and adrenergic block agents have been used to control wheezing and flushing. Control of symptoms seldom is complete, and multiple agents may have to be tried in trial and error fashion to arrive at a successful combination.

Chemotherapy with usual antitumour agents and with streptozotocin most often is unsuccessful. Radiotherapy may produce relief from pain caused by bony metastases. Dietary supplementation with niacin is recommended, especially for patients with skin lesions. Certain foods such as milk and cheese may be found to provoke attacks and should be avoided when they are identified.

PANCREATIC CHOLERA (VIPoma, VERNER–MORRISON, WDHA) SYNDROME

There are two distinct diarrhoeal syndromes associated with pancreatic islet cell tumours. Patients with gastrinoma commonly have diarrhoea as a consequence of the influx of large amounts of acid into the upper intestine. This diarrhoea often is accompanied by steatorrhoea, due to mucosal damage, inactivation of lipase, and precipitation of bile salts, but not by hypokalaemia. The second group of patients present with massive watery diarrhoea not accompanied by gastric acid hypersecretion or steatorrhoea but usually have severe dehydration and hypokalaemia. The first patients with this latter syndrome were reported in 1958 by Verner and Morrison. The name 'pancreatic cholera' has been applied to this condition because of the high faecal excretion of water and electrolytes, the absence of intestinal mucosal lesions, and the pancreatic origin of the neoplasm usually responsible for this disease (Matsumoto et al, 1966). Until recently no specific hormone could be implicated as the cause of this syndrome. Now there is good evidence that tumours in these patients secrete a peptide known as vasoactive intestinal peptide, or VIP, and these tumours have been named 'VIPomas' (Bloom et al, 1973).

Clinical Manifestations

Pancreatic cholera is recognised most often in the fourth to sixth decades of life, affects men and women with similar frequency, and has not been described in a familial form or in association with other endocrine tumours. The interval between onset of symptoms and diagnosis ranges from months to years.

The primary symptom of this disorder is prolonged watery diarrhoea leading to weight loss, dehydration, and severe muscular weakness. Stool output may be maintained at high rates of 1 to 5 litres/day, or there may be periods of high output of watery stool alternating with periods during which the stool is semiformed. During acute episodes of massive diarrhoea it is not uncommon to observe rapid weight loss of several kilograms due to dehydration. Weakness is a prominent symptom. It is caused by dehydration and by severe hypokalaemia. Serum potassium concentrations frequently are less than 2 mmol/litre, and massive doses of oral or intravenous potassium may be required to replenish body potassium stores. Nausea, vomiting, and abdominal cramps are common during periods of severe diarrhhoea.

Peptic ulcer is not associated with pancreatic cholera although a previous history of ulcer does not exclude the diagnosis. Some patients have complained of facial flushing during diarrhoeal attacks but evidence of serotonin hypersecretion has not been obtained.

Diagnosis

General laboratory studies

Stool volume frequently exceeds 2 litres/day. The diarrhoea can be characterised as secretory rather than osmotic because it persists in the absence of oral food intake and because the osmolality of the stool can be accounted for entirely by its electrolyte content (i.e. stool osmolality in mOsm/kg equals twice the sum of faecal sodium and potassium concentrations). Stool volume is related to degree of hydration and tends to increase after replacement of fluid and electrolyte losses. Stool potassium concentration varies inversely with stool volume so that total daily faecal potassium losses tend to remain between 100 and 300 mmol/day regardless of faecal volume. The other faecal cation is sodium, and its concentration and total output increases progressively as stool volume increases. Stool pH usually is alkaline. Since similar stool volume and electrolyte content can be produced by surreptitious laxative ingestion, it is good practice to examine the stool routinely for presence of phenolphthalein. This is done by adding sodium hydroxide to bring stool pH above 10 and observing for presence of a red colour. Laxative abuse is the most common cause of 'idiopathic secretory diarrhoea' in adults, especially women, and early identification of laxative in the stool can prevent exhaustive medical and surgical evaluation. (See Chapter 6.)

Serum electrolyte measurements usually reveal severe hypokalaemia with moderate metabolic acidosis due to faecal losses of potassium and bicarbonate. In the severely dehydrated patient acidosis may become more severe after fluid and electrolyte replacement have been initiated and extracellular fluid volume is restored towards normal. Moderate hypercalcaemia is found in about half of all patients with this syndrome and has not been explained. Usually it is not due to parathyroid adenoma and is corrected by resection of the diarrhoegenic tumour. Abnormal glucose tolerance is common and may be due in part to the effects of prolonged hypokalaemia on the pancreatic beta cells.

Other tests of gastrointestinal function are seldom helpful in establishing a positive diagnosis. Gastric acid secretion may be absent or normal but is not increased. Pancreatic water and bicarbonate secretion usually are normal although basal secretion may be moderately increased. Stool fat excretion is normal or slightly increased. Radiological examination of the gastrointestinal tract usually reveal no abnormality. Negative barium enema and proctoscopic examinations are helpful in excluding the presence of villous tumours of the colon, another cause of watery diarrhoea with hypokalaemia. Prolonged hypokalaemia may lead to renal function abnormalities. Small bowel biopsy reveals normal villi. Gastric biopsy may show normal numbers of parietal cells even in achlorhydric patients suggesting the presence of a circulating inhibitor of gastric acid secretion. Selective coeliac and superior mesenteric arteriography are successful in identifying tumours only in about one-third of patients.

The site of fluid and electrolyte secretion appears to be the small intestine. High rates of water and electrolyte output were observed in one patient who had an ileostomy performed (Rambaud et al, 1975). The colon appears to function almost normally, absorbing water and sodium to the limit of its capacity while increasing faecal potassium output. In unpublished studies (Fordtran, Morawski, and Walsh) we found that patients with pancreatic cholera actively secreted sodium and chloride into the jejunum. There was no evidence of mucosal abnormality since water movement responded appropriately to glucose absorption and to increased osmotic pressure produced in the lumen by addition of mannitol. These studies indicate that the designation 'pancreatic cholera' is an appropriate description of the abnormality in intestinal function. Similar results have been obtained in patients with bacterial cholera.

Hormone measurements

Data presented by Bloom et al (1973) strongly suggest that VIP is the hormone produced in excesses by pancreatic cholera tumours. Subsequently Bloom and Polak (1975) reported plasma VIP concentrations greater than 200 pg/ml in 17 patients with severe watery diarrhoea associated with tumours (15 pancreatic islet cell, 2 ganglioneuroma) contrasted with normal mean values around 20 pg/ml. Circulating concentrations of GIP, secretin, and glucagon were normal in the same patients. Eight other patients with a clinical picture suggestive of pancreatic cholera but with negative pancreatic exploration had normal plasma VIP concentrations. Normal VIP measurements also were obtained in patients with diarrhoea due to other causes. Radioimmunoassay of acid–alcohol extracts of tumours revealed high concentrations of VIP in each tumour examined.

Similar results were reported by Said and Faloona (1975). In their radioimmunoasay, plasma VIP concentrations were less than 200 pg/ml in most normal subjects but were elevated in 26 of 28 patients with diarrhoeogenic tumours, averaging 5100 pg/ml. Tissue diagnosis in 26 of the patients was pancreatic islet cell tumour in 13, islet cell hyperplasia in 5, bronchogenic carcinoma in 6, pheochromocytoma in 1, and ganglioneuroblastoma in 1. High tissue concentrations of VIP were found in one patient with bronchogenic carcinoma and in several pancreatic tumours. Apparently bronchogenic carcinoma and ganglioneuroblastoma can be added to islet cell tumours as tumours responsible for the pancreatic cholera syndrome.

VIP was isolated by Said (Said and Mutt, 1970) who determined the peptide structure of this material. VIP belongs to a family of four peptides which have similarities in amino acid sequence and activities (Table 3.3). These peptides are VIP, secretin, glucagon, and gastric inhibitory peptide or GIP (Brown and Dryburgh, 1971). All are potent inhibitors of gastric acid secretion. Glucagon, VIP and GIP are potent stimulants of intestinal secretion in the dog (Barbezat and Grossman, 1971). VIP is a weak stimulant of pancreatic water and bicarbonate secretion and is a partial agonist of secretin (Makhlouf and Said, 1975). VIP has a glycogenolytic effect which is much weaker than that of glucagon and also may produce mild increases in serum calcium concentration. The most striking systemic effect of VIP is marked vasodilatation with hypotension. At one time or another all four members of this peptide family have been considered leading candidates as the hormone responsible for pancreatic cholera. GIP was reported to be present in diarrhoeogenic tumour tissue when tested by immunofluorescent staining techniques (Elias et al, 1972) but this result appears to have been erroneous and caused by cross-reactivity with VIP in the antiserum employed (Bloom, personal communication). Specific identification of increased concentrations of VIP alone in plasma and tumour tissue appears to have resolved the controversy, but the possibility exists that other tumours may produce diarrhoea through elaboration of one or more of the other hormones. Indeed, Mallinson et al (1974) reported diarrhoea in several patients with glucagon-secreting tumours and Schmitt et al (1975) reported watery diarrhoea and pancreatic hypersecretion in a patient whose tumour secreted multiple hormones, including secretin.

Treatment

Surgical resection of a benign pancreatic islet tumour or ganglioneuroma is optimal treatment for patients with this syndrome and is possible in about half the cases (Verner and Morrison, 1974). In another 20 per cent of cases only diffuse islet cell hyperplasia can be identified. These patients apparently can be cured by pancreatic resection. However, there is little data available on preoperative and postoperative plasma VIP in such patients. Distant meta-

Table 3.3 Amino acid sequences of porcine GIP, glucagon, secretin and VIP

	GIP	Glucagon	Secretin	VIP
Amino acid residues	43	29	27	28
Molecular weight	5104	3484	3055	3326
	Tyr	His	—	—
	Ala	Ser	—	—
	Glu	Gln	Asp	—
	Gly	—	—	Ala
	Thr	—	—	Val
	Phe	—	—	—
	Ile	Thr	—	—
	Ser	—	—	Asp
	Asp	—	Glu	Asn
	Tyr	—	Leu	Tyr
	Ser	—	—	Thr
	Ile	Lys	Arg	—
	Ala	Tyr	Leu	—
	Met	Leu	Arg	—
	Asp	—	—	Lys
	Lys	Ser	—	Gln
	Ile	Arg	Ala	Met
	Arg	—	—	Ala
	Gln	Ala	Leu	Val
	Gln	—	—	Lys
	Asp	—	Arg	Lys
	Phe	—	Leu	Tyr
	Val	—	Leu	—
	Asn	Gln	—	Asn
	Trp	—	Gly	Ser
	Leu	—	—	Ile
	Leu	Met	Val–NH$_2$	Leu
	Ala	Asp		Asn–NH$_2$
	Gln	Thr		
	Gln			
	Lys			
	Gly			
	Lys			
	Lys			
	Ser			
	Asp			
	Trp			
	Lys			
	His			
	Asn			
	Ile			
	Thr			
	Gln			

(−) indicates amino acid residue identical to preceding column.

stasis is present in about 40 per cent of patients at the time of surgery. Partial tumour resection may provide temporary relief in such patients. High dose steroids have provided significant relief of symptoms in some patients with metastatic disease. More recently, good relief of diarrhoea was produced in two patients treated with intra-arterial infusions of streptozotocin (Kahn et al, 1975).

GLUCAGONOMA

In 1942, Becker, Kahn and Rothman described a patient with an unusual necrotising erythaematous migratory skin rash accompanied by stomatitis, weight loss, diabetes mellitus, and anaemia. McGavran et al (1966) described a patient with skin lesions, adult-onset diabetes mellitus, and a glucagon-secreting carcinoma of the pancreatic alpha cells. More recently (Mallinson et al, 1974) a series of patients with glucagon-secreting pancreatic alpha-cell tumours, diabetes, and necrotising skin lesions was reported. Half of the patients in this series also had diarrhoea. Several additional patients have been reported in the literature. These have had increased immunoreactive plasma glucagon concentrations and high glucagon content in tumour extracts. In one patient, insulin-dependent diabetes mellitus was cured by successful tumour resection (Lightman and Bloom, 1974). Tumour resection also has produced rapid resolution of skin lesions and diarrhoea. Glucagon-secreting tumours can be added to the family of apudomas. They also have been found as part of the multiple endocrine neoplasia syndrome (Croughs et al, 1972).

REFERENCES

Barbezat, G. O. & Grossman, M. I. (1971) Intestinal secretion: stimulation by peptides. *Science*, **174**, 442–424.
Becker, S. W., Kahn, D. & Rothman, S. (1942) Cutaneous manifestations of internal malignant tumors. *Archives of Dermatology and Syphilology*, **45**, 1069–1080.
Blair, E. L., Greenwell, J. R., Grund, E. R., Reed, J. D. & Sanders, D. J. (1975) Gastrin response to meals of different composition in normal subjects. *Gut*, **16**, 766–773.
Bloom, S. R. & Polak, J. M. (1975) The role of VIP in pancreatic cholera. In *Gastrointestinal Hormones*, ed. Thompson, J. C., pp. 635–642. Austin and London: University of Texas Press.
Bloom, S. R., Polak, J. M. & Pearse, A. G. E. (1973) Vasoactive intestinal peptide and watery-diarrhoea syndrome. *Lancet*, **2**, 14–16.
Brown, J. C. & Dryburgh, J. R. (1971) A gastric inhibitory polypeptide. II. The complete amino acid sequence. *Canadian Journal of Biochemistry and Physiology*, **49**, 867–872.
Carpena, C., Kay, J. H., Mendez, A. M., Redington, J. V., Zubiate, P. & Zucker, R. (1973) Carcinoid heart disease: surgery for tricuspid and pulmonary valve lesions. *American Journal of Cardiology*, **32**, 229–233.
Creutzfeldt, W., Arnold, R., Creutzfeldt, C., Deuticke, U., Frerichs, H. & Track, N. S. (1973) Biochemical and morphological investigations of 30 human insulinomas. *Diabetologia*, **9**, 217–231.
Creutzfeldt, W., Arnold, R., Creutzfeldt, C. & Track, N. S. (1975) Pathomorphologic, biochemical, and diagnostic aspects of gastrinomas (Zollinger–Ellison syndrome). *Human Pathology*, **6**, 47–76.
Croughs, R. J. M., Hulsmans, H. A. M., Israel, D. E., Hackeng, W. H. L. & Schopman, W. (1972) Glucagonoma as part of the polyglandular adenoma syndrome. *American Journal of Medicine*, **52**, 690–698.
Dockray, G. J. & Walsh, J. H. (1975) Amino terminal gastrin fragment in serum of Zollinger–Ellison syndrome patients. *Gastroenterology*, **68**, 222–230.

Dockray, G. J., Walsh, J. H. & Passaro, E., Jr. (1975) Relative abundance of big and little gastrins in the tumours and blood of patients with the Zollinger–Ellison syndrome. *Gut*, **16**, 353–358.
Elias, E., Bloom, S. R., Welbourn, R. B., Kuzio, M., Polak, J. M., Pearse, A. G. E., Booth, C. C. & Brown, J. C. (1972) Pancreatic cholera due to production of gastric inhibitory polypeptide. *Lancet*, **2**, 791–793.
Fox, P. S., Hofmann, J. W., Decosse, J. J. & Wilson, S. D. (1974) The influence of total gastrectomy on survival in malignant Zollinger–Ellison tumors. *Annals of Surgery*, **180** 558–565.
Grahame-Smith, D. G. (1968) The carcinoid syndrome. *American Journal of Cardiology*, **21**, 376–387.
Grossman, M. I. (1972) Gastrointestinal hormones: some thoughts about clinical applications. *Scandinavian Journal of Gastroenterology*, **7**, 97–104.
Grossman, M. I., Tracy, H. J. & Gregory, R. A. (1961) Zollinger–Ellison syndrome in a Bantu woman, with isolation of a gastrin-like substance from the primary and secondary tumors. II. Extraction of gastrin-like activity from tumours. *Gastroenterology*, **41**, 87–91.
Hajdu, S. I., Winawer, S. J. & Myers, W. P. L. (1974) Carcinoid tumors: a study of 204 cases. *American Journal of Clinical Pathology*, **61**, 521–528.
Isenberg, J. I., Walsh, J. H. & Grossman, M. I. (1973) Zollinger–Ellison syndrome. *Gastroenterology*, **65**, 140–165.
Isenberg, J. I., Walsh, J. H., Passaro, E., Jr., Moore, E. W. & Grossman, M. I. (1972) Unusual effect of secretin on serum gastrin, serum calcium, and gastric acid secretion in a patient with suspected Zollinger–Ellison syndrome. *Gastroenterology*, **62**, 626–631.
Ivey, K. J. & Hansky, J. (1975) Variability of serum gastrin levels in Zollinger–Ellison syndrome: studies with two antisera to gastrin. *Digestive Diseases*, **20**, 513–517.
Johnson, L. R. (1975) Trophic action of gastrointestinal hormones. In *Gastrointestinal Hormones*, ed. Thompson, J. C., pp. 215–230. Austin and London: University of Texas Press.
Kahn, C. R., Levy, A. G., Gardner, J. G., Miller, J. V., Gordon, P. & Schein, P. S. (1975) Pancreatic cholera: beneficial effects of treatment with streptozotocin. *New England Journal of Medicine*, **292**, 941–945.
Kaplan, E. L., Jaffe, B. M. & Peskin, G. W. (1972) A new provocative test for the diagnosis of the carcinoid syndrome. *American Journal of Surgery*, **123**, 173–179.
Kellum, J. M. & Jaffe, B. M. (1975) Radioimmunoassay of serotonin. *Gastroenterology*, **68**, 924 (Abstract).
Kowlessar, O. D. (1973) Carcinoid tumors and the carcinoid syndrome. In *Gastrointestinal Disease*, ed. Sleisenger, M. H. & Fordtran, J. S., pp. 1031–1041. Philadelphia, London, Toronto: W. B. Saunders Co.
Lightman, S. L. & Bloom, S. R. (1974) Cure of insulin-dependent diabetes mellitus by removal of a glucagonoma. *British Medical Journal*, **1**, 367–368.
Lubarsch, O. (1888) Ueber den primaren Krebs des Ileum nebst Bemerkingen uber das gleichzeitige Vorkommen von Krebs und Tuberkulose. *Virchows Archiv für pathologische Anatomie und Physiologie und für bluische Medizin*, III, 280–317.
Makhlouf, G. M. & Said, S. I. (1975) The effect of vasoactive intestinal peptide (VIP) on digestive and hormonal function. In *Gastrointestinal Hormones*, ed. Thompson, J. C., pp. 599–610. Austin and London: University of Texas Press.
Mallinson, C. N., Bloom, S. R., Warin, A. P., Salmon, P. R. & Cox, B. (1974) A glucagonoma syndrome. *Lancet*, **2**, 1–4.
Matsumoto, K. K., Peter, J. B., Schultze, R. G., Hakim, A. A. & Franck, P. T. (1966) Watery diarrhea and hypokalemia associated with pancreatic islet cell adenoma. *Gastroenterology*, **50**, 231–242.
McGavran, M. H., Unger, R. H., Recant, L., Polk, H. C., Kilo, C. & Levin, M. E. (1966) A glucagon-secreting alpha-cell carcinoma of the pancreas. *New England Journal of Medicine*, **274**, 1408–1413.
McGuigan, J. E. & Trudeau, W. L. (1968) Immunochemical measurement of elevated levels of gastrin in the serum of patients with pancreatic tumors of the Zollinger–Ellison variety. *New England Journal of Medicine*, **278**, 1308–1313.
Oates, J. A., Pettinger, W. A. & Doctor, R. B. (1966) Evidence for the release of bradykinin in carcinoid syndrome. *Journal of Clinical Investigation*, **45**, 173–178.

Oberhelman, H. A., Jr & Nelsen, T. S. (1964) Surgical consideration in the management of ulcerogenic tumors of the pancreas and duodenum. *American Journal of Surgery*, **108**, 132–141.

Orloff, M. J. (1971) Carcinoid tumors of the rectum. *Cancer*, **28**, 175–180.

Pearse, A. G. E. (1975) Neurocristopathy, neuroendocrine pathology and the APUD concept. *Zeitschrift für Krebsforschung*, **84**, 1–18.

Pearse, A. G. E., Polak, J. M. & Heath, C. M. (1974) Polypeptide hormone production by 'carcinoid' apudomas and their relevant cytochemistry. *Virchows Archiv für Pathologische Anatomic and Physiologie und für Klinische Medizin*, Abt. B, **16**, 95–109.

Pedersen, A. T., Batsakis, J. G., Vanselow, N. A. & McLean, J. A. (1970) False-positive tests for urinary 5-hydroxyindolacetic acid. Error in laboratory determinations caused by glyceryl guaiacolate. *Journal of the American Medical Association*, **211**, 1184–1188.

Polak, J. M., Stagg, B. & Pearse, A. G. E. (1972) Two types of Zollinger–Ellison syndrome: immunofluorescent, cytochemical and ultrastructural studies of the antral and pancreatic gastrin cells in different clinical states. *Gut*, **13**, 501–512.

Rambaud, J. C., Modigliani, R., Matuchamsky, C., Bloom, S., Said, S., Pessayre, D. & Bernier, J. J. (1975) Pancreatic cholera. Studies on tumoral secretions and pathophysiology of diarrhea. *Gastroenterology*, **69**, 110–122.

Reed, M. L., Kuipers, F. M., Vaitkevicius, V. K., Clark, M. D., Drake, E. H. & Eyeler, W. R. (1963) Treatment of disseminated carcinoid tumors including hepatic artery catherisation. *New England Journal of Medicine*, **269**, 1005–1010.

Rehfeld, J. F., Stadil, F. & Vikelsoe, J. (1974) Immunoreactive gastrin components in human serum. *Gut*, **15**, 102–111.

Richardson, C. T. & Walsh, J. H. (1976) The value of a histamine H$_2$-receptor antagonist in the management of patients with Zollinger–Ellison syndrome. *New England Journal of Medicine*, **294**, 133–135.

Said, S. I. & Faloona, G. R. (1975) Elevated plasma and tissue levels of vasoactive intestinal polypeptide in the watery-diarrhea syndrome due to pancreatic, bronchogenic, and other tumors. *New England Journal of Medicine*, **293**, 155–160.

Said, S. I. & Mutt, V. (1970) Polypeptide with broad biological activity: isolation from small intestine. *Science*, **169**, 1217–1218.

Schmitt, M. G., Jr, Soergel, K. H., Hensley, G. T. & Chey, W. Y. (1975) Watery diarrhea associated with pancreatic islet cell carcinoma. *Gastroenterology*, **69**, 206–216.

Sjoerdsma, A., Weissbach, H., Terry, L. L. & Udenfriend, S. (1957) Further observations on patients with malignant carcinoid. *American Journal of Medicine*, **23**, 5–15.

Soga, J. & Tazawa, K. (1971) Pathologic analysis of carcinoids: histologic re-evaluation of 62 cases. *Cancer*, **28**, 990–998.

Stadil, F., Stage, G., Rehfeld, J. F., Efsen, F. & Fischerman, K. (1976) Treatment of Zollinger–Ellison patients with streptozotocin. *Scandinavian Journal of Gastroenterology* (in press).

Thompson, J. C., Reeder, D. D., Villar, H. V. & Fender, H. R. (1975) Natural history and experience with diagnosis and treatment of the Zollinger–Ellison syndrome. *Surgery, Gynecology and Obstetrics*, **140**, 721–739.

Trudeau, W. L. & McGuigan, J. M. (1969) Effects of calcium on serum gastrin levels in the Zollinger–Ellison syndrome. *New England Journal of Medicine*, **281**, 862–866.

Verner, J. V. & Morrison, A. B. (1958) Islet cell tumor and a syndrome of refractory watery diarrhea and hypokalemia. *American Journal of Medicine*, **25**, 374–380.

Verner, J. V. & Morrison, A. B. (1974) Endocrine pancreatic islet disease with diarrhea: report of a case due to diffuse hyperplasia of nonbeta islet issue with a review of 54 additional cases. *Archives of Internal Medicine*, **133**, 492–500.

Walsh, J. H. & Grossman, M. I. (1975) Gastrin. *New England Journal of Medicine*, **292**, 1324–1332, 1377–1384.

Walsh, J. H., Isenberg, J. I., Ansfield, J. & Maxwell, V. (1976) Clearance and acid-stimulating action of human big and little gastrins in duodenal ulcer subjects. *Journal of Clinical Investigation*, **57**, 1125–1131.

Walsh, J. H., Richardson, C. T. & Fordtran, J. S. (1975) pH dependence of acid secretion and gastrin release in normal and ulcer subjects. *Journal of Clinical Investigation*, **55**, 462–468.

Yalow, R. S. & Berson, S. A. (1960) Immunoassay of endogenous plasma insulin in man. *Journal of Clinical Investigation*, **39**, 1157–1175.

Yalow, R. S. & Berson, S. A. (1965) Dynamics of insulin secretion in hypoglycemia. *Diabetes*, **14**, 341–349.

Yalow, R. S. & Wu, N. (1973) Additional studies on the nature of big big gastrin. *Gastroenterology*, **65**, 19–27.

Zollinger, R. M. & Ellison, E. H. (1955) Primary peptic ulcerations of the jejunum associated with islet cell tumors of the pancreas. *Annals of Surgery*, **142**, 709–728.

4
THE EFFECTS OF MASSIVE SMALL BOWEL RESECTION

E. A. Shaffer   R. A. Brown   J. W. Dutton

The residual absorptive surface following extensive small bowel resection is the key to survival. The minimum length which can sustain life, however, varies considerably between individual patients. Some discrepancy arises from inaccurate measurement of gut length at surgery and/or the presence of disease in the remaining gut. Generally, resections over 200 cm (50–60 per cent of the total length) will result in some disability (Brenizer and Addison, 1929), although exceptional patients have been reported to survive with only 15 cm of small intestine (Anderson, 1965).

The clinical consequences of a surgically shortened midgut with loss of function have been termed 'the short gut syndrome' since the original description almost 100 years ago (Koeberlé, 1881). Modern concepts of the syndrome, derived from a more precise understanding of the pathophysiological disturbances following massive resection, have lead to more rational therapy, specifically nutritional modalities which circumvent the more complex (and hence more readily disturbed) processes in alimentation.

NORMAL DIGESTION AND ABSORPTION

The intact alimentary tract has an enormous capacity to digest and absorb food. Digestion, the hydrolysis of nutrients to smaller molecules, largely occurs in the small intestine although this process may be initiated in the mouth by the secretion of tongue lipase (Hamosh and Scow, 1973) and salivary amylase. The end-products of digestion are then absorbed through the intestinal epithelium by two major transport mechanisms:

Passive diffusion, which proceeds in a 'downhill' direction along electrochemical gradients, is not energy-requiring or carrier-mediated and does not exhibit competitive inhibition. Low molecular weight substances, such as some fat-soluble vitamins and drugs, are absorbed by simple diffusion and the rate of absorption depends on the solute concentration. Simple diffusion probably also accounts for a large portion of carbohydrate and amino acid absorption in the proximal small bowel because postprandial intraluminal concentrations exceed blood levels. 'Non-ionic' diffusion involves the transfer of uncharged molecules, such as weak acids and bases and is relatively more rapid than 'ionic' diffusion which is retarded by lipid membrane impermeability to ionised compounds. Many nutrients present in the intestinal lumen at low concentrations, however, are water soluble, ionised and of a high molecular weight. Simple diffusion through membrane barriers would be inadequate for these, so that specialised transport mechanisms are required.

Active transport occurs 'uphill' against an electrochemical gradient, requires energy, is carrier-mediated and subject to competitive inhibition. This transport system has a rate limiting maximum and is potentially saturable at high concentrations. Active absorption has been demonstrated for most essential nutrients including certain monosaccharides, amino acids, fatty acids, cholesterol, iron, calcium, sodium, bile salts and vitamin B_{12}.

FAT DIGESTION AND ABSORPTION

As steatorrhoea is generally the outstanding clinical feature of maldigestion and malabsorption, a brief summary of the complex processes involved in fat assimilation is appropriate (Hofmann, 1967) (see also Chapter 2).

The average Western adult ingests daily 60 to 100 g of fat, mainly in the form of long-chain triglycerides. This neutral fat is water insoluble (Small, 1970) whereas the bulk phase of intraluminal contents is an aqueous milieu. Triglycerides must therefore undergo an orderly processing, being physically broken into fine lipid droplets (emulsification), undergoing hydrolysis (lipolysis), solubilisation of the split products (micellarisation), and their presentation to the absorptive surface. The churning action of the stomach first produces a crude emulsion which later becomes stabilised in the duodenum by biliary lecithin and also by the products of lipolysis, monoglyceride and fatty acids. Fat droplet size is important in the duodenum because pancreatic lipase, a surface active enzyme, catalyses hydrolysis only at oil–water interfaces. Pancreatic lipase activity is also dependent on the presence of a colipase (Morgan and Hoffman, 1971) plus bile salts which reduce its pH optimum to 6.5. Lipase preferentially hydrolyses the ester bonds of the triglycerides in the α- and α'-positions forming primarily long chain fatty acids and β-monoglycerides. The β-monoglyceride must then isomerise to the α or α' form before lipolysis is completed. None of these lipolytic products is water soluble to any degree (Small, 1970) but must be removed from the oil–water interface for lipolysis to proceed. Bile salts are the biologically active detergent molecules responsible for solubilising these end-products of lipolysis. When secreted into the duodenum above a certain concentration (the 'critical micellar concentration') bile salts form small molecular aggregates called 'micelles' (Hofmann, 1967, 1968). The subsequent addition of phospholipids and certain fatty acids swell the aggregates which are known as 'mixed micelles' and expand their lipid solubilising capacity. Fatty acids, monoglycerides and the fat soluble vitamins (A, D, E and K) are then incorporated into the 'mixed micelles'. In this way they are brought into aqueous solution and hence removed from the oil–water interface thereby promoting further lipolysis.

Membrane uptake now beings. Micellar solubilisation removes the products of lipolysis and presents the long-chain fatty acids and β-monoglycerides to the intestinal epithelial cells. The micelle probably distintegrates at the mucosal cell surface releasing fatty acids and monoglyceride which then traverses an unstirred water layer (Dietschy, Sallee and Wilson, 1971) to penetrate the lipoprotein membrane. Once inside the cell the fatty acids are re-esterified to triglyceride and these neutral lipid molecules coalesce into fat droplets. Covered by protein, cholesterol and phospholipid, large chylomicron particles form and have free access to exit into the lymphatic system. Thus, fat digestion and absorption involves micellar solubilisation and delivery of chylomicrons through intestinal lymphatics, both complex processes which are not involved in protein and carbohydrate assimilation.

Medium-chain triglycerides, composed of fatty acids with C-6 to C-10 carbon chains are assimilated at every step much more readily than long-chain triglycerides and may even be absorbed intact in significant amounts (some 30 per cent of an oral dose). Digestion is facilitated by enhanced susceptibility to pancreatic lipase activity which hydrolyses fatty acids both at the α- and β-positions. The free fatty acids so formed have enhanced water solubility and form micelles more readily with bile salts. Once absorbed medium-chain fatty acids are neither re-esterified to any extent nor incorporated into lipoproteins. Instead they directly enter the portal venous system and are transported bound to protein.

Sites of Normal Absorption

Major regional differences in small bowel absorptive function exist because specific active transport is localised to selective areas (Ingelfinger, 1967). Thus the length of any resection does not solely determine the severity of the resultant absorptive defect although passive diffusion occurs all along the gastrointestinal tract. In the duodenum, calcium and iron are maximally absorbed, whereas the jejunum is the major site for carbohydrate, protein and fat absorption. The ileum is specific for the active absorption of bile salts (Dietschy, 1968; Tyor, Garbutt and Lack, 1971), and vitamin B_{12}. Active sodium absorption increases aborally whereas concomitant passive permeability to sodium decreases distally (Fordtran, Rector and Carter, 1968). Sodium entrance into the epithelial cell is partly passive and partly carrier mediated while sodium exit into the extracellular space is probably active with the sodium pump being located at the basolateral border of the cell (Schultz and Curran, 1968). Water absorption passively follows osmotic gradients created by such active solute transport. Net uptake of sodium then determines residual intraluminal fluid, stool water and volume. Loss of such specific regional differences underlie the clinical features which result from bowel resection.

Bile Salt Absorption and Enterohepatic Circulation

Bile salt absorption is perhaps the best example of regional specialisation (see also Chapter 10). Bile salts promote fat digestion and absorption through their effect on lipolysis and micellar solubilisation, and are essential for absorption of fat-soluble vitamins and cholesterol (Hofmann, 1968; Holt, 1972). Bile salt absorption is largely confined to a specialised transport system in the distal ileum, whereas fat absorption is completed in the proximal small intestine. Passive transport of bile salts occurs to a limited extent throughout

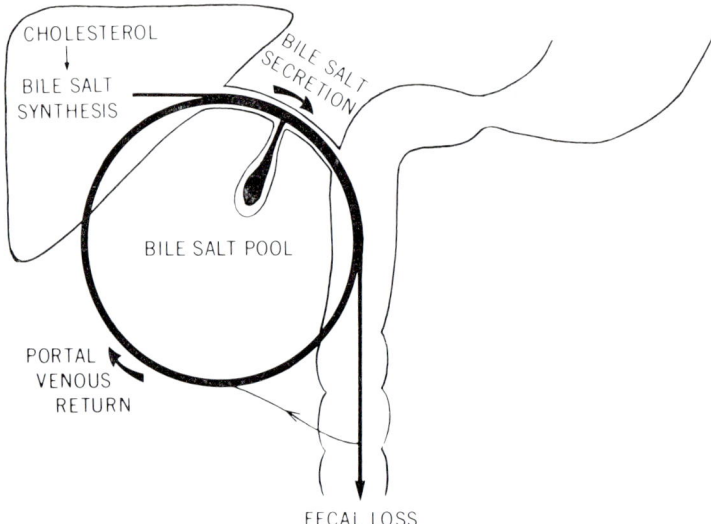

Figure 4.1 The enterohepatic circulation of bile salts

the intestinal length (Tyor et al, 1971), although permeability may be higher in the jejunum (Krag and Phillips, 1974). But even bile salts with higher lipid solubilities are poorly absorbed by passive non-ionic diffusion (Dietschy, 1968). Following their active reabsorption in the terminal ileum bile salts enter the portal vein bound to albumin and are rapidly transported to the liver, where they are efficiently cleared and secreted into bile. Bile salts, thus, undergo an enterohepatic circulation (Fig. 4.1.) which is so efficient that over 95 per cent are reabsorbed during each cycle (Dowling, Mack and Small, 1970). A small bile salt pool, normally about 3 g, is able to recirculate 6 to 10 times a day (Borgström et al, 1957) with a net loss of but 500 mg daily. In a steady state this loss is accurately replaced each day by an equivalent hepatic synthesis from cholesterol. An intact ileum is obviously crucial for maintenance of the integrity of this enterohepatic circulation (Hofmann, 1967). Because bile salt absorption largely occurs at a site distal to fat absorption significant bile salt absorption is delayed until after dietary lipids have been absorbed, allowing the system to economically re-use bile salts and thus maintain adequate micellar solubilisation in the jejunum despite a small bile salt pool.

PATHOPHYSIOLOGICAL CONSEQUENCES OF SMALL INTESTINAL LOSS

Primary Effects

The site of intestinal loss is a major determinant of the resultant digestive–absorptive dysfunction:

Duodenal resection or bypass commonly leads to iron malabsorption and

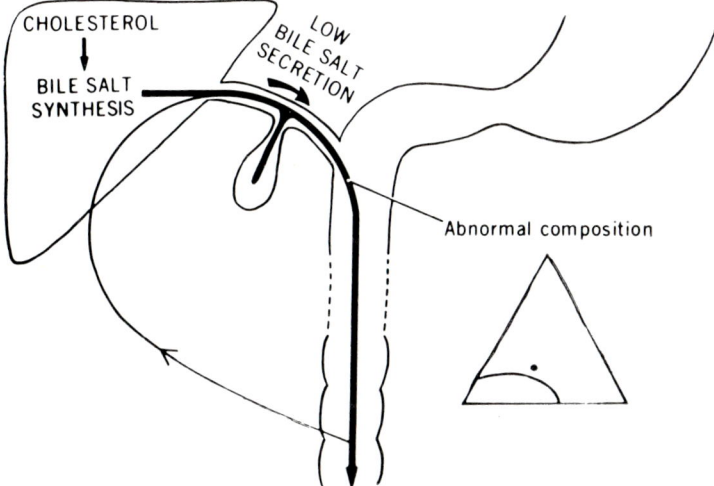

Figure 4.2 The effect of ileal disease or resection on the enterohepatic circulation of bile salts

subsequent anaemia. Osteomalacia may also develop because calcium absorption is most efficient in the more acid milieu of the proximal small intestine.

Midintestinal resection, as in a limited jejunectomy, is usually well tolerated so long as dietary intake is maintained. The residual bowel often has sufficient digestive and absorptive capacity to compensate for even major jejunal loss.

Distal small bowel resection has a more profound effect, causing diarrhoea and steatorrhoea, even if the preferential site for fat absorption, the proximal intestine, remains intact. Loss of the active transport sites in the ileum results in bile salt malabsorption and interruption of the enterohepatic circulation as illustrated in Figure 4.2. Reduction of bile salt return to the liver turns off the negative feedback mechanisms regulating synthesis from cholesterol, but the ensuing increase in hepatic synthesis cannot fully compensate (see also Chapter 10). Although the bile salt pool which collects in the gallbladder following an overnight fast may be nearly normal (Abaurre et al, 1969), it fails to recirculate so that hepatic secretion and duodenal output diminish during the day.

The clinical consequences of altered bile salt metabolism include (Garbutt et al, 1971; Hofmann, 1972):

DIARRHOEA

Excess bile salts passing into the colon cause both impaired absorption and enhanced secretion of water and electrolytes (Mekhjian, Phillips and Hofmann, 1971). This cathartic effect from excess bile salts in the colon can be alleviated by administration of cholestyramine. By binding bile salts, cholestyramine decrease the diarrhoea in patients with limited ileal resection (30–100 cm) although the modest steatorrhoea (< 20 g/day) may be slightly aggravated (Hofmann and Poley, 1969). Patients with more substantial resection (> 100 cm) and steatorrhoea (> 20 g/day) are not improved on cholestryamine and the steatorrhoea worsens with a significant caloric loss.

STEATORRHOEA

Both fat maldigestion and malabsorption result from inadequate bile salt concentration in the jejunum. This effect is the therapeutic rationale behind ileal bypass surgery in patients with morbid obesity (Payne and DeWind, 1969) or hypercholesterolaemia (Buchwald, 1967) leading to malabsorption of bile salts (the end product of cholesterol catabolism) and dietary fat.

CHOLESTEROL GALLSTONE DISEASE

This occurs in one-third of patients with ileal disease (Heaton and Read, 1969; Cohen et al, 1971). Interruption of the enterohepatic circulation reduces the bile salt pool and secretion (Dowling et al, 1970) causing the liver to produce abnormal bile with excess cholesterol (Dowling, Bell and White, 1972). The function of the gallbladder as a reservoir for bile may not be important in subjects with an intact small intestine who handle fats very well after cholecystectomy (Simmons and Bouchier, 1971) but could become critical following loss of the ileum (Jordan, Olsan and Paige, 1968). Indeed, asymptomatic cholelithiasis is perhaps best left alone in those with precarious nutritional balance and generally the largest meal should be breakfast when the gallbladder can eject a sizeable fraction of the bile salt pool into the duodenum.

SPECIFIC ILEAL ABSORPTIVE DYSFUNCTION

Vitamin B_{12} malabsorption follows removal of the specific transport site for the intrinsic factor–vitamin B_{12} complex so that the traditional B_{12} absorption (Schilling) test may disclose this prior to any overt deficiency. More promising techniques to detect ileal dysfunction have evolved from the distortion evoked in bile salt metabolism. There is an alteration in the taurine : glycine ratio. Because taurine-conjugated bile salts are principally absorbed in the terminal ileum and there is a limited supply of taurine in man, this amino acid is easily depleted and conjugation occurs with the more available glycine moiety thereby increasing its proportion in the bile. Rather than the more gross change in bile salt taurine : glycine ratio, a most sensitive breath test has been developed to measure bile salt deconjugation (Fromm, Thomas and Hofmann, 1973). Cholyl (1-^{14}C) glycine is administered; the malabsorbed bile salt is delivered to the colon where deconjugation by gut bacteria release the labelled glycine. The ^{14}C glycine is absorbed, converted to $^{14}CO_2$ and subsequently exhaled. The $^{14}CO_2$ in breath then reflects the extent of deconjugation and hence malabsorption (see also Chapter 9).

NEPHROLITHIASIS

Oxalate stones have been associated with bowel disease for years but only recently has the mechanism been uncovered (Daren, 1974). Acquired hyperoxaluria has been specifically linked to distal small bowel resection, including therapeutic bypass surgery and inflammatory bowel disease (Smith and Hofmann, 1974). The oxaluria originated from increased oxalate absorption and presumably is due to some physicochemical change of oxalate in the lumen. The malabsorbed fat, in the form of fatty acids, may precipitate as calcium soaps, thus decreasing any ionised calcium. Reduced calcium in the lumen allows more oxalate to be in the form of the sodium salt which is more readily soluble and absorbable. Whatever the precise mechanism, oxaluria is reduced by a low oxalate diet or administration of a bonding agent like cholestyramine. Uric acid stones also occur despite the absence of uricosuria probably because of decreased urine volume, the production of a more acid urine, or from coprecipitation with calcium salts.

Secondary Effects

Certain secondary phenomena compound the direct loss of absorptive surface leading to a further deterioration of gut function.

GASTRIC ACID HYPERSECRETION

This commonly occurs following massive resection and has resulted in peptic ulcer disease (Osborne et al, 1967). Increased acid output has been attributed to either a loss of inhibitory hormones normally present in the small intestines, such as secretin, or a heightened postprandial rise in gastrin (Wickbom et al, 1975). Hypersecretion appears proportional to the amount rather than the level (proximal or distal) of resection, but its duration and the underlying mechanism remains obscure.

INTRALUMINAL BACTERIAL OVERGROWTH

Excessive bacterial growth can develop from disordered intestinal motility (stagnation in a blind loop or behind a stricture) or from faecal contamination (through a fistula or enterocolonic anastomosis with free reflux). Bacterial proliferation in the small bowel remnant further aggravates the malabsorption of bile salts, fat and vitamin B_{12}.

CHANGES IN INTESTINAL MOTILITY

These are induced by small bowel resection with more rapid transit occurring following resection of the ileocaecal sphincter especially when combined with ileectomy (Singleton, Redmond and McMurray, 1964). Distal resection may also enhance gastric emptying.

COMPENSATORY ADAPTATION

There is an intimate relationship between the microscopic and histochemical anatomy of the small intestine and all digestive processes. Following partial surgical resection, morphological and functional changes are initiated in an apparent attempt to compensate for the lost digestive–absorptive function (Dowling and Booth, 1966).

Microscopic Anatomy

Three structural designs allow the normal intestine to increase greatly its absorptive surface. These are the valvuli conniventes, the finger-like villi, and the microvilli numbering more than 1700 on the apical surface of each cell (Brown, 1962). In the normal intestine the height of the villus decreases from duodenum to ileum (Altmann and Enesco, 1967). Any disruption of the normal cell production in the crypts or alteration of cell maturation and migration to the tips disturbs the structural–functional integrity of the villus as a unit. A commonly seen response is the loss of the normal finger-like appearance and the adoption of a leaf or tongue shape, as in coeliac disease with consequent steatorrhoea and malabsorption (Creamer, 1967). In contrast, the opposite histological change is noted after resection which primarily reduces the total absorptive area. Each remaining villus elongates, becomes thinner and the number of villi per surface area increases—a true hyperplasia (Dowling, 1973; Porus, 1965). At a subcellular level, there is also a marked increase in the length of the microvilli (Tilson and Wright, 1972). Overall, compensatory increase in absorption comes from the morphological increase in surface area, but the exact role of luminal nutrition, endogenous secretion of hormonal trophic factors and changes in blood flow is unknown.

Different anatomical areas of the small intestine possess variable adaptive capacities in experimental models. The ileal adaptive capacity appears superior to that of jejunum (Dowling and Booth, 1966). When the ileum is transposed proximally to be in continuity with the duodenum it adopts the villus size and indices identical to normal jejunum (Altmann and Leblond, 1970). Conversely if the jejunum is placed next to the caecum, the jejunum will not assume the morphology of normal ileum. Due to such limited adaptation of the remaining jejunum, ileal loss produces more profound malabsorption and steatorrhoea than a comparable loss of jejunum. Some adaptation in the residual jejunum does occur and enhanced bile salt absorption may account for the clinical observation that the diarrhoea of the short gut syndrome abates with time (Dowling, White and Perry, 1973; Weser and Hernandez, 1971). In addition preservation of the ileocaecal sphincter appears protective in enhancing the functional capacity of the remaining small bowel so that significant resections can be tolerated if the terminal ileum and ileocaecal sphincter are retained (Singleton et al, 1964). Removal of the ileocaecal sphincter may alter intestinal bacteria or destroy a barrier effect allowing bacterial contamination to reflux from the colon.

Histochemistry

Histochemical delineation of the number and precise location of digestive enzymes have revealed their close association with the brush border of the villus. Brush border enzymes identified include lactase, maltase, non-specific alkaline phosphatase, adenosine triphosphatase and leucine aminopeptidase (Pearse and Riecken, 1967). All have specific digestive functions and their fate following resection has recently been investigated. Obviously the total complement of enzymes is reduced because of massive mucosal loss (Dowling, 1973). Other subtle effects are produced by ileectomy. Cell turnover is increased (Loran and Crocker, 1963) resulting in more rapid cell migration from their origin in the crypts. Immature cells thus reach the villous tips with reduced enzyme content and decreased availability for intraluminal digestion (Flint, 1912). With increased cell turnover there is also enhanced sloughing of apical cells into the lumen. This endogenous cellular debris contains not only significant amounts of essential nutrients such as iron, but also fat and protein which in turn are poorly digested (Creamer, 1967; Conrad, Weintraub and Crosby, 1964). Thus, more active cell turnover may actually impair digestive function. If a protein deficient state ensues cell turnover will then be reduced and these adverse effects ameliorated (Deo and Ramalingasuami 1965). Such reverse adaptation in gravely malnourished patients explains the survival of some hopeless patients before the advent of ancillary nutrition.

CLINICAL COURSE AND COMPLICATIONS

The clinical course and potential complications following massive small bowel resection can be categorised (Wright and Tilson, 1971) (Table 4.1) as:

1. those which occur immediately following surgical intervention;
2. those which occur during the stage of adaptation; and
3. those which are chronic, remaining once adaptation has taken place.

In the immediate postoperative period a severe extracellular fluid deficit may arise from either inadequate preoperative rehydration or a continuing third space sequestration following resection. Tachycardia, a low central venous pressure, and oliguria are commonly present. Urine specific gravity is high, often in excess of 1.030, while urinary sodium concentration approaches zero. Large volumes of fluid replacement are necessary to correct this deficit.

Sepsis may arise on the second or third postoperative day from either incomplete removal of necrotic bowel or progression of a vascular infarction.

Table 4.1 Complications of massive bowel resection

1. Immediate postoperative phase
    i. Fluid and electrolyte abnormalities particularly hypokalaemia, hypochloraemia
    ii. Sepsis
    iii. Ileus
    iv. Calcium, magnesium, phosphate deficiency
    v. Hypoprothrombinaemia

2. Adaptive phase
    i. Uncontrolled diarrhoea
        (a) due to ↑ acid production
        (b) due to ↑ intestinal secretions
        (c) bile acid diarrhoea
        (d) fatty acid diarrhoea

3. Chronic phase
    i. Malnutrition
    ii. Peptic ulcer
    iii. Cholelithiasis
    iv. Anaemias—Iron deficiency
                —B_{12} deficiency
    v. Osteoporosis—hypocalcaemia
    vi. Hypomagnesaemia
    vii. Hypokalaemia ± nephropathy
    viii. Renal stone formation
    ix. Recurrent dehydration
    x. Perianal disease
    xi. Depression

A severe metabolic acidosis in the presence of ischaemia together with hypovolaemic shock unresponsive to resuscitation is the sine qua non of further bowel infarction requiring re-exploration. The fever, tachycardia and leukocytosis which denote infection can be masked postoperatively by concomitant steroid therapy.

Persistent ileus frequently complicates the course following massive bowel resection. Of many potential causes hypoxaemia often appears to be a factor in older individuals with chronic lung disease, whereas the severe catabolic state in debilitated patients perpetuates the ileus until reversed by ancillary nutrition. Hypokalaemia has long been known to result in prolonged postoperative ileus but only recently has it been realised that severe hypomagnesaemia may similarly retard normal bowel peristalsis. Finally small interloop abscesses require surgical drainage to abate postoperative ileus.

Diarrhoea becomes the most difficult problem once the postoperative ileus has cleared. Hypokalaemia can quickly develop from losses of up to 200 mmol of potassium daily. Hypocalcaemia, hypomagnesaemia and hypophosphataemia can be expected to occur within two to three weeks following resection if no fluid and electrolyte replacement is given. All such complications can be prevented by the addition of the appropriate elements to standard hyperalimentation solutions, and prophylactic vitamin K for hypoprothrombinaemia.

The diarrhoea occurring during the adaptive phase of recovery is discussed on page 91 but the possible mechanisms are re-emphasised in Table 4.1.

More chronic sequelae arise after the three to four week period in which adaptation should have occurred. Inadequate nutrition underscores all the complications spanning the postoperative period, but may be largely circumvented by prophylactic nutritional and electrolyte support.

THERAPEUTIC SMALL BOWEL BYPASS

The 'short bowel syndrome' has been therapeutically induced by the small bowel bypass procedures for treatment of morbid obesity. Intestinal bypass in the form of jejunocolic shunt, the first surgical attempt to short circuit the absorption of calories, had rather catastrophic complications all related to the severe loss of small bowel function. It was subsequently abandoned in favour of the less drastic jejunoileostomy (Payne and DeWind, 1969). This modification alleviated most of the adverse effects of bypass surgery but the unresolved problem of severe fatty liver infiltration and occasional cirrhosis remained (Dudrick et al, 1972). The hepatic dysfunction which develops following bypass surgery has been considered to be secondary to the formation of lithocholic acid, a known hepatotoxin. Lithocholic acid levels in bile and serum, however, are not increased after surgery although accumulation in the liver has not been excluded (Sherr et al, 1973). A more likely explanation for the occasional development of profound liver disease is the occurrence of protein malnutrition with depletion of essential amino acids.

In obesity excess cholesterol is secreted into bile resulting in lithogenic bile formation and probably accounting for the well-established relationship of obesity to cholesterol gallstone disease (Bennion and Grundy, 1975; Shaffer and Small, 1975). The catabolic state during the period of weight loss has also been implicated in lithogenic bile formation (Schreibman et al, 1974), so that the obese patient undergoing weight reduction appears doubly at risk. The bile salt malabsorption caused by loss of ileal function, can also effect lithogenic bile formation (Fig. 4.2), placing these obese subjects further at risk for developing gallstones (see also Chapter 9).

The high operative mortality plus the major risk factors associated with the bypass procedure, especially liver failure, have limited its usefulness in the management of intractable obesity. Similarly ileal bypass for hypercholesterolaemia has had limited success despite an ostensively sound physiological basis—the induction of bile salt malabsorption and increased catabolism of cholesterol to bile salts.

TREATMENT

Nutritional Support

Patients suffering from the short gut syndrome have benefited immensely from the intense research into clinical nutritional support that has been ongoing since Dudrick's classic observations on intravenous hyperalimentation (Dudrick, Vars and Rhoads, 1967). The earliest hypertonic intravenous

Table 4.2 Caloric distribution of elemental diet

	g/1000 kcal		kcal/litre	
Protein equivalent[a]	24.07	(23.3 minimum)	56	92
Casein hydrolysate powder		22.94 (22.2 minimum)		92
Added amino acids		1.13		4
Fat	34.29		304	
Soy oil (lightly hydrogenated)		26.63		240
MCT (75% Ca 25% C_{10})		6.66		35
Lecithin		1.00		9
Carbohydrate	149.93		600	
Sucrose		77.34		309
Corn syrup solids		63.20		253
Arrowroot starch		9.39		38
Product 'Flexical' powder	233		1000	

[a] $N \times 6.25$ (N : kcal = 1 : 250).

solution contained amino acids, sugars, electrolytes and vitamins and was infused through a major venous channel as blanket therapy to cover all body needs. Controversy subsequently arose from the critical observation by Blackburn et al (1973) that more efficient nitrogen balance could be realised by omitting glucose and using a peripheral vein for the infusion of amino acids mainly in the L-form.

'Elemental diet' is the term applied to an oral nutritional source containing in a simplified form all the factors essential to normal growth and development (Russell, 1975). Research into efficient diets of this kind was originally spurred by the aerospace race in the 1960s in an attempt to find the ideal oral diet for space flight. It had to fulfil three criteria. The nutritionally complete diet had to be acceptable to the astronaut, of low residue, and simple to reconstitute. The composition of the aerospace or elemental diet was amino acids, glucose and fat with appropriate electrolytes and vitamins and with an energy equivalent of 1 kcal/ml (Table 4.2). The absence of significant complex residue was expected to dramatically reduce faecal bulk. Although frequency of elimination decreases, the average stool weight may not be reduced (Brown, unpublished data), but a watery dark stool may result. The astronauts further rejected the diet due to its abnoxious taste and smell.

Fortunately experimental progress on the nutritional benefits of refined diets came with the report by Bounous et al (1967) concerning the protective effect of the elemental diet on canine intestine in low flow shock states. This work culminated in the successful treatment of patients suffering from the short bowel syndrome (Thompson et al, 1969; Stephens and Randall, 1969) and other disease states associated with severe malnutrition (Voitk et al, 1972). The rationale for the use of such a refined diet in nutritional support lies in its near total absorption in the upper small intestine with minimal digestive requirements. Fat may be present in the form of medium chain triglycerides (Flexical, Mead-Johnson), which obviates many of the complex steps in assimilation.

The weakness in parenteral and oral nutritional support lies in their non-specificity, both in requirements and response to therapy. Deficiencies have arisen in serum amino acids, fats and copper in patients managed by the standard parenteral solutions (Dudrick et al, 1972). The emergence of the aminogram focusing on the deficiencies noted has offered hope that ancillary nutrition can become as specific as fluid and electrolyte therapy (Fischer et al, 1974). Monitoring of nutritional gains and losses is presently a cumbersome task when nitrogen balances are used. Recent work by Shizgal, Kurtz and Spanier (1976) employing radioisotopes and calculating total body composition offers hope that a more facile and precise method will become available as an index of success of any nutritional programme. A plethora of pharmaceutical parenteral fluids as well as oral elemental diets have further clouded the therapeutic approach to this group of patients.

A rational therapeutic approach which has proven successful will be outlined (Voitk et al, 1973a and b). The primary indication for ancillary alimentation in massive small bowel resection is malnutrition which presents in three specific clinical situations:

1. Preoperatively associated with the primary intestinal disease.
2. Postoperatively during the stage of compensatory adaptation.
3. Postoperatively with failure of compensatory adaptation.

Preoperative

Inflammatory bowel disease is the major clinical setting in which patients must be preoperatively assessed for ancillary nutritional support. The extensively diseased intestine functionally produces a short bowel which may be further compromised by an operative procedure. Two simple determinations which identify those patients requiring ancillary nutritional support prior to surgery are weight loss greater than 10 per cent of ideal body weight and a serum albumin level at or below 2.5 g/dl on two occasions. The serum albumin level will not return rapidly to normal despite appropriate supportive therapy. A positive nitrogen balance is easily attained in the preoperative period and can be re-established postoperatively, thus minimising the obligatory catabolic effects of surgery (Voitk et al, 1973a and b). The patient illustrated in Figure 4.3 demonstrates a markedly negative nitrogen balance preoperatively which dramatically responded to oral elemental diet. Arbitrarily 10 to 14 days of nutritional support prior to surgery is a reasonable guideline

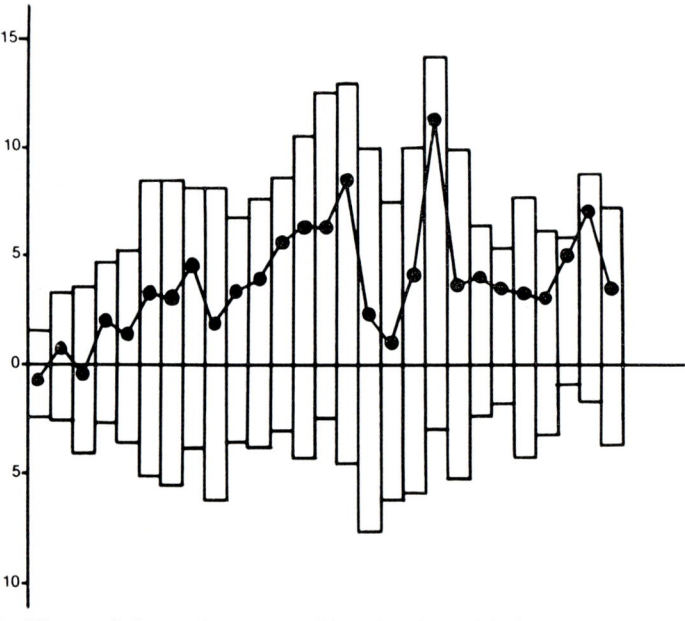

Figure 4.3 Nitrogen balance of a woman with regional enteritis. Each bar represents one day; area above zero line is daily intake and area below is output. Net balance is represented by joined dots. Her weight fell from 45.2 to 23.5 kg before elemental diet therapy. Three weeks of elemental diet resulted in a 4 kg weight gain and enabled her to withstand surgery without complication

and in this patient two days were required to achieve a positive nitrogen balance. If complications such as severe sepsis or toxic megacolon ensue during this period of supportive treatment then any high risks involved must be accepted, and surgery immediately undertaken.

The caloric load that should be reached with nutritional support is 3000 kcal/day, a level at which most patients will be in positive balance. Two exceptions must be recognised. Patients with sepsis will need a higher caloric load of approximately 4000 kcal/day. Secondly, patients on steroids require an enormous caloric intake to attain a positive nitrogen balance. In fact, achievement of a positive nitrogen balance preoperatively solely by means of the elemental diet is nearly impossible in the presence of glucocorticoids unless a minimum of 5000 kcal is administered (Dudrick, personal communication). Currently any adult patient being treated with glucocorticoids or ACTH and in need of nutrition should be treated by the Dudrick method of hypertonic glucose and amino acids rather than any peripheral infusion of amino acids, or fat solutions. Lipid infusions have been successfully used as the nutritional source in the paediatric age group (Grace, Beardmore and Cummings, 1976).

Nutritional therapy should be tailored to the individual in the absence of steroid therapy or bacterial infection. In regional enteritis without obstruction, adequate calories can often be delivered via a small Levin tube employing a pump to continuously infuse an elemental diet. During any such supplemental alimentation, patient tolerance is improved when other oral intake is stopped except for sips of water and the occasional hard candy. If severe diarrhoea or subjective intolerance of the diet occurs then intravenous alimentation should be used.

Postoperative compensatory adaptation

Nutritional support, the number one priority in postoperative therapy, should be maintained for approximately 21 days which is the time necessary for compensatory adaptation to occur in the residual healthy intestine. A standard hyperalimentation solution with glucose should be parenterally infused although this substrate may not be optimally utilised in the immediate postoperative period following anaesthesia (Wright, Henderson and Johnstone, 1974). As noted previously a daily intake of at least 3000 kcal is ideal but must be markedly increased with concomitant steroid therapy or sepsis.

The elemental diet has a marked advantage over normal food in the short gut syndrome during the subsequent postoperative period when bowel function is returning (Voitk et al, 1973a). Endogenous fluid entering the proximal small intestine is reduced because of diminished gastric acid output (Bury and Jambunathan, 1973) and a marked decrease in pancreatic secretion (McArdle et al, 1972) and general output of succus entericus (Voitk, 1973c). The elemental diet appears not only to protect the intestinal mucosa in low flow states, but also to initiate the adaptive changes in the microvilli identical to that seen after bowel resection (Brown, unpublished data), including increased intestinal mucosal growth (Feldman et al, 1974). Studies in animal models given the elemental diet have noted that the villi become taller and thinner. Morphological elongation of the microvilli (as demonstrated by the electron photomicrographs in Figures 4.4.a, b) may be induced by either a change in the amino acid content of intraluminal chyme or alterations in bacterial flora (Bounous et al, 1967; Bounous and Devroede, 1974). Finally, nitrogen balance in a postoperative patient with the short gut syndrome (Fig. 4.5) will become positive when placed on an elemental diet despite persistent disease and continued bowel adaptation. Thus the elemental diet is beneficial in promoting compensatory adaption while still supplying nutritional requirements despite the intestinal dysfunction.

Routine ward diet should not be started until the patient has finished a period of 21 days or more of elemental diet. A trial of clear fluids at this time when the elemental diet is still being infused will help to determine if a normal diet can be tolerated during the stage of compensatory adaptation. If the ileostomy or diarrhoea exceeds 2.5 litres/day with concomitant crampy abdominal pain then clear fluids should be stopped. Conversely in the absence of any adverse effects during this initial trial routine ward diet may be increased while the volume of the elemental diet is gradually tapered.

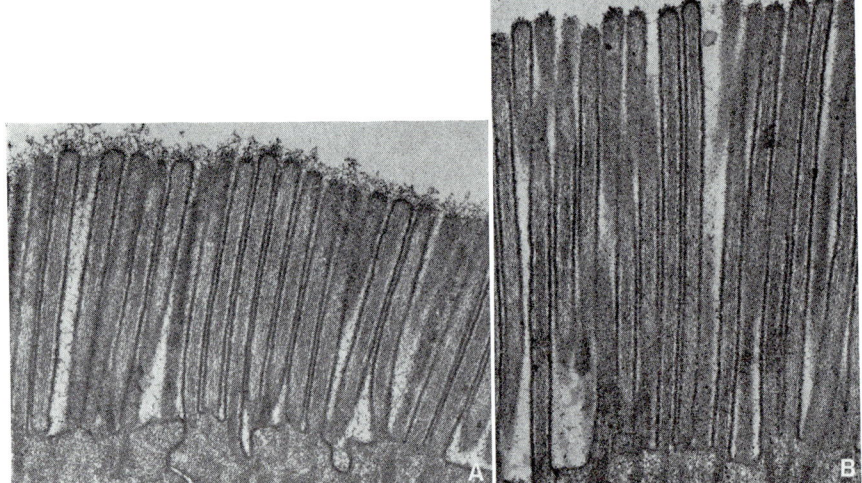

Figure 4.4A Ileal microvilli of dog fed a chow diet. Photomicrograph demonstrates normal microvillous architecture

Figure 4.4B Ileal microvilli of dog fed elemental diet. Note elongation of these organelles

Composition of the diet may be altered in accordance with patient tolerance, especially as regards volume and osmolarity. In general the use of medium-chain triglycerides and the reduction of the amount of fat will not only improve the steatorrhoea but may also reduce the fatty-acid-induced diarrhoea.

Postoperative adaptive failure

It is fortunate that most patients who survive massive small bowel resection have sufficient intestine to support life. Conversely, it may appear obvious at the time of resection—especially after a mesenteric vascular occlusion—that there may be inadequate residual bowel for survival under ordinary circumstances. Ambulatory home care has recently evoked a new optimistic approach in which patients are taught to administer their own parenteral nutrition via vascular catheters for circulatory access over prolonged periods (Broviac and

Scribner, 1974; Jeejeebhoy, Langer and Zahrab, 1972). The technical difficulties associated with the preparation and administration of these vital solutions has largely been overcome. Maintenance of adequate nutrition, including growth in children, has been demonstrated. Such benefits offset the risk factors including thromboembolic and septic complications, and the occasional severe anaemia due to acute copper deficiency. Although the quality of life and the moral implications may be questioned, alternatives previously were dismal.

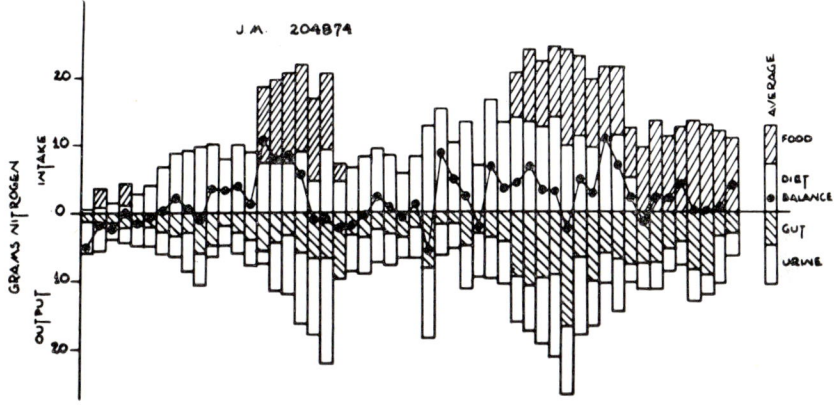

Figure 4.5 Nitrogen balance of patient while on elemental diet. Bars above zero line represent daily nitrogen intake, the shaded portion being derived from food, and the upper portion representing nitrogen from elemental diet. Nitrogen losses are shown below zero line, with enteric losses being shaded. This woman, with active regional enteritis, postoperatively had only 130 cm of small bowel ending in a jejunostomy. Note that attempts at feeding some two weeks after the surgery resulted in diarrhoea, malaise and increased urinary nitrogen losses with a negative balance. On institution of an elemental diet instead of food, positive nitrogen balance was restored. After an additional two weeks, elemental diet was gradually withdrawn while a well-tolerated ward diet was reintroduced with an ensuing mildly positive nitrogen balance on food alone

This problem of inadequate residual bowel despite adaptation was demonstrated by a recent patient who underwent complete resection of the small intestine for desmoid tumour invasion plus a colectomy for Gardner's syndrome (Voitk et al, 1973a). Only a functioning stomach and duodenum remained, with drainage through a permanent fistula. In hospital his nutrition was maintained alternatively by an elemental diet and by parenteral feeding and at times a combination of both, but this led to a bedridden stage with severe psychological depression. The patient was therefore allowed to eat as desired, but this resulted in drainage, 14 litres/day, from the fistula. A renal dialysis-type shunt was then constructed in order to maintain electrolyte balance. Instead of permanent intravenous hyperalimentation a nutritional regime was instituted, consisting of an oral intake during the day of about 1500 ml and 18 g of fat, supplemented by 1500 ml of an elemental diet infused via a gastrostomy tube throughout the hours of sleep. Immediately the fistula drainage dropped to approximately 2 to 4 litres/day and at present, eight months later, he has gained weight and works a full day as an insurance broker. This is an alternate way to handle the most difficult problem of no small intestine and no colon.

Ancillary nutritional support by either the parenteral or oral route constitues a vitally important advance in the treatment of the patient with massive bowel loss. In many instances this is the only hope for a return to an acceptable existence. Ancillary nutritional support on a temporary basis is usually sufficient to allow return to a relatively normal state but in a few instances permanent support has been necessary even in the home environment. All the nutritional needs, including the fat soluble vitamins, are supplied except for iron, copper and vitamin B_{12} which may require supplementation.

Psychological Support

Many of these patients become severely depressed during this time and their overall status is only complicated by the use of antidepressant drugs alone. In the overall management of the patient the often forgotten but extremely important role of the family should be utilised. The patients should be encouraged to participate in dietary planning and a well-informed imaginative wife can often make an otherwise unpalatable and depressing diet much more tolerable (Wright and Tilson, 1971). Diarrhoea itself may be the most depressing and debilitating symptom to the patient and can often be controlled with cholestyramine. Every effort should be made to prevent perianal excoriation and secondary infection. The patients should be instructed to use absorbent cotton balls rather than toilet paper after each bowel movement and sitz baths in warm water to which sodium bicarbonate has been added may be particularly soothing. The intertriginous area should be kept dry between bowel movements by use of talcum powder without additives and by wearing clean, loose fitting cotton under-garments. Local treatment with Xylocaine and/or antibiotic-containing creams should not be used as it can evoke secondary skin irritation.

Surgical Treatment

At the time of surgery every attempt must be made to preserve absorptive capacity while retaining healthy bowel. End-to-end anastomosis should be performed to prevent blind loops and insure that all remaining bowel will remain in continuity with the enteric stream. The ileocaecal sphincter should be spared if at all possible although it may predispose to some degree of functional obstruction. In vascular insufficiency, direct revascularisation of ischaemic but not necrotic bowel has been performed albeit with only limited success. Massive venous thrombosis and infarction presents an even more complex problem. The abdomen should be closed and the patient placed on anticoagulant therapy (Williams, 1971). The use of the second look operation 12 to 48 h following initial resection has also been used when the viability of the bowel cannot be adequately assessed or when the extent of the resection appears incompatible with life.

Gastric hypersecretion following bowel resection has been recognised since 1914 (Stassoff, 1914) and is known to result in jejunal inflammation and decreased absorption of simple sugars from the intestine. Before vagotomy and pyloroplasty or other acid decreasing operations are undertaken every effort must be made to prove that gastric acid secretion is increased, that it is uncontrollable by medical means, and that it is a significant factor in the patients' malabsorption and diarrhoea. No prophylactic ulcer surgery should therefore be undertaken at the time of initial resection (Wright and Tilson, 1971). Vagotomy, when used for control of peptic ulcer disease is known to result in diarrhoea in a small but significant number of patients. The division of the pyloric sphincter may also be detrimental as it normally regulates the passage of gastric contents into the small bowel. The use of medical therapy such as potent H_2 (histamine) receptor (Black et al, 1972) blocking agents, may prove to effectively control the acid hypersecretion secondary to small bowel resection.

The management of intestinal hypermotility has been attempted by a number of ingenuous surgical techniques including reversed intestinal segments (Saho and Blackman, 1962; Baldwin-Price and Singleton, 1965), circular loops, formation of artificial sphincters (Waddell et al, 1970) and intestinal smooth muscle oblation (Hidalgo et al, 1973). Such sophisticated surgery should be considered only when all other methods of treatment have failed. None of these procedures has produced exceptional results and all tend to further shorten the bowel. In fact, any surgical manoeuvre which jeopardises the remaining small bowel should be delayed until full adaptation has taken place and all other methods of therapy have failed.

As for the future, bowel transplantation may be the key to restoring digestive function, but little clinical advancement appears possible until rejection factors are better understood (Lillehei et al, 1967).

CONCLUSION

Extirpation of dysfunction from intrinsic disease involving more than 200 cm of small intestine causes the short gut syndrome. Since its description over 100 years ago the attitude towards the patient has evolved from despair to guarded optimism. Accounting for this change has been a vast improvement in prognosis, the result of a more basic comprehension of altered gastrointestinal physiology, specifically bile salt and fat metabolism. Conceptual amalgamation of structure, function and the clinical setting has provided the basis for three clinical phases necessitating nutritional support: preoperatively associated with the primary intestinal disease, postoperatively during compensatory adaptation and postoperatively if adaptation fails. At each instance, either oral elemental or parenteral hyperalimentation fluid will eliminate malnutrition and its sequelae.

REFERENCES

Abaurre, R., Gordon, S. G., Mann, J. G. & Kern, F. (1969) Fasting bile salt pool size and composition after ileal resection. *Gastroenterology*, **57**, 679.

Altmann, G. G. & Enesco, M. (1967) Cell number as a measure of distribution and removal of epithelial cells in the small intestine of growing and adult rats. *American Journal of Anatomy*, **121**, 319.

Altmann, G. G. & Leblond, C. P. (1970) Factors influencing villus size in the small intestine of adult rats as revealed by transposition of intestinal segments. *American Journal of Anatomy*, **127**, 15.

Anderson, C. M. (1965) Long-term survival with six inches of small intestine. *British Medical Journal*, **1**, 419.

Baldwin-Price, H. K. & Singleton, A. O. (1965) Reversed intestinal segments in the management of amenteric malabsorption syndrome. *Annals of Surgery*, **161**, 225.

Bennion, L. J. & Grundy, S. M. (1975) Effects of obesity and caloric intake on biliary lipid metabolism in man. *Journal of Clinical Investigation*, **56**, 996.

Black, J. W., Duncan, W. A. M., Durant, C. J., Ganellin, C. R. & Parsons, E. M. (1972) Definition and antagonism of histamine H_2-receptors. *Nature*, **236**, 385.

Blackburn, G. L., Flatt, J. P., Clowes, G. H. & O'Donnell, T. F. (1973) Peripheral intravenous feeding with isotonic amino acid solutions. *American Journal of Surgery*, **125**, 447.

Borgström, B., Dahlquist, A., Lundh, G. & Sjövall, J. (1957) Studies of intestinal digestion and absorption in the human. *Journal of Clinical Investigation*, **36**, 1521.

Bounous, G. & Devroede, G. J. (1974) Effect of an elemental diet on human fecal flora. *Gastroenterology*, **66**, 210.

Bounous, G., Sutherland, N. G., McArdle, A. H. & Gurd, F. N. (1967) The prophylactic use of an elemental diet in experimental hemorrhagic shock and intestinal ischemia. *Annals of Surgery*, **166**, 312.

Brenizer, A. G. & Addison, G. (1929) Extensive resections of the small intestine. *Annals of Surgery*, **89**, 675.

Broviac, J. W. & Scribner, B. H. (1974) Prolonged parenteral nutrition in the home. *Surgery, Gynecology and Obstetrics*, **139**, 24.

Brown, A. L., Jr (1962) Microvilli of the human jejunal epithelial cell. *Journal of Cell Biology*, **12**, 623.

Buchwald, H. (1967) The development of the subtotal ileal bypass operation as a therapeutic approach to hypercholesterolemia and atherosclerosis: a review. *Disease of the Chest*, **51** 459.

Bury, K. D. & Jambunathan, G. (1973) Effects of elemental diets on gastric emptying and gastric secretion in man. *American Journal of Surgery*, **127**, 59.

Cohen, S., Kaplan, M., Gottlieb, L. et al (1971) Liver disease and gallstones in regional enteritis. *Gastroenterology*, **60**, 237.

Conrad, M. E., Weintraub, L. R. & Crosby, W. H. (1964) The role of the intestine in iron kinetics. *Journal of Clinical Investigation*, **43**, 963.

Creamer, B. (1967) The turnover of the epithelium of the small intestine. *British Medical Bulletin*, **23**, 226.

Daren, J. J. (1974) Renal lithiasis in gastrointestinal disease. *Annals of Internal Medicine*, **80**, 550.

Deo, M. G. & Ramalingasuami, V. (1965) Reaction of the small intestine to induced protein malnutrition in Rhesus monkeys, a study of cell population kinetics. *Gastroenterology*, **49**, 150.

Dietschy, J. M. (1968) Mechanism for the intestinal absorption of bile acids. *Journal of Lipid Research*, **9**, 297.

Dietschy, J. M., Sallee, V. L. & Wilson, F. A. (1971) Unstirred water layers and absorption across the intestinal mucosa. *Gastroenterology*, **61**, 932.

Dowling, R. H. (1973) Intestinal adaptation. *New England Journal of Medicine*, **288**, 520.

Dowling, R. H., Bell, C. D. & White, J. (1972) Lithogenic bile in patients with ileal dysfunction. *Gut*, **13**, 415.

Dowling, R. H. & Booth, C. C. (1966) Functional compensation after small bowel resection in man. *Lancet*, **2**, 146.

Dowling, R. H., Mack, E. & Small, D. M. (1970) Effects of controlled interruption of the enterohepatic circulation of bile salts by biliary diversion and by ileal resection on bile salt secretion, synthesis and pool size in the Rhesus monkey. *Journal of Clinical Investigation*, **49**, 232.

Dowling, R. H., White, J. & Perry, P. M. (1973) Conservation of intestinal bile acid concentration after ileal resection. *Helvetica medica acta*, **37**, 103.

Dudrick, S. J., Macfadyen, B. V., Jr, Van Buren, C. T., Ruberg, R. L. & Maynard, A. T. (1972) Parenteral hyperalimentation, metabolic problems and solutions. *Annals of Surgery*, **176**, 259.

Dudrick, S. J., Vars, H. M. & Rhoads, J. E. (1966, 1967) Growth of puppies receiving all nutritional requirements by vein. *Fortschritte Ernähraney, Symposium of the International Society of Parenteral Nutrition, 1966*, West Germany, 1967.

Feldman, E. J., Peters, T. J., McNaughton, J. & Dowling, R. H. (1974) Adaptation after small bowel resection, comparison of oral versus intravenous nutrition. *Gastroenterology*, **66**, 691.

Fischer, J. E., Yoshimura, N., Aquirre, A., James, J. H., Cummings, M. G., Abel, R. M. & Deindoerfer, F. (1974) Plasma amino acids in patients with hepatic encephalopathy—effects of amino acid infusions. *American Journal of Surgery*, **127**, 40.

Flint, J. M. (1912) The effect of extensive resections of the small intestine. *Bulletin of the Johns Hopkins Hospital*, **23**, 127.

Fordtran, J. S., Rector, F. C., Jr & Carter, N. W. (1968) The mechanisms of sodium absorption in the human small intestine. *Journal of Clinical Investigation*, **47**, 884.

Fromm, H., Thomas, P. J. & Hofmann, A. E. (1973) Sensitivity and specificity in tests of distal ileal function: prospective comparison of bile acid and vitamin B_{12} absorption in ileal resection patients. *Gastroenterology*, **64**, 1077.

Garbutt, J. T., Lack, L. & Tyor, M. P. (1971) The enterohepatic circulation of bile salts in gastrointestinal disorders. *American Journal of Medicine*, **51**, 627.

Grace, A. E. N., Beardmore, H. E. & Cummings, G. I. N. (1976) Supportive use of total peripheral and parenteral alimentation with severe pancreatic injury. *Journal of Paediatric Surgery*, **11** (in press).

Hamosh, M. & Scow, R. O. (1973) Lingual lipase and its role in the digestion of dietary lipid. *Journal of Clinical Investigation*, **52**, 88.

Heaton, K. W. & Read, A. E. (1969) Gallstones in patients with disorders of the terminal ileum and disturbed bile salt metabolism. *British Medical Journal*, **3**, 494.

Hidalgo, H., Cortes, M. L., Salas, J. S. & Zavala, J. (1973) Intestinal muscular layer ablation in short-bowel syndrome. *Archives of Surgery*, **188**, 106.

Hofmann, A. F. (1972) Bile acid malabsorption caused by ileal resection. *Archives of Internal Medicine*, **130**, 597.

Hofmann, A. F. (1968) Functions of bile in the alimentary canal. In *Handbook of Physiology*, Section 6: Alimentary Canal, ed. C. F. Code, Vol. III, pp. 2507–2533. Washington DC: American Physiological Society.

Hofmann, A. F. (1967) The syndrome of ileal disease and the broken enterohepatic circulation: cholerheic enteropathy. *Gastroenterology*, **52**, 752.

Hofmann, A. F. & Poley, J. R. (1969) Cholestyramine treatment of diarrhea associated with ileal resection. *New England Journal of Medicine*, **281**, 397.

Holt, P. R. (1972) The role of bile acids during the process of normal fat and cholesterol absorption. *Archives of Internal Medicine*, **130**, 574.

Ingelfinger, F. (1967) Regional absorption. *American Journal of Surgery*, **114**, 388.

Jeejeebhoy, K. N., Langer, B. & Zahrab, W. J. (1972) Total parenteral alimentation at home. *Annals of the College of Physicians and Surgeons of Canada*, **5**, 26.

Jordan, P. H., Olson, R. & Paige, R. (1968) Is the gallbladder's reservoir function important after small bowel resection? *Surgery*, **64**, 446.

Koeberlé, P. (1881) Résection de L,intestin grête. *Bullitin de l'Académie de Médicine*, **10**, 128.

Krag, E. & Phillips, S. F. (1974) Active and passive bile acid absorption in Man. *Journal of Clinical Investigation*, **53**, 1686.

Lillehei, R. C., Idezuki, Y., Freemester, J. A., Dietzman, R. H., Kelly, W. D., Merkel, F. K., Goetz, F. C., Lyons, G. W. & Manax, W. G. (1967) Transplantation of stomach, intestine, and pancreas: experimental and clinical observations. *Surgery*, **62**, 721.

Loran, M. R. & Crocker, T. T. (1963) Population dynamics of intestinal epithelia in the rat two months after partial resection of the ileum. *Journal of Cell Biology*, **19**, 285.

McArdle, A. H., Brown, R. A., Echave, V., Rivilis, J. & Thompson, A. G. (1972) Alterations in gastric and pancreatic secretion induced by the feeding of an elemental diet. *Archives Françaises des Maladies de L'appareil Digestif*, **61**, 115C.

Mekhjian, H. S., Phillips, S. F. & Hofmann, A. F. (1971) Colonic secretion of water and electrolytes induced by bile acids: perfusion studies in man. *Journal of Clinical Investigation*, **50**, 1569.

Morgan, R. & Hoffman, N. (1971) The interaction of lipase cofactor and bile salts in triglyceride hydrolysis. *Biochimica et biophysica acta*, **248**, 143.

Osborne, M. P., Sizer, J., Frederick, P. L. & Zamcheck, N. (1967) Massive bowel resection and gastric hypersecretion. *American Journal of Surgery*, **114**, 393.

Payne, J. H. & DeWind, L. T. (1969) Surgical treatment of obesity. *American Journal of Surgery*, **118**, 141.

Pearse, A. G. E. & Riecken, O. E. (1967) Histology and cytochemistry of the cells of the small intestine, in relation to absorption. *British Medical Bulletin*, **23**, 217.

Porus, R. L. (1965) Epithelial hyperplasia following massive small bowel resections in man. *Gastroenterology*, **48**, 753.

Russell, R. I. (1975) Progress report: elemental diets. *Gut*, **16**, 68.

Saho, K. & Blackman, G. E. (1962) The use of a reversed jejunal segment after massive resection of the small bowel. *American Journal of Surgery*, **103**, 202.

Schultz, S. G. & Curran, P. F. (1968) Intestinal absorption of sodium chloride and water. In *Handbook of Physiology*, Section 6: Alimentary Canal, ed. C. F. Code, Vol. III, pp. 1245–1275. Washington, DC: American Physiological Society.

Schreibman, P. H., Pertsemilidis, D., Liu, G. C. K. & Ahrens, E. H. (1974) A consequence of weight reduction. *Journal of Clinical Investigation*, **53**, 72a.

Shaffer, E. A. & Small, D. M. (1975) Biliary lipid secretion in cholesterol gallstone disease: the effect of cholecystectomy and obesity. *Clinical Research* (Abstract), 23.

Sherr, H. P., Nair, P. P., Banwell, J. G., White, J. J. & Lockwood, D. H. (1973) The role of bile acids in liver disease following small bowel bypass for obesity. *Gastroenterology*, **64**, 800.

Shizgal, H. M., Kurtz, R. S. & Spanier, A. M. (1976) The effect of total parenteral nutrition on body composition in critically ill patients. *American Journal of Surgery*, January (in press).

Simmons, F. & Bouchier, I. A. D. (1971) Intraluminal bile salt concentration and fat digestion after cholecystectomy. *South African Medical Journal*, **46**, 2089.

Singleton, A. O., Redmond, D. C. & McMurray, J. E. (1964) Ileocecal resection and small bowel transit and absorption. *Annals of Surgery*, **159**, 690.

Small, D. M. (1970) Surface and bulk interactions of lipids and water with a classification of biologically active lipids based on these interactions. *Federation Proceedings, Federation of American Societies for Experimental Biology*, **29**, 1320.

Smith, L. H. & Hofmann, A. F. (1974) Acquired hyperoxaluria, urolithiasis and intestinal disease: a new digestive disorder. *Gastroenterology*, **66**, 1257.

Stassoff, B. (1914) Experimentelle Untersuchungen uber die kompensatorischen vorgange bei darmresektionen. *Bruns Beiträge zur klinischen Chirurgie*, **89**, 527.

Stephens, R. V. & Randall, H. T. (1969) Use of concentrated balanced liquid elemental diet for nutritional management of catabolic states. *Annals of Surgery*, **170**, 642.

Thompson, W. R., Stephens, R. V., Randall, H. T. & Bowen, J. R. (1969) Use of the 'space diet' in the management of a patient with extreme short bowel syndrome. *American Journal of Surgery*, **117**, 449.

Tilson, M. D. & Wright, K. H. (1972) The effect of resection of the small intestine upon the fine structure of the intestinal epithelium. *Surgery, Gynecology and Obstetrics*, **134**, 992.

Tyor, M. P., Garbutt, J. T. & Lack, L. (1971) Metabolism and transport of bile salts in the intestine. *American Journal of Medicine*, **51**, 614.

Voitk, A. J., Brown, R. A., McArdle, A. H., Hinchey, E. J. & Gurd, F. N. (1972) Clinical uses of an elemental diet—preliminary studies. *Candian Medical Association Journal*, **107**, 123.

Voitk, A. J., Echave, V., Brown, R. A. & Gurd, F. N. (1973a) Use of elemental diet during the adaptive state of short gut syndrome. *Gastroenterology*, **65**, 419.

Voitk, A. J., Echave, V., Feller, J. M., Brown, R. A. & Gurd, F. N. (1973b) Experience with elemental diet in treatment of inflammatory bowel disease, is this primary therapy? *Archives of Surgery*, **107**, 329.

Voitk, A. J., Echave, V., Brown, R. A., McArdle, R. H. & Gurd, F. U. (1973c) Elemental diet in the treatment of fistulas in the alimentary tract. *Surgery, Gynecology & Obstetrics*, **137**, 68.

Waddell, W. R., Kern, F., Halgrimson, C. G. & Woodbury, J. J. (1970) A simple jejunocolic valve for relief of rapid transit and the short bowel syndrome. *Archives of Surgery*, **100**, 438.

Weser, E. & Hernandez, M. H. (1971) Studies of small bowel adaptation after intestinal resection in the rat. *Gastroenterology*, **60**, 69.

Wickbom, G., Landor, J. H., Bushkin, F. L. & McGuigan, J. E. (1975) Changes in canine gastric acid output and serum gastrin levels following massive small intestinal resection. *Gastroenterology*, **69**, 448.

Williams, L. F. (1971) Vascular insufficiency of the intestines. *Gastroenterology*, **61**, 757.

Wright, P. D., Henderson, R. & Johnstone, D. A. (1974) Glucose utilisation and insulin secretion during surgery in man. *British Journal of Surgery*, **61**, 5.

Wright, H. K. & Tilson, M. D. (1971) The short gut syndrome. In *Current Problems in Surgery*. Chicago: Year Book Medical Publishers, Inc.

5
CONNECTIVE TISSUE DISORDERS AFFECTING THE GASTROINTESTINAL TRACT

A. M. Hoare   C. F. Hawkins

Disorders of connective tissue often affect the viscera, and the gut is at risk more in some than in others. The rare hereditary forms, where there is structural derangement rather than chronic inflammation, damage the gut because of the weakness and fragility of elastic and other tissues which support it. The acquired disorders, associated with disturbed immunity and inflammatory reactions especially in joints, share arteritis as a common denominator. This arteritis can affect the alimentary tract at any point. Erosions, ulceration, bleeding, perforation, infarction and gangrene may result; the lesion depends upon the speed of onset and degree to which the blood supply is reduced.

RHEUMATOID ARTHRITIS

Eating may be difficult because of arthritis of the temporo-mandibular joints. This impedes biting and opening the jaw is painful. Its incidence varies from 53 per cent (Franks, 1969) to 71 per cent (Chalmers and Blair, 1973). Sjögren's syndrome also causes problems with mastication because of the dry mouth (xerostomia). Both of these may worsen the already poor nutrition of rheumatoid patients.

No specific lesion of the oesophagus or stomach has been ascribed to rheumatoid arthritis. Yet dyspepsia—the mechanism of which is unknown—is common and often makes drug therapy difficult. Anti-inflammatory drugs themselves cause gastric irritation; the more potent their effect, the more likely the damage to the gastric mucosa. The problem as to whether gastric and duodenal ulcers are more common in these patients is complicated not only by this effect of drugs but also because many articles in the literature deal with ulcers as one disease—peptic ulcer. However, their cause and prognosis is different. Gastric ulcer is probably more likely to be due to ingested ulcerogenic agents whereas duodenal ulcer could be caused by endogenous factors. If ulcers are taken together, a small increase in the incidence of gastric ulcer might be obscured in the total data. Indeed, in a study of 140 rheumatoid patients, Sun et al (1974) found a 27.8 per cent incidence of gastric and duodenal ulcer with the ratio of gastric to duodenal ulcer increased. Ivey and Clifton (1974) measured back diffusion of hydrogen ions across the gastric mucosa. This was increased across the mucosa of patients with rheumatoid arthritis to the same extent as in those with just gastric ulcer; the change was greatest in those with the most active disease and not in those receiving the most therapy. Emmanuel and Montgomery (1971) suggested that the antrum is the most likely site of drug-induced ulcer.

Aspirin may cause slow blood loss in anyone but is probably an uncommon cause of haematemesis or melaena from erosions (Langman, 1970). It could be a factor in causing chronic ulcer as well as erosions. Patients with analgesic abuse are more likely to have an ulcer, especially in the stomach (Gault et al, 1968); but gastric ulcer is more likely in those with poor nutrition and this may be a factor. Billington (1965) showed a great increase in gastric ulcer in young Australian women. Chapman and Duggan (1969) also presented a strong case that aspirin causes gastric ulcer. However, in all these studies the matter is complicated because analgesic abuse could be secondary to the chronic discomfort of the ulcer.

The role of corticosteroids in ulcerogenesis is controversial (Cooke, 1967). Peptic ulcer is more common in patients with rheumatoid arthritis receiving steroids (Atwater et al, 1965) but not in steroid-treated patients with asthma (Rees and Williams, 1962), ulcerative colitis (Palmer and Kirsner, 1959) and chronic skin diseases (Spiro and Milles, 1960). These ulcers are commonly antral, equally common in both sexes and often silent, just presenting with complications. They are uncommon with a dose of prednisone less than 15 mg daily and can heal despite continued prednisone therapy. Prednisone increases acid output, though it has no effect on the mucosal barrier (Murray, Strottman and Cooke, 1974). Apart from bleeding ulcers, prednisone does not cause gastrointestinal blood loss (Scott et al, 1961b). Phenylbutazone and indomethacin may also cause ulcers and blood loss.

There is no evidence that gastritis is more common in rheumatoid patients. Rooney (1976) describes 25 volunteer patients examined by endoscopy with biopsies being taken in 18; these did not differ from the normal. Pentagastrin studies of maximal gastric output were performed in 16 and acid outputs were normal both during the basal hour and in the poststimulated hour. He undertook this study because of his observation (Rooney et al, 1973) that immunoreactive gastrin was elevated in some patients with rheumatoid arthritis. In 1976, he found that patients with rheumatoid arthritis seemed to belong to two distinct populations in regard to their gastrin level. No correlation was found between this hypergastrinaemia and gastric output nor could it be attributed to anti-inflammatory drug therapy. No other clinical aspect of rheumatoid disease could be incriminated but other inflammatory arthritides failed to show a similar increase of immunoreactive gastrin. There was no evidence that it was an artifact in measurement or caused by any of the known immunological or biochemical abnormalities present in the sera of rheumatoid patients.

Radiological hiatus hernia is said to occur in 54 per cent of these patients

(Sun et al, 1974) though such findings depend so much upon radiological criteria. These workers reported that manometry demonstrated decreased amplitude of contraction in the lower third of the oesophagus, and reduced lower oesophageal sphincter pressures in addition to hiatus hernia.

The other gastrointestinal complications of rheumatoid arthritis are caused by vasculitis. Three types of arteritis are seen (Scott et al, 1961a). The commonest is *obliterative endarteritis* affecting digital vessels. Characteristic nail bed infarcts are found in 15 per cent, being commoner in sero-positive patients and those with severe disease (Gordon, Stein and Broder, 1973). Visceral involvement is rare, but 4 of 35 patients in the series of Bywaters and Scott (1963) had visceral infarcts. *Subacute inflammatory arteritis* of the small vessels of the muscles, heart and nerve sheafs, also occurs. It is associated with peripheral neuropathy and other organs are rarely affected. A third form is a *necrotising arteritis* similar to polyarteritis nodosa; indeed, it is usually impossible to know whether this is polyarteritis nodosa developing in a rheumatoid patient or a more aggressive form of rheumatoid vasculitis. The gastrointestinal tract is affected in the same way as in polyarteritis nodosa. So, if the rheumatoid patient develops abdominal pain and there is no obvious diagnosis, complications due to arteritis must be considered. Commonest is multiple ischaemic ulcers of the intestine, which may cause severe haemorrhage and perforate. Lesions in larger arteries may cause segmental or extensive bowel gangrene, mesenteric infarctions or alimentary or intraperitoneal haemorrhage (Parker and Thomas, 1959; Alder, Norcross and Lockie, 1962; Webb and Payne, 1970) or pancreatitis (Lindsay et al, 1973). Perisplenitis and splenic infarct cause left hypochondrial pain in rheumatoid patients (Sinclair and Cruickshank, 1956). Acute arteritis of hepatic, cystic, pancreatic, and renal vessels and of the peritoneum itself has been recorded. Apart from unavoidable operation, corticosteroids offer the best chance of controlling the arteritis.

Malabsorption has been found in 40 per cent of 28 patients with rheumatoid arthritis (Dyer, Kendall and Hawkins, 1971). Jejunal biopsy was carried out in 28 and was always normal apart from three who showed increased infiltration of round cells. The malabsorption was slight and may have been non-specific as might occur in any ill patient. It was unlikely to be the cause of the various biochemical abnormalities found in 100 consecutive patients with rheumatoid disease (Cockel et al, 1971); these included hypoproteinaemia. Recently gastrointestinal protein loss was demonstrated in patients with rheumatoid arthritis by Plantin and Stranberg (1974) using labelled chromic chloride. Schneider and Dobbins (1968) found arteritis on rectal biopsy in 6 of 36 patients with rheumatoid arthritis and 5 of 22 were sero-positive. Necrotising colitis has been reported in rheumatoid arthritis (Mogadam et al, 1962). Hepatosplenomegaly occurs commonly in juvenile rheumatoid arthritis (Still's disease); systemic symptoms may occur in 20 per cent before the arthritis and these cause difficulties in diagnosis (Svantesson and Garwicz, 1970).

Amyloidosis complicates rheumatoid arthritis and is the most lethal sequela of Still's disease (Tribe, 1966). Proteinuria is the commonest symptom though diarrhoea (Sinclair and Cruickshank, 1956) or malabsorption can occur (Babb et al, 1967). Jejunal biopsy often proves amyloid when this is suspected in rheumatoid arthritis. Petterson and Wegelius (1972) found evidence of amyloid disease on jejunal biopsy in all 12 patients tested but only 10 of 15 examined by rectal biopsy; seven of these had some malabsorption. Jejunal biopsy is a simpler way of diagnosing amyloid disease than renal biopsy and without its attendant risk (Sfikakis and Giamarellou, 1971).

Minor changes of liver function tests have been found in patients with rheumatoid arthritis (Kendall et al, 1970; Cockel et al, 1971). Twenty-six of 100 patients were found to have a raised serum alkaline phosphatase and this was often associated with increased 5-nucleotidase, an enzyme considered specific to liver disease. The activity of the rheumatoid process correlated with alkaline phosphatase, implying that hepatic dysfunction is not uncommon in active rheumatoid disease. Despite this evidence of liver disease, the bilirubin and glutamic oxaloacetic transaminase were consistently normal. Whether or not these abnormalities which are symptomless and of no obvious significance are specific to rheumatoid patients or occur in others with chronic disease is not clear. They are more common in those who have Sjögren's syndrome with rheumatoid arthritis than rheumatoid arthritis alone (Webb et al, 1975). Kornreich, Malouf and Hanson (1971) reported seven children with Still's disease with acute changes suggestive of hepatic dysfunction. Two had infectious hepatitis, and one infectious mononucleosis. In four the cause was unknown. As with the adult disease, the arthritis improved with the onset of hepatitis. Aspirin has been blamed for causing liver damage in rheumatoid patients (Seaman, Platz and Ishak, 1974).

SJÖGREN'S SYNDROME

Sjögren's syndrome is defined as a triad of dry mouth (xerostomia), dry eyes (xerophthalmia) and a connective tissue disorder—usually rheumatoid arthritis. The characteristic lymphoid infiltration occurs not only in the salivary and lachrymal glands but also in the respiratory tract, sweat glands, and kidney, causing epistaxis, chest infection and renal tubular abnormality as well. Immunological changes include hypergammaglobulinaemia and the presence of various circulating auto-antibodies, both organ and non-organ specific. These and its clinical features have been reviewed in a monograph by Shearn (1971). Whaley and his colleagues (1973) reported a six-year study of 171 patients with Sjögren's syndrome. Ninety-four had rheumatoid arthritis, four systemic lupus erythematosus, one progressive systemic sclerosis and one psoriatic arthritis. In 71, the syndrome was unassociated with rheumatoid arthritis or other connective tissue diseases (the so-called Sicca syndrome). The Schirmer test for secretion of tears is useful but also positive in hot dry atmospheres and in the elderly. Biopsy of labial salivary glands is diagnostic. The dry mouth makes eating difficult and lack of saliva may cause severe dental caries. Dysphagia may occur and oesophageal webs similar to those found in the Plummer–Vinson syndrome are occasionally seen on barium swallow (Doig et al, 1971). Atrophic gastritis and absence of free acid after stimulation is common (Buchanan et al, 1966). Clinical evidence of pancreatitis may occur (Fenster et al, 1964) or it may present subclinically as shown by decreased volume and bicarbonate in pancreatic secretion (Hradsky, Bartos and Keller, 1967); but correlation of the functional abnormalities with histological changes is lacking, and no significant pancreatic lymphocytosis has been found. A link between Sjögren's syndrome and liver disease, especially chronic active hepatitis, has been shown (Golding et al, 1970). Also mitochondrial antibodies have been detected in the sera of about six per cent of patients with the Sicca syndrome in titres normally present in liver disease, together with histological evidence of liver disease (Whaley et al, 1970; Walker, Doniach and Doniach, 1970). In a review of patients with primary biliary cirrhosis, Alarcón-Segovia, Diaz-Jouanen and Fishbein (1973) found some features of Sjögren's syndrome in all patients tested.

SYSTEMIC LUPUS ERYTHEMATOSUS (SLE)

The prevalence of systemic lupus erythematosus is increasing according to recent reports. Fessel (1974) estimated its occurrence at 1 in 1959 of the population. He found it commoner in the black population although this has not been the experience of others (Dubois, 1974; Estes and Christian, 1971). Many drugs can cause it though usually without the potentially lethal renal lesion; a recent addition to the list of drugs is penicillamine (Harpey et al, 1971).

Sjögren's syndrome occurs in SLE and oesophageal abnormalities are reported. Ramirez-Mata et al (1974) found abnormalities of oesophageal peristalsis in 32 per cent of 50 patients. However, dysphagia was very mild though all but two had some difficulty in swallowing solid food and two with liquids. The upper third of the oesophagus was involved in seven, the lower two-thirds in five, the entire oesophagus in two and lower oesophageal sphincter in two. Ulceration of the oesophagus due to arteritis is rare (Harvey et al, 1954).

Involvement of the gut occurs commonly in SLE, though not as frequently as in polyarteritis nodosa. In a review of 520 cases, Dubois and Tuffaneli (1967) found anorexia in 59 per cent, nausea or vomiting in 53 per cent, diarrhoea in 5.9 per cent, dysphagia 1.5 per cent, haemorrhage in 6.3 per cent, abdominal pain in 19.2 per cent, hepatomegaly in 23.2 per cent, jaundice in 3.8 per cent, and ulcerative colitis in 0.4 per cent. But these symptoms were not prominent and only 0.4 per cent presented with gastrointestinal symptoms. The main complaints were anorexia (0.2 per cent), nausea (0.2 per cent), haemorrhage (0.4 per cent), abdominal pain (1.3 per cent) and jaundice (0.8 per cent). Lymphadenopathy was found in 58.6 per cent patients and may be so pronounced as to simulate lymphoma (Dubois, 1974). Enlarged abdominal lymph nodes similar to reticulosis occurred in eight patients on whom a lymphangiogram was performed (Wiljasalo and Ikkala, 1971). Ascites occurred in 11.3 per cent of the 520 cases, usually due to a nephrotic syndrome or congestive cardiac failure. Dubois does not consider that serositis alone causes ascites, although Estes and Christian (1971) found an incidence of 16 per cent of peritoneal serositis in 150 patients. Gastrointestinal bleeding is not common, most often being due to peptic ulcer. Although gastrointestinal complaints are not prominent, severe lesions do occur as in polyarteritis. The arteritis can lead to small and large bowel ulcers which may bleed (Harvey et al, 1954). Bleeding due to shallow ulcers caused by arteritis can be diagnosed by mesenteric angiography. In addition to finding the site of bleeding, Phillips and Howland (1968) found diffuse irregularities of the small vessels but not the aneurysms seen in polyarteritis nodosa. Massive bleeding can occur without cause being found at necropsy (Chatterjee, 1973). Localised areas of ileus due to vasculitis may cause pain or obstruction and a dilated loop may be seen on a plain x-ray of the abdomen. It usually responds to conservative management (Brown, Shirey and Haserick, 1956; Dubois, 1974; Shapeero et al, 1974).

An 'acute abdomen' may occur in SLE due to ischaemia, infarction or perforation. Serious surgical problems are less common than in polyarteritis and conservative treatment can be successful (Shapeero et al, 1974). Parencentesis may help in the diagnosis: the fluid is sterile and contains less than 450 wbc/µl (Musher, 1972). Providing bowel sound are present, conservative treatment may succeed even if tenderness with guarding is present. The response to steroids is usually within 24 to 48 h (Pollock et al, 1958). SLE may simulate appendicitis but terminal ileitis similar to Crohn's disease is found at laparotomy (Shafer and Gregory, 1970; Dubois, 1974). Intussusception caused by arteritis has been reported in children (Hermann, 1967). Pancreatitis is another cause of abdominal emergency. It is usually caused by vasculitis (Seifert, Heinz and Ruffmann, 1967) and responds to steroids (Sparberg, 1967). However, steroids themselves may cause pancreatitis in children (Dubois, 1974). One case associated with type I hyperlipoproteinaemia has been reported (Glueck et al, 1969). A symptomless rise in amylase may occur in active SLE (Dubois, 1974). Perirenal haematoma has been reported (Castleman and Kibbee, 1962).

Siurala et al (1965) found malabsorption in 3 of 28 patients with SLE. Two had villous atrophy on jejunal biopsy and three a low bicarbonate output in response to secretin. That these findings are not just incidental has been supported by two further reports (Bazinet and Martin, 1971; Pachas, Linscheer and Pinali, 1971). Many cases of ulcerative colitis and non-specific inflammatory bowel disease have been associated with SLE (Kurlander and Firsner,

1964; Alarćon-Segovia et al, 1965). This may be a true association though Alarćon-Segovia et al have suggested that sulphonamides used for treating ulcerative colitis may have caused the SLE, but Skinner and Fernandez-Herlihy (1966) found no case of SLE among 500 patients with ulcerative colitis. Malignancy may be more common in patients with SLE (Miller, 1967; Canoso and Cohen, 1974).

Hepatomegaly occurred in 23.2 per cent of patients with SLE and abnormalities of liver function tests are found though jaundice occurred in only 3.8 per cent of the 520 cases described by Dubois and Tuffaneli (1967). The commonest cause of jaundice was haemolytic anaemia and next was viral hepatitis; only one had cirrhosis. The so-called 'lupoid hepatitis' is a different disease from SLE (Mackay, Taft and Cowling, 1959) and patients with features of both diseases have only been reported rarely (Fung, Chew and Tan, 1969). Patients with chronic active hepatitis and positive LE cells behave the same as those without LE cells but the prognosis is worse (Solway et al, 1972). Recently Seaman, Ishak and Platz (1974) reported three patients with SLE who developed liver function abnormalities when taking aspirin. These tests all returned to normal when the aspirin was stopped and recurred when it was begun again. Two had biopsies which showed changes suggestive of active chronic hepatitis and smooth muscle and antimitochondrial antibodies were positive. Australia antigen has been found in 25 per cent of patients with SLE (Alarćon-Segovia and Fishbein, 1971). A case of liver rupture in SLE has been reported (Haslock, 1974).

Diagnosis is made because of the typical clinical picture and serological findings. Antinuclear factor is nearly always positive. Homogeneous stain in a titre greater than 1/640 is found only in SLE (Parker and Kerby, 1974). Peripheral stain is specific for SLE and homogeneous less so. Reticulated and speckled stains are found more widely, in particular speckled is seen in mixed connective tissue disease. Nuclear stain is found in scleroderma. Immunoassays of anti-double stranded DNA antibodies are more specific for SLE, being found in 83 per cent with SLE and 100 per cent of patients with active disease (Hughes, 1973). A high titre is only found in a small percentage of other collagen diseases (Webb and Whaley, 1974; Hughes, 1974). Davis and Read (1975) found positive double-stranded anti-DNA antibodies in 15 of 36 patients with chronic active hepatitis. Life is prolonged by treatment with prednisone (Dubois et al, 1974) and a 10 years survival of over 90 per cent has been reported (Fessel, 1974). The position of immunosuppressive drugs is not clearly defined at present. The main cause of death is neurological involvement and renal failure, gastrointestinal lesions being only responsible for a few fatalities (Feng, Cheah and Lee, 1973). In the 249 patients reported by Dubois et al (1974), gastrointestinal causes of death were as follows: malignant neoplasm, 4 per cent; hepatic coma, 4.0 per cent; gastrointestinal bleeding, 2 per cent; bleeding peptic ulcer, 1 per cent and perforated peptic ulcer, 1 per cent.

SYSTEMIC SCLEROSIS (SCLERODERMA)

The underlying lesion is probably a vasculitis affecting the capillary bed (Norton and Narda, 1970). An increased synthesis of collagen by fibroblasts in skin culture (Carwile LeRoy, McGuire and Chen, 1974) and a high proportion of reducible aldimine bond links in patients have also been demonstrated; these links are responsible for the high tensile strength of collagen (Herbert et al, 1974).

Systemic sclerosis affecting the skin around the mouth can cause difficulty in eating and at intubation for anaesthesia (Birkhan, Heifetz and Haim, 1972). The lower two-thirds of the oesophagus is often involved. Oesophageal symptoms were present in 42 per cent of 727 patients reported by Tuffanelli and Winkelman (1961). Dysphagia is commonest, though symptoms of reflux also occur; the dysphagia is rarely disabling and swallowing is more difficult for solids than liquids. Radiological changes were present in 66.9 per cent of Tuffanelli and Winkelman's series: barium swallow showed reduced or absent peristalsis in the lower two-thirds; these changes together with tertiary contraction are best seen by cine-radiography in the head-down position, and the oesophagus may be dilated. On the lateral chest x-ray air may be seen in the oesophagus (Martinez, 1974). Hiatus hernia is found in about half of patients (Garrett et al, 1971) but the most important cause of reflux is incompetence of the lower oesophageal sphincter (Atkinson and Summerling, 1966) (see Chapter 1). Uncommonly, diffuse spasm associated with intermittent dysphagia and substernal pain is found (Garrett et al, 1971). The metacholine test is negative. Manometry reveals abnormalities more often than radiology, and these occur in asymptomatic patients. At an early stage weak incoordinated pressure waves are found and later the oesophagus is paralysed with no pressure at the cardia. Changes were found in 89 of 103 patients by Garrett et al (1971) affecting only the lower third, although 5 of 22 patients described by Atkinson and Summerling (1966) had no contractions anywhere in the oesophagus. Unlike achalasia, there is no association with carcinoma of the oesophagus, except for one report (Johnson and Munroe, 1973). Patients are treated symptomatically as for hiatus hernia though nothing affects progress of the oesophageal disease and it never improves (Garrett et al, 1971). Dysphagia may also be due to a peptic stricture and this should be excluded by endoscopy and radiology. Once a stricture has developed, dilatation will be necessary and operation is best avoided (Barnett, 1974). Results of simple hiatus hernia repair are usually disappointing at a late stage (Brain, 1973) though Henderson and Pearson (1973) found good results in 8 of 11 patients who had a Collis gastroplasty and Belsey hiatus hernia repair.

The main cause of the oesophageal lesion is not infiltration by collagen but smooth muscle atrophy with secondary fibrosis (Atkinson and Summerling, 1966; D'Angelo et al, 1969). Cohen and his colleagues (1972) found that patients with early abnormal peristalsis had a normal response to metacholine and abnormal response to edrophonium and gastrin, suggesting that a neural element was causing the muscular atrophy. Two late cases showed no response to any substance including metacholine.

The stomach is rarely involved by systemic sclerosis. Tuffanelli and Winkelman (1961) found only five instances of delayed emptying in 727 patients. Peachey, Creamer and Pierce (1969) described marked sclerosis of the stomach, though the patient also had a prepyloric ulcer. Valignat, Lambert and Moulin (1973) studied 29 patients by endoscopy, gastric biopsy and acid studies. All were normal apart from four who had Sjögren's syndrome as well; these had chronic atrophic gastritis and hypochlorhydria. Thompson and Mackay (1971) described one patient with systemic sclerosis and diffuse haemorrhagic gastritis, histological section showing atrophic gastritis and endarteritis affecting the vessels of the gastric mucosa; the bleeding was partially controlled by prednisone.

The small intestine can be involved in systemic sclerosis and the incidence depends on how carefully a search is made for it. There were only 15 in Tuffanelli and Winkelman's series of 727 patients (1961), though Reinhaardt and Barry (1962) found radiological abnormality in 44 per cent of 52, and Bluestone, MacMahon and Dawson (1969) in 12 of 21 patients. Barium studies (Fig. 5.1) show dilated loops of bowel with lack of tone, thickened folds, a wire-spring appearance and succulations like colonic haustra (Queloz and Woloshin, 1972). The intervalvular distance is narrowed and transient non-obstructive intussusception may occur (Horowitz and Meyers, 1973). The patient is often asymptomatic though distension, nausea, vomiting, constipation, pain and diarrhoea or malabsorption may occur (Reinhaardt and Barry, 1962; Barnett and Coventry, 1969). Sometimes the first symptoms in systemic sclerosis may be caused by small intestinal involvement (Leneman et al, 1962). Malabsorption was found in 7 of 31 cases by Barnett and Coventry (1969). It is usually due to excessive growth of organisms in the small bowel— a stagnant bowel syndrome—from deficient peristalsis, and can be treated by antibiotics (Kahn, Jeffries and Sleisender, 1966; Atlas, 1968). Pancreatic insufficiency is also found in some patients with malabsorption (Scudamore et al, 1968). Obstruction is usually due to paralytic ileus, although stenosis has been reported (Barnett, 1974). Episodes of obstruction usually respond to intravenous fluids and nasogastric suction but rarely it persists. Operation is only likely to be successful if the dilated area is limited (Herrington, 1959). The mucosa looks normal; collagenous encapsulation of Brunner's glands reported by Rosson and Yesner (1965) has not been found by all workers (Barnett and Coventry, 1969). The muscle is atrophied and replaced with fibrosis but fibrosis is not prominent (D'Angelo et al, 1969); and normal nexial connections have been demonstrated (Greenberger et al, 1961). The muscular atrophy distinguishes systemic sclerosis of the small bowel from intestinal pseudo-obstruction where the muscle is normal (Maldonadu et al, 1970). Motility studies have shown a reduced number of slow waves associated with spikes when duodenal pressure is measured after distension with water (Dimarino et al, 1973); in some they found fewer spike bursts in response to gastrin and secretin, suggesting that motor dysfunction is due to impaired activation by mechanical and hormonal stimuli. Pneumatosis intestinalis has been reported and reviewed recently by Mueller et al (1972). There are 13 cases in the literature and it is associated with poor prognosis and may cause pneumoperitoneum.

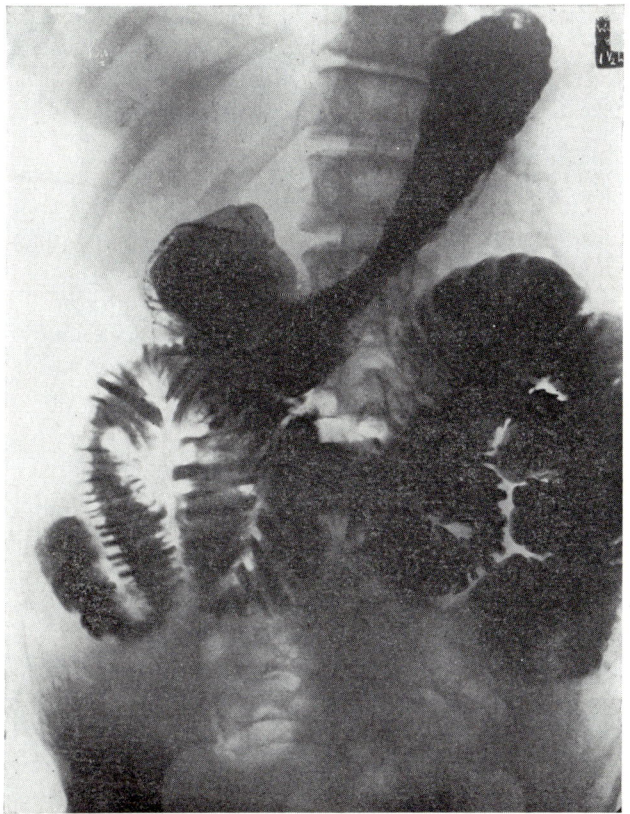

Figure 5.1 Small bowel in systemic sclerosis showing sacculations like colonic haustra

The frequency of colonic involvement, which is similar to that of the small bowel, is difficult to assess as barium enemas are not undertaken in asymptomatic patients. Barium enemas were performed in 50 patients (Tuffanelli and Winkelman, 1961) and only two were abnormal. However, those with bowel symptoms often have colonic disease; Harper and Jackson (1965) reported colonic involvement in 20 of 39 such patients. Constipation is common and stercoral ulceration and perforation may occur (Robinson and Teitelbaum, 1974). This is usually fatal though one patient has survived (Jayson et al,

1972). Large diverticula may lead to obstruction (Compton, 1969). A case of infarction associated with systemic sclerosis was reported by Edwards et al (1960) and believed to be due to ischaemia from intimal proliferation in the arteries. Ulcerative colitis has been reported though it is probably incidental (Barnett, 1974). Dilatation and wide diverticula with rigidity between the sacculations and later a dilated atonic colon are seen on barium radiographs. Histological examination shows patchy muscular atrophy with normal areas, and later atrophy of all the muscles (Harper and Jackson, 1965).

The liver is rarely involved in systemic sclerosis though mild changes in liver function tests may be found (Barnett and Coventry, 1969). Primary biliary cirrhosis has been reported sporadically (Murray-Lyon et al, 1970; O'Brien, Eddy and Krawitt, 1972; Uhl, Baldwin and Arnett, 1974) but is more commonly seen in the CRST syndrome (calcinosis, Raynaud's phenomenon, sclerodactyly and telangiectasia) and many have features of this syndrome (Morris, Htut and Read, 1972). However, seven cases only of liver disease were found in 727 patients (Bartholomew et al, 1964) so there may be little or no association of systemic sclerosis and liver disease. MacMahon (1972) reported one case of massive infarction of the liver and intestine.

Systemic sclerosis is usually diagnosed by the skin changes and can be proved by skin biopsy. The nuclear type of antinuclear factor is frequently positive (Parker and Kerby, 1974). Effective treatment is not yet possible.

CRST SYNDROME

Variants of systemic sclerosis occur though whether these represent one or many diseases is uncertain. The Thiebierge–Weissenbach syndrome consists of sclerodactyly with calcinosis. Recently a syndrome consisting of calcinosis, Raynaud's phenomenon, sclerodactyly and telangiectasia has been recognised and christened the CRST syndrome (Winterbauer, 1964; Schimke, Kirkpatrick and Deip, 1967). This has a more benign course than systemic sclerosis. Oesophageal involvement does occur (Winterbauer, 1964) and Frayha, Scarola and Shulman (1973) suggested that the syndrome should be renamed the CREST syndrome, because of this 'esophageal' aperistalsis. They also pointed out that intestinal bleeding occurred commonly, probably from telangiectasia. A patient with megaduodenum has also been reported (Oaks and O'Malley, 1969). Reynolds et al (1971) found an association of the CREST syndrome with primary biliary cirrhosis. Most reported as having systemic sclerosis and primary biliary cirrhosis do in fact have some or all of the features of the CREST syndrome.

MIXED CONNECTIVE TISSUE DISEASES

Sharp and his colleagues (1972) described an apparently distinct disease with features both of systemic sclerosis and SLE and cases have been seen in this country (Thompson, 1974). Polyarthralgia occurs in 95 per cent and

Raynaud's phenomenon in 85 per cent. Swollen hands, myositis, rashes and scleroderma of the hands are commonly found. Diminished oesophageal motility similar to that found in systemic sclerosis occurs in 67 per cent of those tested. Splenomegaly was found in 19 and hepatomegaly in 15 per cent. Definite renal involvement only occurred in 5 per cent (Sharp, 1975); as renal involvement is less common, the prognosis is better than that of SLE. All have a high titre of antinuclear antibody producing a speckled immunofluorescence. They have a specific antibody in high titre to a RNA-sensitive component of extractable nuclear antigen (ENA). Patients respond favourably to corticosteroids but it is not known whether this affects the oesophageal lesion.

DERMATOMYOSITIS

Dermatomyositis consists of a proximal myopathy and rash. Lilac discolouration of the eye-lids and peri-orbital oedema and telangiectasia are typical. Striated muscle of the upper third of the oesophagus is affected in 50 per cent of patients. This leads to dysphagia and pooling of barium in the valleculae and piriform sinuses on barium meal; in addition 30 per cent have oesophageal hypomotility and atonicity (Pearson, 1966). Pharyngeal biopsy may confirm the diagnosis even if skeletal biopsy is negative (Porubsky, Murray and Pratt, 1973). In adults dermatomyositis is reputed to be associated with malignancy (Curtis, Blaylock and Harrell, 1952). Forty per cent of those over 40 years have been found to have malignant disease (Mills, 1963). But, though there are reports of 5 to 34 per cent overall incidence of malignancy, doubt exists about the association (Bohan and Peter, 1975). The dermatomyositis may improve after resection of the carcinoma (Curtis et al, 1952); however, only a few of these reports included biopsy and the patients were all treated with corticosteroids as well (Bohan and Peter, 1975). An exhaustive search for malignancy is unnecessary.

The disease in children is quite different, as the underlying defect is widespread vasculitis (Banker and Victor, 1966). Contractures, muscle atrophy and subcutaneous calcification are common in children. In addition to oesophageal involvement, present in 3 of 22 described by Steiner et al (1974), children commonly develop abdominal pain. Ulceration and perforation are the commonest causes of death; in the seven patients reported by Banker and Victor (1966) vasculitis caused lesions from the oesophagus to the colon with or without ulceration and perforation. Perforation is frequently preceded by melaena (Cook, Rosen and Banker, 1963). Megaduodenum and sacculations of the colon are also found, and episodes of pseudo-obstruction may occur (Feldman and Marshak, 1963; Kleckner, 1970).

High doses of prednisone are used in treatment, though its value is not proved (Bohan and Peter, 1975). Prognosis is worse in children but it is not as gloomy as originally thought (Sullivan et al, 1972).

POLYARTERITIS NODOSA (PERI-ARTERITIS NODOSA)

Medium and small arteries are affected (Fig. 5.2), the organs most commonly involved being the skin, gut, liver, kidney, central nervous system and peripheral nerves. It is rare under 20 or over 65 years. The cause is unknown. Recently, some patients have been described who are positive for hepatitis B antigen; they develop circulating immune complexes in their blood which deposit in the walls of blood vessels where they can be detected by immunofluoresence (Gocke et al, 1970, 1971; Baker et al, 1972; Trepo et al, 1974). This was shown to occur in animals (Henson, Gorham and Leader, 1963) and

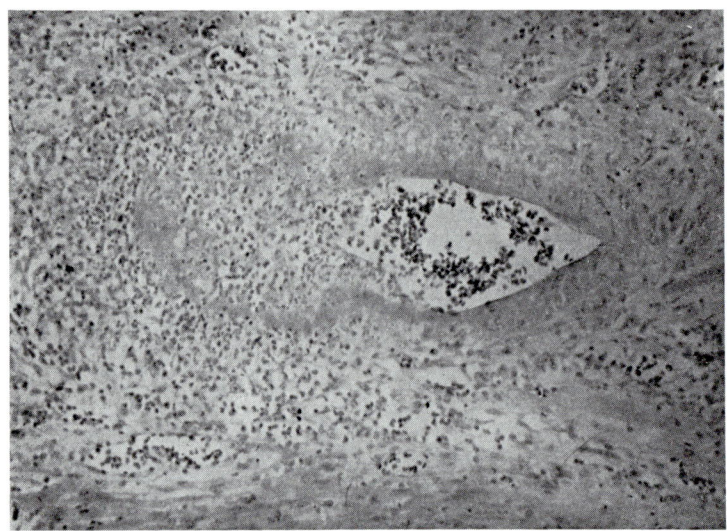

Figure 5.2 Histology of the small bowel in a patient with polyarteritis nodosa showing involvement of blood vessel. (We are grateful to Dr E. L. Jones for permission to use this photograph)

immune complexes are involved in the arthralgia (Alpert, Isselbacher and Schur, 1971) and renal lesions (Knieser et al, 1974) of hepatitis B in man. Drug addicts may also develop polyarteritis, often with pancreatitis (Citron et al, 1970; Halpern and Citron, 1971); these patients take multiple drugs but metamphetamine and lysergic acid diethylamide (LSD) are common factors. Hepatitis B antigen may also be the cause of polyarteritis in these drug addicts (Koff, Widrich and Robbins, 1973).

Polyarteritis nodosa often causes ischaemia in the gut which may lead to ulcers or gangrene (Fig. 5.3), with bleeding or perforation. The incidence of these complications is shown in Tables 5.1 and 5.2. Differences in various reports are due to varying definitions and the inclusion of necropsy studies which tends to select the worst patients. The best series is probably that of

Frohert and Sheps (1967) who defined polyarteritis nodosa as a necrotising arteritis of unknown aetiology unassociated with other collagen disease. The incidence of gastrointestinal complications amongst 130 patients seen at the Mayo Clinic was 14 per cent and this is unusually low. Abdominal pain is extremely common, aching or colicky and usually in the right upper quadrant or epigastrium, though it may be felt anywhere in the abdomen. This pain may simulate peptic ulcer (Norman and Wilkins, 1957), appendicitis or cholecystitis (Livolsi, Perzia and Porter, 1973). Anorexia, nausea and vomiting occur commonly and there is associated diarrhoea or constipation. When small vessels are involved a condition similar to ulcerative colitis may result and inflammatory masses may mimic regional ileitis (Hart, 1969). Malabsorption

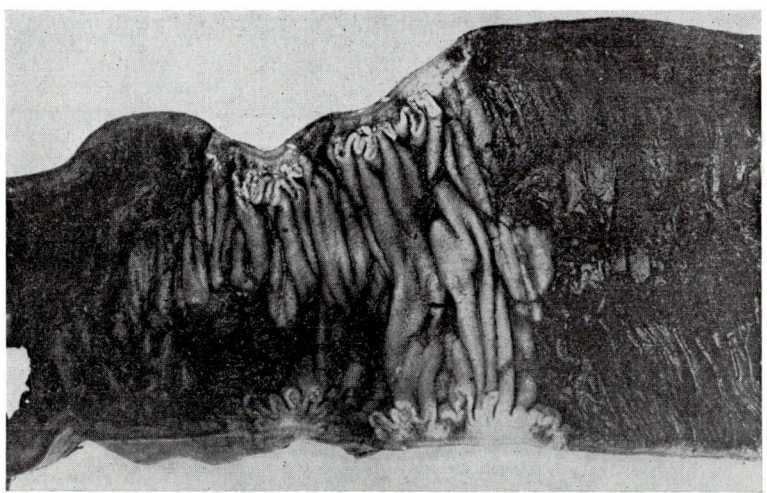

Figure 5.3 Resected specimen of small bowel with infarction due to polyarteritis nodosa. (We are grateful to Dr E. L. Jones for permission to use this photograph)

was found in 3 of 13 patients by Carron and Douglas (1965); this was mainly symptomless though it may contribute to the weight loss.

In the series described by Wold and Baggenstoss (1949) 17 per cent had melaena and 10 per cent haematemesis. The bleeding may come from shallow ischaemic ulcers anywhere in the gut, though the small bowel is the commonest site. These ulcers are often not seen by barium meal, but angiography may show the bleeding point as well as make the diagnosis (Cabal and Holtz, 1971). Resection of the diseased portion of the bowel may control the bleeding but recurrence can occur (Painter, 1971). Haemorrhage may also occur into the peritoneum (Akbarian, 1966), retroperitoneally (Scully and McNeely, 1974) or into the mesocolon (Buranasiri et al, 1973). Submucosal haemorrhages which ulcerate into the bowel are also seen (Drake, LeFeber and Patterson, 1964). The initial presentation may be with an 'acute abdomen' and if this is due to ischaemia alone corticosteroid treatment may be successful. However, it may be caused by cholecystitis, appendicitis or pancreatitis. The arterial lesions are seen by histological examination of the appendix or gallbladder. Perforation may occur anywhere in the alimentary tract but the small bowel is the commonest site, and gastric perforation is surprisingly rare though one case has been reported (Gourgoutis, Paguirigan and Berzins, 1971). Multiple sites of infarction (O'Neil, 1961) and multiple ulcers are not uncommon (Finkbiner and Decker, 1963; Sethi and Thomas, 1973). Intestinal obstruction is less common but can be caused by haematoma or ischaemic

Table 5.1 Organs involved in polyarteritis nodosa at necropsy

	Mowrey and Lundberg (1954)	Nazum and Nazum (1954)
Gut	47%	—
Pancreas	50%	—
Liver	42%	—
Spleen	37%	—
Gallbladder	16%	2%
Mesenteric arteries	—	25%
Number of patients	230	175

Table 5.2 Abdominal symptoms and signs in polyarteritis nodosa

	Frohert and Sheps (1967)	Mowrey and Lundberg (1954)	Nazum and Nazum (1954)
Abdominal pain	14%	48%	62%
Other GI symptoms	—	45%	—
Peptic ulcer	11%	—	—
GI bleeding	3%	—	—
Mouth ulcers	3%	—	—
Small bowel infarct	0.8%	—	—
Jaundice	0.8%	—	—
Hepatomegaly	—	21%	—
Number of patients	130	607	175

adynamic ileus (Drake et al, 1964) or intussusception caused by granulomas (Lowerstein and Heeb, 1955). Perinephric haematomas may mimic the acute abdomen (Ostrum and Soder, 1960). A trial of steroids is justified if there are no signs of perforation or peritonitis, but laparotomy should not be deferred unnecessarily and then the diagnosis can be confirmed histologically. The mortality rate with perforation may be as low as 27.2 per cent (Couris, Block and Rupe, 1964) but recurrent perforation may occur (McKeown and Ganguli, 1956).

Diagnosis of polyarteritis nodosa is difficult. Muscle biopsy is positive in only 35 per cent and random biopsies are of little value (Maxeiner, McDonald and Kirklin, 1952). Rectal (Rosenmann and Levis, 1971) and testicular biopsies (Dahl, Baggenstoss and Deweerd, 1960) have been suggested as possibly helpful. Diagnostic help may also come from selective coeliac axis and renal angiography (Bron, Strott and Shapiro, 1965; Dornfield, Lecky and Peter, 1971; Robins and Bookstein, 1972); arterial obstruction is a common finding but this is non-specific. The diagnostic accuracy of arteriograms may be improved by infusion of the vasodilator drug tolazoline (Bron, Stilley and Shapiro, 1971). Multiple aneurysms are virtually conclusive of polyarteritis nodosa, if subacute bacterial endocarditis has been excluded.

OTHER FORMS OF ARTERITIS

The *localised arteritis* of the skin which has a similar histological appearance to polyarteritis nodosa, causes no systemic involvement but may be associated with ulcerative colitis (McGovern, 1971) or Crohn's disease (Verbov and Stansfeld, 1972). *Drug-induced arteritis* affects vessels of the skin, kidneys, lung and spleen, and the gastrointestinal tract uncommonly. However, there is doubt about the existence of this condition, for the histology of hypersensitivity angiitis attributed to drugs is the same as that of Henoch–Schönlein purpura, and the two diseases are very similar in adults (Braverman, 1970).

Wegener's granuloma only involves the gut in the terminal stage and this is not normally the cause of death. Then there may be widespread vasculitis with liver involvement in 18.5 per cent, intestine in 24.1 per cent, pancreas in 9.3 per cent, gallbladder in 7.4 per cent and granuloma of the liver in 16.7 per cent (Walton, 1958).

Temporal arteritis (giant cell arteritis, cranial arteritis) generally only occurs in patients over 60 years; although vessels of the aortic arch and coronary arteries can be affected, the mesenteric vessels are spared. The condition may mimic gastric carcinoma because of anorexia, weight loss and anaemia. Eating may be difficult because of claudication of the masseter muscles (Hamilton, Shelley and Tumulty, 1971). Abnormalities of liver function occur and may improve with corticosteroid therapy (Dickson et al, 1973). The erythrocyte sedimentation rate is invariably high and diagnosis is confirmed by temporal or facial artery biopsy. It is commonly associated with polymyalgia rheumatica. These patients may have a high instance of hepatitis B antigen so that sometimes there may be an abnormal immunological response to the virus in the elderly (Bacon, Doherty and Zuckerman, 1975). Treatment of temporal arteritis with prednisone should not be delayed because of the risk of blindness.

Takayasu's disease (pulseless disease, aortic arch syndrome) is a rarity affecting the aortic arch and its branches, especially in young women. Early in the disease pyrexia and arthralgia may be prominent and abdominal pain may occur due to abdominal aneurysm. Mesenteric vessels may be involved (Roberts et al, 1969); 3 of 54 patients who had aortograms showed stenosis of the mesenteric arteries and one of the hepatic artery (Nakao et al, 1967). Gastric ulcer, intestinal angina and melaena may occur (Strachan, 1966).

Angiography is diagnostic (Sano, Aiba and Saito, 1970). Corticosteroids may be successful early in the disease.

Henoch–Schönlein purpura (anaphylactoid purpura) should, according to Cream, Gumpel and Peachey (1970) include all patients with crops of purpura and a normal platelet count but with no known cause of purpura. Streptococcal sore throats have preceded it (Bywaters, Isdale and Kempton, 1957). The purpura especially affects the legs and buttocks. In a review of 77 adults, 44 were reported as having gastrointestinal involvement, 26 of 77 suffered abdominal pain, 12 of 77 passed fresh blood, 11 had minor gastrointestinal bleeding, 12 had diarrhoea, 10 nausea and vomiting, 3 constipation and 5 of the 7 patients tested with ^{131}I has gastrointestinal protein loss (Cream et al, 1970). Patients may present with obstruction and pain (Yentis, 1973) though at laparotomy oedema and haemorrhage only are found. Intussusception is uncommon in adults. Perforation is rare. Purpura usually starts before the gastrointestinal symptoms though this is not always so. Intussusception may occur especially in children aged five to seven and operation may have to be performed, for delay may make resection necessary instead of simple reduction. Radiographs may show filling defects, oedema, thumb-printing, ulceration or spasm and these are reversible (Roderiguez-Erdmann and Levitan, 1968). Endoscopy may show mucosal haemorrhage similar to the purpura (Akdamar, Agrawal and Varela, 1973). C3 complement levels are normal, unlike those in acute streptococcal nephritis or SLE. Treatment by corticosteroids reduces systemic and gastrointestinal symptoms including abdominal pain and bleeding (Borges, 1972) but does not improve the renal lesion (Meadow et al, 1972).

HEREDITARY DISORDERS OF CONNECTIVE TISSUE

Pseudoxanthoma elasticum, a dystrophy of elastic fibres (McKusick, 1972), causes gastrointestinal haemorrhage and is easily missed. Indeed, many patients have several haemorrhages and some operations because of incidental findings such as hiatus hernia before the correct diagnosis is made. Bleeding often occurs from the stomach but the exact site is not evident (McKusick, 1972). An incidental peptic ulcer may bleed because of the arterial disease (Altman et al, 1974) or superficial ulceration may be found. Hence endoscopy is essential to exclude possible treatable causes of haemorrhage. Changes similar to pseudoxanthoma in the skin are usually seen in the stomach (Cocco et al, 1969). Diffuse bleeding from the jejunum can occur (Sames, 1961). Recurrent tortion of the stomach which responds to conservative treatment has been reported (Linnemann, 1975). An instant diagnosis can be made by picking up the skin especially of the upper trunk (Fig. 5.4). The skin is lax and relatively inelastic; it is thickened and grooved and between the grooves are elevated yellow areas, hence the name pseudoxanthoma. The characteristic angioid streaks can be seen in the retina and are clearly demonstrated by fluorescent studies even if invisible through an ophthalmoscope (Kadri, Rosen and Harcourt, 1973). Degeneration of the elastic tissues of the arteries, with changes indistinguishable from atherosclerosis, and resulting calcification cause weak peripheral pulses, arterial occlusion, hypertension and coronary insufficiency. Abdominal pain may be due to abdominal angina from coeliac artery stenosis. Recently four types of pseudoxanthoma have been described—two inherited as a dominant and two recessive (Pope, 1974a, b). The common recessive form is associated with gastrointestinal bleeding.

The Ehlers–Danlos syndrome is characterised by loose-jointedness, hyperextensibility, fragility and easy bruising of the skin with 'cigarette paper' scarring and general friability of the tissues. The defect is thought to concern

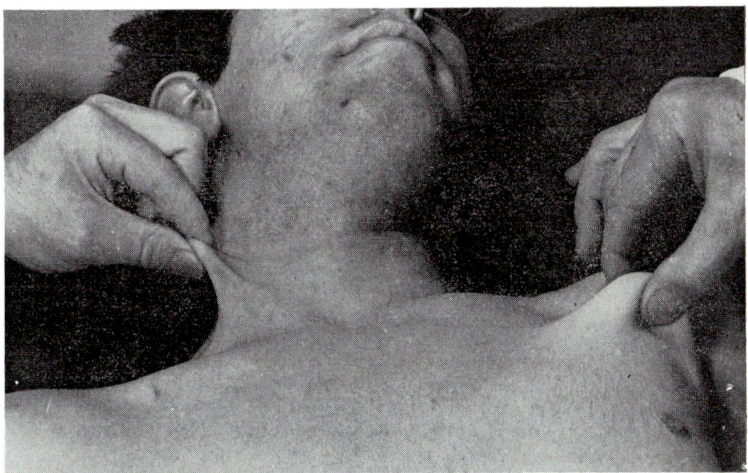

Figure 5.4 Pseudoxanthoma elasticum with lax skin. This patient presented with recurrent gastrointestinal haemorrhage

the organisation of collagen bundles into an intermeshing network (McKusick, 1972). McKusick (1974) distinguishes several forms of the disease according to inheritance and clinical features. The Sack–Barabas variety is most commonly associated with gastrointestinal complications.

The skin is hyperextensible, thin and fragile. It bruises easily and bleeding after dental extractions and operations may occur though a coagulation defect is usually not detectable. The commonest gastrointestinal problem are hernias: hiatus, umbilical, inguinal, femoral and incisional which despite the fragile tissues, can usually be repaired successfully. Surgical difficulties include suturing, bleeding, friable bowel and wound dehiscence. Haemorrhoids and bleeding from splits of anal skin are also common. Rectal prolapse may occur in childhood and usually resolves spontaneously (Beighton, 1970) though it may persist into adult life (Grant and Alder, 1967). The most severe complications are gastrointestinal bleeding and perforation. Beighton, Murdoch and

Votteler (1969) found bleeding in 8 of 125 patients reviewed: three from peptic ulcer, one from hiatus hernia, two from colonic diverticula and in two the cause of bleeding was unknown. Uncontrollable haemorrhage can also occur from multiple bleeding sites in the jejunum as a result of the friable bowel. Diagnosis is difficult. Angiography is dangerous because of the friable arteries and one death has been reported (Schoolman and Kepes, 1967). We know of no reports of endoscopy which presumably would also be hazardous. Diverticula have been reported in the stomach, duodenum, jejunum and colon and these may bleed or perforate (Aldridge, 1967; Grant and Alder, 1967; McKusick, 1972). Megacolon and megaoesophagus have also been described and recently dilatation of the whole small bowel was found in an asymptomatic patient (Harris, 1974). Dilatation of the duodenum may lead to malabsorption from bacterial overgrowth (Hines and Davies, 1973). Dissecting aorta and rupture of a major vessel should be included in the differential diagnosis of the acute abdomen (Beighton, 1968).

Cutis Laxa causes a striking laxity of the skin also due to defective elastic tissues and occasionally there are abnormalities of the lungs and arteries. Hernias or diverticula of the gastrointestinal tract are reported (Goltz et al, 1965). The recently described wrinkley skin syndrome which is related has not been known to affect the gut (Gazit et al, 1973).

Homocystinuria, an inborn error of metabolism, leads to secondary changes in connective tissue resulting in skeletal abnormalities, ectopia lentis and disruption of the arterial tunica media. The arterial lesion may cause gastrointestinal bleeding and radiographs may show small wedge-shaped ulcerations in the gastric mucosa consistent with local infarction. Mesenteric artery occlusion and intestinal infarction have been reported (McKusick, 1972). Diagnosis is made by demonstrating homocystinuria by urine tests.

REFERENCES

Akbarian, M. (1966) Abdominal apoplexy in polyarteritis nodosa. Report of a case. *American Journal of Digestive Diseases*, **11**, 63–67.

Akdamar, K., Agrawal, N. M. and Varela, P. Y. (1973) The endoscopic appearances of anaphylactoid purpura. *Gastrointestinal Endoscopy*, **20**, 68–69.

Alarćon-Segovia, D., Diaz-Jouanen, E. & Fishbein, E. (1973) Features of Sjögren's syndrome in primary biliary cirrhosis. *Annals of Internal Medicine*, **79**, 31–36.

Alarćon-Segovia, D. & Fishbein, E. (1971) Australian antigen in systemic lupus. *New England Journal of Medicine*, **284**, 448.

Alarćon-Segovia, D., Herskovic, T., Dearing, W. H., Bartholomew, L. G., Cain, J. C. & Shorter, R. G. (1965) Lupus erythematosus cell phenomenon in patients with chronic ulcerative colitis. *Gut*, **6**, 39–47.

Alder, R. H., Norcross, B. M. & Lockie, L. M. (1962) Arteritis and infarction in the intestine in rheumatoid arthritis. *Journal of the American Medical Association*, **180**, 922–926.

Aldridge, R. T. (1967) Ehlers–Danlos syndrome causing intestinal perforation. *British Journal of Surgery*, **54**, 22–25.

Alpert, E., Isselbacher, K. J. & Schur, P. H. (1971) The pathogenesis of arthritis associated with viral hepatitis complement component studies. *New England Journal of Medicine*, **285**, 185–189.

Altman, L. A., Fialkow, P. J., Parker, F. & Sagebiel, R. W. (1974) Pseudoxanthoma elasticum: an underdiagnosed heterogenous disorder with protean manifestations. *Archives of Internal Medicine*, **134**, 1048–1054.
Atkinson, M. & Summerling, M. D. (1966) Oesophageal changes in systemic sclerosis. *Gut*, **7**, 402–408.
Atlas, E. (1968) Intestinal scleroderma with malabsorption. *Journal of the American Medical Association*, **205**, 939.
Atwater, E. L., Mongan, E. S., Wieche, D. R. & Jacox, R. F. (1965) Peptic ulcer and rheumatoid arthritis: a prospective study. *Archives of Internal Medicine*, **115**, 184–189.
Babb, R. B., Alarćon-Segovia, D., Diessner, G. I. R. & McPherson, J. R. (1967) Malabsorption in rheumatoid arthritis: an unusual complication caused by amyloidosis. *Arthritis and Rheumatism*, **10**, 63–68.
Bacon, P. A., Doherty, S. M. & Zuckerman, A. J. (1975) Hepatitis B antibody in polymyalgia rheumatica. *Lancet*, **2**, 476–478.
Baker, A. L., Kaplan, M. M., Berz, W. C., Sidel, J. S. & Wolfe, H. J. (1972) Polyarteritis associated with Australia antigen-positive hepatitis. *Gastroenterology*, **62**, 105–110.
Banker, B. Q. & Victor, M. (1966) Dermatomyositis (systemic angiopathy) in childhood. *Medicine*, **45**, 261–289.
Barnett, A. J. (1974) *Scleroderma*. Springfield: C.C. Thomas.
Barnett, A. J. & Coventry, D. A. (1969) Scleroderma: 2. Incidence of systemic disturbance and assessment of possible aetiological factors. *Medical Journal of Australia*, **1**, 1040–1047.
Bartholomew, L. G., Cain, J. C., Winkleman, R. K. & Baggenstoss, A. H. (1964) Chronic disease of the liver associated with systemic scleroderma. *American Journal of Digestive Diseases*, **9**, 43–55.
Bazinet, P. & Martin, G. A. (1971) Malabsorption in systemic lupus erythematosus. *American Journal of Digestive Diseases*, **16**, 460–466.
Beighton, P. (1968) Lethal complications of the Ehlers–Danlos syndrome. *British Medical Journal*, **3**, 656–659.
Beighton, P. (1970) *The Ehlers–Danlos Syndrome*, London: Heinemann.
Beighton, P. H., Murdock, J. A. & Votteler, T. (1969) Gastrointestinal complications of Ehlers–Danlos syndrome. *Gut*, **10**, 1004–1008.
Billington, B. P. (1965) Observation from New South Wales on the changing incidence of gastric ulcer in Australia. *Gut*, **6**, 121–133.
Birkhan, J., Heifetz, M. & Haim, S. (1972) Diffuse cutaneous scleroderma: an anaesthetic problem. *Anaesthesia*, **27**, 89–90.
Bluestone, R., MacMahon, M. & Dawson, J. M. (1969) Systemic sclerosis and small bowel involvement. *Gut*, **10**, 185–193.
Bohan, A. & Peter, J. B. (1975) Polymyositis and dermatomyositis. *New England Journal of Medicine*, **292**, 344–347, 403–407.
Borges, W. H. (1972) Anaphylactoid purpura. *Medical Clinics of North America*. **56**, 201–206.
Brain, R. H. F. (1973) Surgical management of hiatal herniae and oesophageal strictures in systemic sclerosis. *Thorax*, **28**, 515–520.
Braverman, I. M. (1970) *Skin Signs of Systemic Disease*, Ch. 8. Philadelphia: Saunders.
Bron, K. M., Stilley, J. W. & Shapiro, A. P. (1971) Renal arteriography enhanced by tolazoline. Value in the diagnosis of polyarteritis nodosa complicated by perinephric haematoma. *Radiology*, **99**, 295–301.
Bron, K. M., Strott, C. A. & Shapiro, A. P. (1965) The diagnostic value of angiographic observations in polyarteritis nodosa: a case of multiple aneurysms of the visceral organs. *Archives of Internal Medicine*, **116**, 450–454.
Brown, C. H., Shirey, E. K. & Haserick, J. R. (1956) Gastrointestinal manifestations of systemic lupus erythematosus. *Gastroenterology*, **31**, 649–666.
Buchanan, W. W., Cox, A. G., Harden, R. McG., Glen, A. I. M., Anderson, J. R. & Gray, K. G. (1966) Gastric studies in Sjögren's syndrome. *Gut*, **7**, 351–354.
Buranasiri, S., Baum, S., Nusbaum, M. & Finkelstein, D. (1973) Periarteritis of the middle colic artery: arteriographic, surgical and pathological correlation. *American Journal of Gastroenterology*, **59**, 73–76.
Bywaters, E. G. L., Isdale, I. & Kempton, J. J. (1957) Schönlein–Henoch purpura. Evidence for a group of A β-haemolytic streptococcal aetiology. *Quarterly Journal of Medicine*, **26**, 161–175.

Bywaters, E. G. L. & Scott, J. T. (1963) The natural history of vascular lesions in rheumatoid arthritis. *Journal of Chronic Diseases*, **16**, 905–914.

Cabal, E. & Holtz, S. (1971) Polyarteritis as a cause of intestinal haemorrhage. *Gastroenterology*, **61**, 99–105.

Canoso, J. & Cohen, A. S. (1974) Malignancy in a series of seventy patients with systemic lupus erythematosus. *Arthritis and Rheumatism*, **17**, 383–388.

Carron, D. B. & Douglas, A. P. (1965) Steatorrhoea in vascular insufficiency of the small intestine: 5 cases of polyarteritis nodosa and allied diseases. *Quarterly Journal of Medicine*, **34**, 331–340.

Carwile LeRoy, E., McGuire, M. & Chen, N. (1974) Increased collagen synthesis by scleroderma skin fibroblasts in vitro. *Journal of Clinical Investigations*, **54**, 880–889.

Castleman, B. & Kibbee, B. U. (1962) Case records of the Massachusett's General Hospital No. 1—1962. *New England Journal of Medicine*, **266**, 42–49.

Chalmers, I. M. & Blair, G. S. (1973) Rheumatoid arthritis and the temporo-mandibular joint. *Quarterly Journal of Medicine*, **42**, 369–382.

Chapman, B. L. & Duggan, J. M. (1969) Aspirin and uncomplicated peptic ulcer. *Gut*, **10**, 443–450.

Chatterjee, C. R. (1973) Massive gastrointestinal haemorrhage due to systemic lupus erythematosus. *Journal of the Irish Medical Association*, **66**, 517–518.

Citron, B. P., Halpern, M., McCarron, M., Lundberg, G. P., McCormick, R., Pincus, I., Tatter, D. & Haverback, B. J. (1970) Necrotising angiitis associated with drug abuse. *New England Journal of Medicine*, **282**, 1003–1015.

Cocco, A. E., Grayer, D. I., Walker, B. A & Marryn, L. J. (1969) The stomach in pseudoxanthoma elasticum. *Journal of American Medical Association*, **210**, 2381–2382.

Cockel, R., Kendall, M. J., Becker, J. F. & Hawkins, C. F. (1971) Serum biochemical values in rheumatoid disease. *Annals of Rheumatic Diseases*, **30**, 166–170.

Cohen, S., Fisher, R., Lipshutz, W., Turner, R., Myers, A. & Schumacher, R. (1972) The pathogenesis of oesophageal dysfunction in scleroderma and Raynaud's disease. *Journal of Clinical Investigation*, **51**, 2663–2668.

Compton, R. (1969) Scleroderma with diverticulosis and colonic obstruction. *American Journal of Surgery*, **118**, 602–606.

Cook, C. O., Rosen, F. S. & Banker, B. Q. (1963) Dermatomyositis and focal scleroderma. *Pediatric Clinics of North America*, **10**, 979–1016.

Cooke, A. R. (1967) Corticosteroids and peptic ulcer: is there a relationship? *American Journal of Digestive Diseases*, **12**, 323–329.

Couris, G. D., Block, M. A. & Rupe, C. E. (1964) Gastrointestinal complications of collagen diseases. Surgical implications. *Archives of Surgery*, **89**, 695–700.

Cream, J. J., Gumpel, J. M. & Peachey, R. D. G. (1970) Schönlein–Henoch purpura in the adult. *Quarterly Journal of Medicine*, **39**, 461–484.

Curtis, A. C., Blaylock, H. C. & Harrell, E. R. (1952) Malignant lesions associated with dermatomyositis. *Journal of the American Medical Association*, **150**, 844–846.

Dahl, E. V., Baggenstoss, A. H. & Deweerd, J. H. (1960) Testicular lesions of periarteritis nodosa with special reference to diagnosis. *American Journal of Medicine*, **28**, 222–228.

D'Angelo, W. A., Fries, J. F., Mass, A. T. & Shulman, L. E. (1969) Pathologic observations in systemic sclerosis (scleroderma). *American Journal of Medicine*, **46**, 428–440.

Davis, P. & Read, A. E. (1975) Double-stranded DNA in chronic active hepatitis. *Gut*, **16**, 413–415.

Dickson, E. R., Maldonado, M. A., Sheps, S. G. & Cain, J. A. (1973) Systemic giant cell arteritis: polymyaglia rheumatica: reversible abnormalities of liver function. *Journal of the American Medical Association*, **224**, 1496–1498.

Dimarino, D. J., Carlson, G., Myers, A., Schumacher, H. R. & Cohen, S. (1973) Duodenal myoelectric activity in scleroderma. *New England Journal of Medicine*, **289**, 220–223.

Doig, J. A., Whaley, K., Dick, W. C., Nuki, G., Williamson, J. & Buchanan, W. W. (1971) Otolaryngological aspects of Sjögren's syndrome. *British Medical Journal*, **4**, 460–463.

Dornfield, L., Lecky, J. W. & Peter, J. B. (1971) Polyarteritis and intrarenal renal artery aneurysms. *Journal of the American Medical Association*, **215**, 1950–1952.

Drake, A. M., LeFeber, E. J. & Patterson, M. (1964) Collagen disease primarily affecting the gastrointestinal tract. *American Journal of Digestive Diseases*, **9**, 872–879.

Dubois, E. L. (1974) *Lupus Erythematosus*, 2nd edn. Los Angeles: University of Southern California Press.
Dubois, E. L. & Tuffaneli, D. L. (1967) Clinical manifestations of systemic lupus erythematosus. Computer analysis of 520 cases. *Journal of the American Medical Association*, **190**, 104–111.
Dubois, E. L., Wierzchowiecki, M., Cox, M. B. & Weiner, J. M. (1974) Duration and death in systemic lupus erythematosus. An analysis of 249 cases. *Journal of American Medical Association*, **227**, 1399–1402.
Dyer, N. H., Kendall, M. J. & Hawkins, C. F. (1971) Malabsorption in rheumatoid disease. *Annals of Rheumatic Diseases*, **30**, 626–630.
Edwards, D. A. W., Lennard-Jones, J. E., Lockhart-Mummery, H. E. & Jones, F. A. (1960) Diffuse systemic sclerosis presenting as infarction of the colon. *Proceedings of the Royal Society of Medicine*, **53**, 877–879.
Emmanuel, J. H. & Montgomery, R. D. (1971) Gastric ulcer and the anti-arthritic drugs. *Postgraduate Medical Journal*, **47**, 227–232.
Estes, D. & Christian, C. L. (1971) The natural history of systemic lupus erythematosus by prospective analysis. *Medicine*, **50**, 85–95.
Feldman, F. & Marshak, R. H. (1963) Dermatomyositis with significant involvement of the gastrointestinal tract. *American Journal of Roentgenology, Radium Therapy and Nuclear Medicine*, **90**, 746–752.
Feng, P. H., Cheah, P. S. & Lee, Y. K. (1973) Mortality in systemic lupus erythematosus: a 10 year review. *British Medical Journal*, **4**, 772–774.
Fenster, L. F., Buchanan, W. W., Laster, L. & Bunim, J. J. (1964) Studies of pancreatic function in Sjögren's syndrome. *Annals of Internal Medicine*, **61**, 498–508.
Fessel, W. J. (1974) Systemic lupus erythematosus in the community. *Archives of Internal Medicine*, **134**, 1027–1033.
Finkbiner, R. B. & Decker, J. P. (1963) Ulceration and perforation of the intestine due to necrotising arteriolitis. *New England Journal of Medicine*, **286**, 14–18.
Franks, A. S. T. (1969) Temporomandibular joint in adult rheumatoid arthritis. *Annals of the Rheumatic Diseases*, **28**, 139–145.
Frayha, R. A., Scarola, J. A. & Shulman, L. E. (1973) Calcinosis in scleroderma. A re-evaluation of the 'CRST' syndrome. *Arthritis and Rheumatism*, **16**, 542.
Frohert, P. P. & Sheps, J. G. (1967) Long-term follow-up study of periarteritis nodosa. *American Journal of Medicine*, **43**, 8–14.
Fung, W. P., Chew, B. K. & Tan, V. K. (1969) Active chronic hepatitis with positive lupus erythematosus cell test and lupus nephritis. *Australian Annals of Medicine*, **18**, 288–291.
Garrett, J. M., Winkelman, R. K., Schlegel, J. F. & Cope, C. F. (1971) Esophageal deterioration in scleroderma. *Mayo Clinic Proceedings*, **46**, 92–96.
Gault, M. H., Rudwell, T. C., Engles, W. P. & Dossetor, J. B. (1968) Syndrome associated with abuse of analgesics. *Annals of Internal Medicine*, **68**, 906–925.
Gazit, E., Goodman, R. M., Katznelson, M. B. & Rotem, Y. (1973) The wrinkley skin syndrome: a new heritable disorder of connective tissue. *Clinical Genetics*, **4**, 186–192.
Glueck, C. J., Levy, R. I., Glueck, H. I., Gralnick, H. R., Greten, H. & Frederickson, D. S. (1969) Acquired type I hyperlipoproteinaemia with systemic lupus erythematosus, dysglobulinaemia and heparin resistance. *American Journal of Medicine*, **47**, 318–324.
Gocke, D. J., Morgan, C., Lockshin, M., Hsu, K., Bombardieri, S. & Christian, C. L. (1970) Association between polyarteritis and Australia antigen. *Lancet*, **2**, 1149–1153.
Gocke, D. J., Hsu, K., Bombardieri, S., Lockshin, M. & Christian, C. L. (1971) Vasculitis in association with Australia antigen. *Journal of Experimental Medicine*, **134**, Suppl. 330s–336s.
Golding, P. L., Brown, R., Mason, A. M. S. & Taylor, E. (1970) 'Sicca complex' in liver disease. *British Medical Journal*, **4**, 340–342.
Goltz, R. W., Hult, A. M., Goldfarb, M. & Garlin, R. J. (1965) Cutis laxa: a manifestation of generalised elastolysis. *Archives of Dermatology*, **92**, 373–387.
Gordon, D. A., Stein, J. L. & Broder, I. (1973) The extra-articular features of rheumatoid arthritis. A systemic analysis of 127 cases. *American Journal of Medicine*, **54**, 445–452.
Gourgoutis, G. D., Paguirigan, A. A. & Berzins, T. (1971) Gastric perforation in polyarteritis nodosa: report of a patient. *American Journal of Digestive Diseases*, **16**, 171–177.

Grant, A. K. & Alder, T. A. M. (1967) Haemorrhage into the upper part of the gastrointestinal tract in three patients with heritable disorders of connective tissue. *Australian Annals of Medicine*, **16**, 75–79.

Greenberger, N. J., Dobbins, W. D., Ruppert, R. D. & Jesseph, J. E. (1961) Intestinal atony in progressive systemic sclerosis (scleroderma). *American Journal of Medicine*, **45**, 301–308.

Halpern, N. & Citron, B. P. (1971) Necrotising angiitis associated with drug abuse. *American Journal of Roentgenology, Radium Therapy and Nuclear Medicine*, **113**, 663–672.

Hamilton, C. R., Shelley, W. M. & Tumulty, P. A. (1971) Giant cell arteritis: including temporal arteritis and polymyalgia rheumatica. *Medicine*, **50**, 1–27.

Harper, R. A. K. & Jackson, P. C. (1965) Progressive systemic sclerosis. *British Journal of Radiology*, **38**, 825–834.

Harpey, J. P., Caille, B., Moulias, R. & Goust, J. M. (1971) Lupus-like syndrome induced by D-penicillamine in Wilson's disease. *Lancet*, **1**, 291–292.

Harris, R. D. (1974) Small bowel dilation in Ehler's–Danlos syndrome—an unexpected gastrointestinal manifestation. *British Journal of Radiology*, **47**, 623–627.

Hart, F. D. (1969) Diffuse collagen diseases. In *Text Book of the Rheumatic Diseases*, 4th edn, ed. Copeman, W. S. L., Ch. 11. Edinburgh and London: Livingstone.

Harvey, A. M., Shulman, L. E., Tumulty, P. A., Conley, C. L. & Schoenrich, E. H. (1954) Systemic lupus erythematosus: review of the literature and clinical analysis of 138 cases. *Medicine*, **33**, 291–437.

Haslock, I. (1974) Liver rupture in systemic lupus erythematosus. *Annals of Rheumatic Diseases*, **33**, 483–484.

Henderson, R. D. & Pearson, F. G. (1973) Surgical management of oesophageal scleroderma. *Journal of Thoracic and Cardiovascular Surgery*, **66**, 686–691.

Henson, J. B., Gorham, J. R. & Leader, R. W. (1963) Hypergammaglobulinaemia in mink initiated by a cell-free infiltrate. *Nature*, **197**, 206–207.

Herbert, C. M., Lindberg, K. A., Jayson, M. I. V. & Bailey, A. J. (1974) Biosynthesis and maturation of skin collagen in scleroderma and effect of D-penicillamine. *Lancet*, **1**, 187–192.

Hermann, G. (1967) Intussusception secondary to mesenteric arteritis. Complication of systemic lupus erythematosus in a 5 year old child. *Journal of American Medical Association*, **200**, 74–75.

Herrington, J. L. (1959) Scleroderma as a cause of small bowel obstruction: successful treatment of a case by intestinal resection. *Archives of Surgery*, **78**, 17–24.

Hines, C. & Davies, W. D. (1973) Ehlers–Danlos syndrome with megaduodenum and malabsorption syndrome secondary to bacterial overgrowth. *American Journal of Medicine*, **54**, 539–543.

Horowitz, A. L. & Meyers, M. A. (1973) The 'hide-bound' small bowel of scleroderma: characteristic mucosa fold patterns. *American Journal of Roengenology, Radium Therapy and Nuclear Medicine*, **119**, 332–334.

Hradsky, M., Bartos, V. & Keller, O. (1967) Pancreatic function in Sjögren's syndrome. *Gastroenterologia*, **108**, 252–260.

Hughes, G. R. V. (1973) The diagnosis of systemic lupus erythematosus. *British Journal of Haematology*, **25**, 409–413.

Hughes, G. R. V. (1974) Measurement of DNA antibodies—a three year clinical survey. *Annals of Rheumatic Diseases*, **33**, 402–403.

Ivey, K. J. & Clifton, J. A. (1974) Back diffusion of hydrogen ions across the gastric mucosa of patients with gastric ulcer and rheumatoid arthritis. *British Medical Journal*, **1**, 16–19.

Jayson, M. I. V., Gough, J., Salmon, P. R., Poliness, T. & Bishton, R. L. (1972) Spontaneous bowel perforation in intestinal scleroderma: first report of a non-fatal case. *Postgraduate Medical Journal*, **48**, 56–58.

Johnson, R. B. & Munroe, L. S. (1973) Carcinoma of the oesophagus developing in progressive systemic sclerosis. *Gastrointestinal Endoscopy*, **19**, 189–191.

Kadri, W., Rosen, E. & Harcourt, B. (1973) Intraretinal changes in Groenblad–Strandberg syndrome. *British Journal of Ophthalmology*, **57**, 588–592.

Kahn, I. J., Jeffries, G. H. & Sleisender, M. H. (1966) Malabsorption in intestinal scleroderma: correction by antibiotics. *New England Journal of Medicine*, **274**, 1339–1344.

Kaplan, L. & Hartman, S. W. (1954) Elastica disease, case of Grönblad–Strandberg syndrome with gastrointestinal haemorrhage. *Archives of Internal Medicine*, **94**, 489–492.

Kendall, M. J., Cockel, R., Becker, J. & Hawkins, C. F. (1970) Raised serum alkaline phosphatase in rheumatoid disease. An index of liver dysfunction? *Annals of Rheumatic Diseases*, **29**, 537.
Kleckner, F. S. (1970) Dermatomyositis and its manifestations in the gastrointestinal tract. *American Journal of Gastroenterology*, **53** 141–146.
Knieser, M. R., Jenis, E. H., Lowenthal, D. T., Bancroft, W. H., Burns, W. & Shalhoub, R. (1974) Patholgenesis of renal disease associated with viral hepatitis. *Archives of Pathology*, **97**, 193–200.
Koff, R. S., Widrich, W. C. & Robbins, A. H. (1973) Necrotising angiitis in a methampetamine user with hepatitis B; angiographic diagnosis, 5 month follow-up results and localisation of bleeding site. *New England Journal of Medicine*, **288**, 946–947.
Kornreich, H., Malouf, N. N. & Hanson, V. (1971) Acute hepatitis dysfunction in juvenile rheumatoid arthritis. *Journal of Pediatrics*, **79**, 27–35.
Kurlander, D. L. & Kirsner, J. B. (1964) The association of chronic 'non-specific' inflammatory bowel disease with lupus erythematosus. *Annals of Internal Medicine*, **60**, 799–813.
Langman, M. J. (1970) Epidemiological evidence for the association of aspirin and acute gastrointestinal bleeding. *Gut* **11**, 627–634.
Leneman, F., Fierst, S., Gabriel, J. & Ingegno, A. P. (1962) Progressive systemic sclerosis of the intestine presenting as malabsorption syndrome. *Gastroenterology*, **42**, 175–180.
Lindsay, M. K., Tavadia H. B., White, A. S., Lee, R. & Webb, J. (1973) Acute abdomen in rheumatoid arthritis due to necrosing arteritis. *British Medical Journal*, **2**, 592–593.
Linnemann, M. P. (1975) Ehlers–Danlos syndrome presenting with torsion of the stomach. *Proceedings of the Royal Society of Medicine*, **68**, 330–332.
Livolsi, V. A., Perzia, K. R. & Porter, M. (1973) Polyarteritis nodosa of the gallbladder presenting as acute cholecystitis. *Gastroenterology*, **65**, 115–123.
Lowenstein, P. S. & Heeb, M. A. (1955) Intestinal obstruction secondary to periarteritis nodosa. *Angiology*, **6** 417–426.
Mackay, I. R., Taft, L. I. & Cowling, D. C. (1959) Lupoid hepatitis and the hepatic lesions of systemic lupus erythematosus. *Lancet*, **1**, 65–67.
MacMahon, H. E. (1972) Systemic scleroderma and massive infarction of intestine and liver. *Surgery, Gynecology and Obstetrics*, **134**, 10–14.
Maldonadu, J. E., Gregg, J. A., Green, P. A. & Brown, A. L. (1970) Chronic idiopathic intestinal pseudo-obstruction. *American Journal of Medicine*, **49**, 203–212.
Martinez, L. O. (1974) Air in the oesophagus as a sign of scleroderma. *Journal of Canadian Association of Radiology*, **25**, 234–237.
Maxeiner, S. R., McDonald, J. R. & Kirklin, J. W. (1952) Muscle biopsy in the diagnosis of periarteritis nodosa. *Surgical Clinics of North America*, **32**, 1223–1225.
McGovern, V. J. (1971) Livedo reticularis. In *The Skin*, ed. Helwig, E. B. & Mostofi, F. K., Ch. 17. Baltimore: Williams and Wilkins.
McKeown, K. C. & Ganguli, A. K. (1956) Gastrointestinal symptoms in polyarteritis nodosa. Report of a case. *British Journal of Surgery*, **44**, 308–312.
McKusick, V. A. (1972) *Heritable Disorders of Connective Tissue*, 2nd edn. Louis: Mosby.
McKusick, V. A. (1974) Multiple forms of Ehlers–Danlos syndrome. *Archives of Surgery*, **109**, 475–476.
Meadow, S. R., Glasgow, E. F., White, R. H. R., Moncrieff, M. W., Cameron, J. S. & Ogg, C. S. (1972) Schönlein–Henoch nephritis. *Quarterly Journal of Medicine*, **41**, 241–257.
Miller, D. G. (1967) The association of immune disease and malignant lymphoma. *Annals of Internal Medicine*, **66**, 507–521.
Mills, J. A. (1963) Connective tissue disease associated with malignant neoplastic disease. *Journal of Chronic Diseases*, **16**, 797–811.
Mogadam, M., Schuman, B. M., Duncan, H. & Patton, R. B. (1962) Necrotising colitis associated with rheumatoid arthritis. *Gastroenterology*, **57**, 168–172.
Morris, J. S., Htut, T. & Read, A. E. (1972) Scleroderma and portal hypertension. *Annals of Rheumatic Diseases*, **31**, 316–318.
Mowrey, F. H. & Lundberg, E. A. (1954) The clinical manifestations of essential polyangiitis (periarteritis nodosa) with emphasis on hepatic manifestations. *Annals of Internal Medicine*, **40**, 1145–1164.

Mueller, C. F., Moehead, R., Alter, A. J. & Michener, W. (1972) Pneumatosis intestinalis in collagen disorders. *American Journal of Roentenology, Radium Therapy and Nuclear Medicine*, **115**, 300–305.

Murray, H. S., Strottman, M. P. & Cooke, A. R. (1974) Effect of several drugs on gastric potential difference in man. *British Medical Journal*, **1**, 19–20.

Murray-Lyon, I. M., Thomson, R. P. H., Ansell, I. D. & Williams, R. (1970) Scleroderma and primary biliary cirrhosis. *British Medical Journal*, **3**, 258–259.

Musher, D. R. (1972) Systemic lupus erythematosus. A cause of 'medical peritonitis'. *American Journal of Surgery*, **124**, 368–372.

Nakao, K., Ikeda, M., Kimata, S., Niitani, H., Miyahara, M., Ishimi, Z., Kuramochi, M., Matsushita, S., Ozawa, T., Takeda, Y. & Hashira, K. (1967) Takayasu's arteritis. Clinical report of 84 cases and immunological studies of seven. *Circulation*, **35**, 1141–1155.

Nazum, J. W. & Nazum, J. W. (1954) Polyarteritis nodosa. *Archives of Internal Medicine*, **94**, 942–955.

Norman, A. G. & Wilkins, P. S. (1957) Acute abdomen in periarteritis nodosa. *British Medical Journal*, **1**, 445–446.

Norton, W. L. & Narda, J. M. (1970) Vascular disease in progressive systemic sclerosis (scleroderma). *Annals of Internal Medicine*, **73**, 317–324.

Oaks, W. W. & O'Malley, J. F. (1969) Systemic involvement in CRST syndrome. *Postgraduate Medicine*, **45**, 94–99.

O'Brien, S. T., Eddy, W. M. & Krawitt, E. L. (1972) Primary biliary cirrhosis associated with scleroderma. *Gastroenterology*, **62**, 118–121.

O'Neill, P. B. (1961) Gastrointestinal abnormalities in the collagen diseases. *American Journal of Digestive Diseases*, **6**, 1069–1083.

Ostrum, B. J. & Soder, P. D. (1960) Periarteritis nodosa complicated by spontaneous perinephric haematoma. *American Journal of Roentgenology, Radium Therapy and Nuclear Medicine*, **84**, 849–860.

Pachas, W. N., Linscheer, W. G. & Pinali, R. J. (1971) Protein-losing enteropathy in systemic lupus erythematosus. *American Journal of Gastroenterology*, **55**, 162–167.

Painter, R. W. (1971) Sequential gastrointestinal complications of polyarteritis nodosa. *American Journal of Gastroenterology*, **55**, 383–386.

Palmer, W. L. & Kirsner, J. B. (1959) Therapeutic and side-effects of the anti-inflammatory steroids on the gastrointestinal tract. *Annals of the New York Academy of Sciences*, **82**, 947–956.

Parker, M. D. & Kerby, G. P. (1974) Combined titre and fluorescent pattern of IgG antinuclear antibodies using cultured cell monolayers in evaluating connective tissue disease. *Annals of Rheumatic Diseases*, **33**, 465–472.

Parker, R. A. & Thomas, P. M. (1959) Intestinal perforation and widespread arteritis in rheumatoid arthritis during treatment with cortisone. *British Medical Journal*, **1**, 540–542.

Peachey, R. G., Creamer, B. & Pierce, J. W. (1969) Sclerodermatous involvement of the stomach, and the small and large bowel. *Gut*, **10**, 285–292.

Pearson, C. M. (1966) Polymyositis and dermatomyositis. In *Modern Trends in Rheumatology*, ed. Hill, A. G. S., Vol. 1, Ch. 21. London: Butterworths.

Petterson, T. & Wegelius, O. (1972) Biopsy diagnosis of amyloidosis in rheumatoid arthritis. Malabsorption caused by intestinal amyloid deposits. *Gastroenterology*, **62**, 22–27.

Phillips, J. C. & Howland, W. J. (1968) Mesenteric arteritis in systemic lupus erythematosus. *Journal of the American Medical Association*, **206**, 1569–1570.

Plantin, L. O. & Strandberg, O. (1974) Gastrointestinal protein loss in rheumatoid arthritis, studied with Cr^{15} chromic chloride and I^{251} albumin. *Scandinavian Journal of Rheumatology*, **3**, 169–173.

Pollock, V. E., Grove, W. J., Karl, R. M., Meuhreke, R. C., Piram, C. L. & Steck, I. E. (1958) Systemic lupus erythematosus similating acute surgical condition of the abdomen. *New England Journal of Medicine*, **259**, 258–266.

Pope, F. M. (1974a) Two types of autosomal recessive pseudoxanthoma elasticum. *Archives of Dermatology*, **110**, 209–212.

Pope, F. M. (1974b) Autosomal dominant pseudoxanthoma elasticum. *Journal of Medical Genetics*, **11**, 152–157.

Porubsky, E. S., Murray, J. P. & Pratt, L. L. (1973) Cricopharyngeal achalasia in dermatmyositis. *Archives of Otorhinolaryngology*, **98**, 428–429.

Queloz, J. M. & Woloshin, H. J. (1972) Sacculation and the small intestine in scleroderma. *Radiology*, **105**, 513–515.

Ramirez-Mata, M., Reyes, P. A., Alarćon-Segovia, D. & Garza, R. (1974) Esophageal motility in systemic lupus erythematosus. *American Journal of Digestive Diseases*, **19**, 132–136.

Rees, H. A. & Williams, D. A. (1962) Long-term steroid therapy in thoracic intractable asthama. *British Medical Journal*, **1**, 1575–1579.

Reinhaardt, J. F. & Barry, W. F. (1962) Scleroderma of the small bowel. *American Journal of Roentgenology, Radium Therapy and Nuclear Medicine*, **88**, 687–692.

Reynolds, T. B., Denison, E. K., Frankl, H. D., Lieberman, F. L. & Peters, R. L. (1971) Primary biliary cirrhosis with scleroderma, Raynaud's phenomenon and telangectasia. *American Journal of Medicine*, **50**, 302–312.

Roberts, W. C., MacGregor, R. R., DeBlanc, H. J., Beiser, G. D. & Wolff, S. M. (1969) The prepulseless phase of pulseless disease or pulseless disease with pulses. *American Journal of Medicine*, **46**, 313–324.

Robins, J. M. & Bookstein, J. J. (1972) Regressing aneurysms in periateritis nodosa. *Radiology*, **104**, 39–42.

Robinson, J. C. & Teitelbaum, S. L. (1974) Stercoral ulceration and perforation of the sclerodermatous colon: report of two cases and review of the literature. *Diseases of the Colon and the Rectum*, **17**, 622–632.

Roderiguez-Erdmann, F. & Levitan, R. (1968) Gastrointestinal and roentgenological manifestations of Henoch–Schönlein purpura. *Gastroenterology*, **54**, 260–264.

Rooney, P. J. (1976) Personal communication.

Rooney, P. J., Vince, J., Kennedy, A. C., Webb, J., Lee, P., Dick, W. C., Buchanan, K. D., Hayes, J. R., Ardill, J. & O'Connor, F. (1973) Hypergastrinaemia in rheumatoid arthritis: disease or iatrogenesis. *British Medical Journal*, **2**, 752–753.

Rosenmann, E. & Levis, I. S. (1971) Rectal biopsy as a diagnostic aid in periarteritis nodosa. *Israel Journal of Medical Sciences*, **7**, 1082–1084.

Rosson, R. S. & Yesner, R. (1965) Peroral duodenal biopsy in progressive systemic sclerosis. *New England Journal of Medicine*, **272**, 391–394.

Sames, C. P. (1961) Pseudoxanthoma elasticum: severe melanena from the jejunum treated by resection. *Proceedings of the Royal Society of Medicine*, **54**, 519–520.

Sano, K., Aiba, T. & Saito, I. (1970) Angiography in pulseless disease. *Radiology*, **94**, 69–74.

Schimke, R. N., Kirkpatrick, C. H. & Deip, M. H. (1967) Calcinosis, Raynaud's phenomenon, sclerodactyly and telangiectasia—the CRST syndrome. *Archives of Internal Medicine*, **119**, 365–370.

Schneider, R. E. & Dobbins, W. O. (1968) Suction biopsy of the rectal mucosa for diagnosis of arteritis in rheumatoid arthritis and related diseases. *Annals of Internal Medicine*, **68**, 561–568.

Schoolman, A. & Kepes, J. J. (1967) Bilateral spontaneous carotid-cavenous fistulae in Ehlers–Danlos syndrome. *Journal of Neurosurgery*, **26**, 82–86.

Scott, J. T., Hourihane, D. O., Doyle, F. H., Steiner, R. E., Laws, J. W., Dixon, A. St. J. & Bywaters, E. G. L. (1961a). Digital arteritis in rheumatoid disease. *Annals of Rheumatic Diseases*, **20**, 224–234.

Scott, J. T., Porter, I. H., Lewis, S. M. & Dixon, A. St. J. (1961b) Studies of gastrointestinal bleeding caused by corticosteroids, salicylates and other analgesics. *Quarterly Journal of Medicine*, **30**, 167–188.

Scudamore, H. H., Green, P. A., Hoffman, N. N., Rosevear, J. W. & Tauxe, W. N. (1968) Scleroderma (progressive systemic sclerosis) of the small intestine with malabsorption; evaluation of intestinal absorption and pancreatic function. *American Journal of Gastroenterology*, **49**, 193–208.

Scully, R. E. & McNeely, B. U. (1974) Case records of the Massachusetts General Hospital, Case 45—1974. *New England Journal of Medicine*, **291**, 1073–1080.

Seaman, W. E., Ishak, K. G. & Platz, P. H. (1974) Aspirin-induced hepatotoxicity in patients with systemic lupus erythematosus. *Annals of Internal Medicine*, **80**, 1–8.

Seamen, W. E., Platz, P. H. & Ishak, K. G. (1974) Aspirin-induced hepatotoxicity in patients with rheumatoid arthritis or systemic lupus erythematosus. *Arthritis and Rheumatism*, **17**, 325.

Seifert, V. G., Heinz, N. & Ruffmann, A. (1967) Pankreatitis bei Visceralem Lupus Erythematodes. *Gastroenterologia*, **107**, 317–327.
Sethi, G. K. & Thomas, T. V. (1973) Unusual manifestations of polyarteritis nodosa. *Postgraduate Medicine*, **54**, 245–246.
Sfikakis, P. & Giamarellou, H. (1971) Amyloidosis complicating Still's disease. *Lancet*, **1**, 348.
Shafer, R. B. & Gregory, P. H. (1970) Systemic lupus erythematosus presenting as regional ileitis. *Minnesota Medicine*, **53**, 789–792.
Shapeero, L. G., Myers, A., O'Berkircher, P. E. & Miller, W. T. (1974) Acute reversible lupus vasculitis of the gastrointestinal tract. *Radiology*, **112**, 569–574.
Sharp, G. L. (1975) Mixed connective tissue disease. *Bulletin of Rheumatic Diseases*, **25**, 828–831.
Sharp, G. I.., Irwin, W. S., Tan, E. M., Gould, R. G. & Holman, H. R. (1972) Mixed connective tissue disease. An apparently distinct rheumatic disease syndrome associated with a specific antibody to an extractable nuclear antigen. *American Journal of Medicine*, **52**, 149–159.
Shearn, M. A. (1971) *Sjögren's Syndrome*, Philadelphia: Saunders.
Sinclair, R. J. G. & Cruickshank, B. (1956) A clinical and pathological study of sixteen cases of rheumatoid arthritis with extensive visceral involvement. *Quarterly Journal of Medicine*, **25**, 313–332.
Siurala, M., Julkunen, H., Toivonen, S., Pelkonen, R. & Saxen, E. (1965) Digestive tract collagen diseases. *Acta medica scandinavia*, **178**, 13–25.
Skinner, M. & Fernandez-Herlihy, L. (1966) Entero-arthropathy. The co-existence of articular and gastrointestinal manifestations in systemic disease. *Medical Clinics of North America*, **50**, 417–425.
Solway, R. D., Summerskill, W. H. J., Baggenstoss, A. H. & Schoenfield, L. J. (1972) 'Lupoid' hepatitis, a nonentity in the spectrum of chronic active liver disease. *Gastroenterology*, **63**, 458–465.
Sparberg, M., (1967) Recurrent acute pancreatitis associated with systemic lupus erythematosus. *American Journal of Digestive Diseases*, **12**, 522–525.
Spiro, A. M. & Milles, S. S. (1960) Clinical physiologic implication of the steroid-induced peptic ulcer. *New England Journal of Medicine*, **263**, 286–294.
Steiner, R. M., Glassman, L., Schwartz, W. M. & Vanace, P. (1974) The radiological findings in dermatomyositis of childhood. *Radiology*, **111**, 385–393.
Strachan, R. W. (1966) Prepulseless and pulseless Takayasu's arteritis. *Postgraduate Medical Journal*, **42**, 464–468.
Sullivan, D. B., Cassidy, J. T., Petty, R. E. & Burt, A. (1972) Prognosis in childhood dermatomyositis. *Journal of Pediatrics*, **80**, 555–563.
Sun, D. C. H., Roth, S. H., Mitchell, C. S. & England, D. W. (1974) Upper gastrointestinal disease in rheumatoid arthritis *American Journal of Digestive Diseases*, **19**, 405–410.
Svantesson, H. & Garwicz, S. (1970) Extra-articular manifestations in juvenile rheumatoid arthritis. Diagnostic difficulties. *Acta paediatrica scandinavia*, Suppl. 206, 118.
Thompson, D. M. (1974) Mixed connective tissue disease. *Proceedings of the Royal Society of Medicine*, **67**, 26–28.
Thompson, P. L. & Mackay, I. R. (1971) Diffuse haemorrhagic gastritis in scleroderma. *Medical Journal of Australia*, **2**, 373–375.
Trepo, C. G., Zuckerman, A. J., Bird, R. C. & Prince, A. M. (1974) The role of circulating hepatitis B antigen/antibody immune complexes in the pathogenesis of vascular and hepatic manifestations in polyarteritis nodosa. *Journal of Clinical Pathology*, **27**, 863–868.
Tribe, C. R. (1966) Amyloidosis and rheumatoid arthritis. In *Modern Trends in Rheumatology* ed. Hill, A. G. S., Vol. 1, Ch. 7. London: Butterworths.
Tuffanelli, D. L. & Winkelman, R. K. (1961) Systemic scleroderma: a clinical study of 727 cases. *Archives of Dermatology*, **84**, 359–371.
Uhl, G. S., Baldwin, J. L. & Arnett, F. C. (1974) Primary biliary cirrhosis in systemic sclerosis and polymyositis. *Johns Hopkins Medical Journal*, **135**, 191–198.
Valignat, P., Lambert, R. & Moulin, G. (1973) La muqueuse gastrique au cours de la sclerodermie. *Nouvelle Presse Medicale*, **2**, 3023–3026.
Verbov, J. & Stansfeld, A. G. (1972) Cutaneous polyarteritis nodosa and Crohn's disease. *Transactions of the St John's Hospital Dermatological Society*, **58**, 261–268.

Walton, E. W. (1958) Giant-cell granuloma of the respiratory tract (Wegener's granulomatosis). *British Medical Journal*, **2**, 265–270.
Walker, J. G., Doniach, D. & Doniach, I. (1970) Mitochondrial antibodies and subclinical liver disease. *Quarterly Journal of Medicine*, **39**, 31–48.
Webb, J. & Payne, W. H. (1970) Abdominal apoplexy in rheumatoid arthritis. *Australian Annals of Medicine*, **19**, 168–170.
Webb, J. & Whaley, K. (1974) Evaluation of the native DNA-binding assay for DNA antibodies in systemic lupus erythematosus and other connective tissue disorders. *Medical Journal of Australia*, **2**, 324–328.
Webb, J., Whaley, K., MacSween, R. N. M., Nuki, G., Carson-Dick, W. & Watson Buchanan, W. (1975) Liver disease in rheumatoid arthritis and Sjögren's syndrome. Prospective study using biochemical and serological markers of hepatic dysfunction. *Annals of Rheumatic Diseases*, **34**, 70–81.
Whaley, K., Goudie, R. B., Williamson, J., Nuki, G., Dick, W. C. & Buchanan, W. W. (1970) Liver disease in Sjögren's syndrome and rheumatoid arthritis. *Lancet*, **1**, 861–863.
Whaley, K., Williamson, J., Chisholm, D. M., Webb, J., Mason, D. K. & Buchanan, W. W. (1973) Sjögren's syndrome. Sicca components. *Quarterly Journal of Medicine*, **42**, 279–302.
Wiljasalo, M. & Ikkala, E. (1971) Lymphography in systemic lupus erythematosus. *Annals of Clinical Research*, **3**, 231–235.
Winterbauer, R. H. (1964) Multiple telangiectasia, Raynaud's phenomenon, sclerodactyly and subcutaneous calcinosis: a syndrome mimicking hereditary haemorrhagic telangiectasia. *Bulletin of Johns Hopkins Hospital*, **114**, 361–383.
Wold, L. E. & Baggenstoss, A. H. (1949) Gastrointestinal lesions of periarteritis nodosa. *Staff Meetings Mayo Clinic*, **24**, 28–35.
Yentis, I. (1973) Henoch–Schönlein purpura mimicking acute appendicitis and Crohn's disease. *British Journal of Radiology*, **46**, 555–556.

6
THE USE AND ABUSE OF LAXATIVES

John H. Cummings

What's new about laxatives? The view that laxatives are a relic of the more primitive days of medicine and therapeutics is not unreasonable seen against the background of sophisticated modern patient care and community health programmes. Few really new laxative preparations have been developed in recent years and many of the older more drastic purges have disappeared from the pharmacopoeia. Should we then relegate this topic to the small print of medical teaching and leave the dispensation of laxatives to the nursing staff?

The answer must be no. Laxative consumption in Britain is still substantial and may well be increasing. Earlier concepts of how laxatives produce their effects are probably obsolete and are being slowly revised. The syndrome of laxative abuse remains a diagnostic challenge, is changing in character and is being increasingly recognised.

LAXATIVE CONSUMPTION

Prescriptions and proprietary preparations

The number of prescriptions for laxatives and allied compounds dispensed by chemists' shops for the Health Service has risen steadily over the past 10 years (Fig. 6.1). In 1973 8.2 million were dispensed in England and Wales at a cost to the Treasury approaching £6 million. This rising trend, however, must be seen against a general rise of about 36 per cent in the number of prescriptions dispensed for all drugs when the period 1961 to 1963 is compared to 1971 to 1973. Laxative prescriptions rose 62 per cent when calculated on the same basis, which is ahead of the overall trend although even this rise is small when compared to the 200 per cent increase in prescriptions for tranquillisers. Prescriptions for some drugs have fallen during this period, notably for barbiturates, by 32 per cent.

Whether this trend in laxative prescribing represents a real rise in consumption or merely an increasing reliance by the public on the state to provide their weekly purge is not clear. Laxatives are of course available from sources other than by prescription. In fact the choice of preparations available on prescription is relatively limited when compared to those available 'over the counter'. The 1974 to 1976 *British National Formulary* lists 16 laxative preparations whilst *MIMS* (September 1975) details 48 medications of various sorts under 'laxatives, purgatives and lubricants' all of which are available on prescription. However 108 different proprietary medicines containing laxatives are available over the counter without prescription (Martindale, 1972). Some of these proprietary remedies are well known, e.g. Andrew's Liver Salts, Beecham's Pills, Carter's Little Liver Pills, and Ex-Lax. Others conceal their true nature behind a variety of names, e.g. Father Pierre's Monastery Herbs (contain senna, frangula and ispaghula), Obesettes (phenolphthalein, cascara, frangula), Potter's Herbal Blood Compound (senna, cascara, magnesium sulphate, etc)

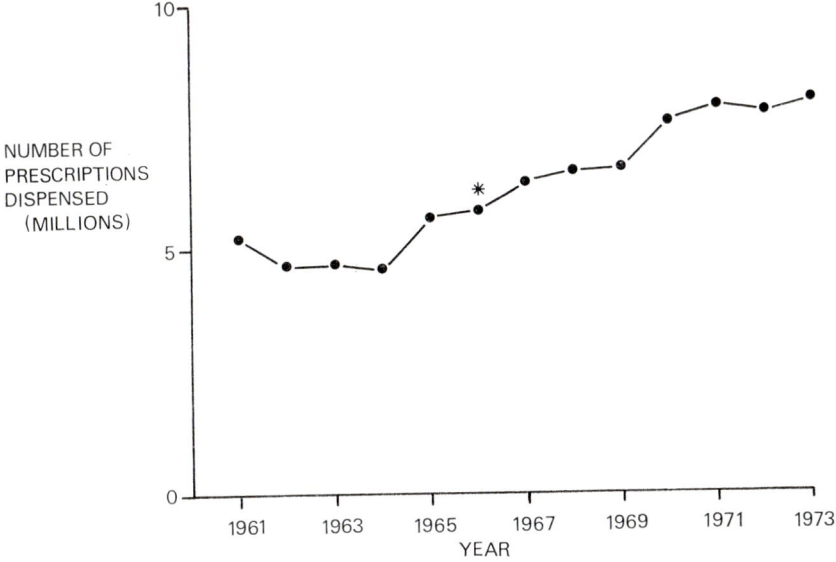

Figure 6.1 Number of prescriptions dispensed annually in England and Wales for 'Laxatives and purgatives, evacuant enemas and suppositories, other preparations acting locally on the rectum and anti-infective agents acting locally on the gastrointestinal tract'. From Health and Personal Social Services Statistics for England, 1972 to 1974, and for Wales, 1974, and Annual Reports of the Department of Health and Social Security, 1961 to 1969.

* After 1966 the Department of Health's system for classifying pharmaceutical preparations changed. Prior to this, laxatives and purgatives are listed separately from preparations acting locally on the rectum. The figure shows the combined data prior to 1966.

and even Stonecracker brand Medicamentum Miraculosa Coronata (aloes and rhubarb).

Whilst only those laxative preparations listed in the *BNF* and *MIMS* are available on prescription all are freely available over the counter and it is this 'proprietary' end of the market which is difficult to quantitate. It has been reported that in 1970 £4 million were spent on laxatives for 'self-medication' (*British Medical Journal*, 1972). Total spending on laxatives must therefore be considerably in excess of £10 million each year particularly when hospital laxative prescribing is also taken into account.

Trends in laxative consumption are also difficult to assess. Over the past 10 years there may well have been an overall increase whilst in the previous two decades laxative consumption apparently fell off (Connell et al, 1965).

Who takes laxatives and why?

Evidence for substantial laxative consumption by the population was found in the community study of Connell et al (1965). Sixteen per cent of an industrial community and 29 per cent of a general practice population took laxatives. A striking increase in laxative consumption was shown with age, over 50 per cent of people aged 60 or more taking them, 28 per cent of the over 60s taking them more than once a week. It has also been reported that the people of South-east England consume 9000 gallons of liquid paraffin annually (*Nursing Times*, 1969).

Laxative consumption is not confined to the British Isles. Darlington (1966) reported that $200 million were spent in the USA on laxatives in 1966 and in 1969 one US company sold over 100 000 gallons of phospha-soda, a sodium phosphate preparation (McConnell, 1971). In Denmark in 1972, 266 kg of oxyphenisatin was consumed, partly as a compound analgesic preparation (Dietrichson et al, 1974); this is enough for a cathartic dose of this one laxative alone every two weeks for all the Danish population over 25. Perhaps even more remarkable is the involvement in the habit of the rural Bantu of South Africa. Bremner (1964) reports that 20 per cent of a selected group used laxatives habitually and a further 20 per cent used enemata.

The taking of laxatives to relieve constipation is only one facet of the picture. Much folklore, custom and cultural mystique surround the workings of the bowels making ritual rather than therapeutic purgation often the norm. Children particularly suffer because of the long-held belief that irregular or infrequent bowel habit is a source of ill health. Furthermore the rather grandiose names of many proprietary laxative preparations indicates their use for a variety of ill-defined conditions associated with the liver, kidney, back and blood. A dose of a laxative-containing medicine is often the first action many people take to obtain relief from abdominal discomfort, malaise, hangover or when feeling generally 'out of sorts'. Laxatives are also present in some slimming pills and some analgesics. To the Zulu, however, must go the prize for an original use of laxatives for seemingly they find them both aperient and aphrodisiac (Bremner, 1964).

Type of laxatives available

The past 10 years has seen a significant change in the type of laxative available and also a reduction in the number of different preparations being marketed. Standard texts of proprietary laxatives now contain fewer preparations than previously particularly those containing mixtures of cathartic substances. In addition many of the old herbal and vegetable extracts are going from *The Extra Pharmacopoeia*, perhaps because of the Medicines Act

(1968). Some of the more drastic agents such as croton oil, podophyllum and other irritant resins have also been dropped.

A more notable change has been the shift in emphasis to 'bulk' laxatives. These laxatives which are composed of various plant polysaccharides (or fibre) are present in 33 per cent of the preparations listed in *MIMS* (Table 6.1), where they are now equal in number to the anthracene purgatives (senna, etc). Overall, however, the anthracene group still remain by far the most widely available cathartic principal (57 per cent of all preparations) with the phenylmethanes (phenolphthalein, etc) following a long way behind at 19 per cent. 'Others' still account for a significant proportion and include liquid paraffin, lactulose, and a host of other 'traditional' ingredients. Of these liquid paraffin is the most widely used especially in hospital practice. Its true

Table 6.1 The percentage of laxative medicines listed in *MIMS* (September 1975), *The Extra Pharmacopoeia* (Martindale, 1972; proprietary or 'over-the-counter' preparations) and the *British National Formulary* (1974–1976), which contain the different types of cathartic substance. (Many preparations contain several different cathartic substances)

	Anthracene	Salts	Phenyl-methanes	Polysac-charides	Detergents	Miscellaneous
MIMS (48)[a]	33	15	17	33	27	23
Martindale (108)[b]	70	11	19	3	0	7
BNF (16)[a]	44	25	25	6	0	38
Overall (%)	57	14	19	12	8	14

[a] Total number of laxative preparations listed.
[b] Total number of laxative-containing preparations listed.

availability is not readily apparent from lists of pharmaceutical preparations as it is usually prescribed by its approved name and is not known by any particular brand name. Formulations containing bile salts are now far fewer and those containing oxyphenisatin have gone.

HOW DO LAXATIVES WORK?

The traditional view

The classic textbook description of laxatives has altered little over the years. Traditionally laxatives are described using terms such as irritant, bulk, stimulant, lubricant, emollient and colloid, and are classified into groups according to their alleged mode of action (Table 6.2) (*British Medical Journal*, 1964; Fingl, 1970). This view must now be modified for several reasons. The precise mechanism by which individual laxatives produce their cathartic effect is far from being fully documented or understood.

The traditional grouping of laxatives which led to the inclusion of such dissimilar substances as senna and phenolphthalein under one heading arose to some extent out of the clinical response produced by these substances in patients when compared with that due to other laxatives such as the saline purges. Differences in the delay before purgation occurred, its duration, extent and the altered character of the stool have been coupled with early pharmacological data to produce a manageable scheme for the bedside use of these drugs. However, in the light of present knowledge both of pharmacology and intestinal physiology some rearrangement is probably justifiable. Furthermore the use of words like 'irritant' implies the production of redness, swelling and inflammation in the gut which if it were so would have precluded the use of these agents long ago. Laxatives are not irritant in this sense and such a term is not helpful in conveying their likely effect on the gut.

In the absence of comprehensive knowledge about the way laxatives work how is one to group them? The pharmacological effect of a particular substance

Table 6.2 Traditional classification of laxatives

	Type	Example
1.	Irritant	Anthraquinones (senna, cascara, etc) Phenolphthalein Castor oil
2.	Bulk	Salts ($MgSO_4$, Na_2SO_4, etc) Plant mucilages, gums (Sterculia, Psyllium)
3.	Lubricant	Liquid paraffin Dioctyl sodiumsulphosuccinate

can usually be related to its chemical structure. The structure of most laxatives is known and many show marked similarities. It would seem appropriate therefore to group them according to their structure. Such a grouping has some backing in experimental pharmacology.

Current Views of Laxative Action

Anthracene derivatives

The best known, most widely investigated and most widely used group of laxatives are the anthracene derivatives which include such familiar names as senna, cascara, aloes, rhubarb and danthron. (Rhubarb in this instance does not refer to the domestic plant but to a plant of the Polygonaceae sp. called *Rheum palmatum* found in China from the rhizome of which laxative substances are extracted.) They are often referred to as the anthraquinones but include a variety of active cathartic substances derived from the 1,8-dihydroxyanthracene nucleus including anthraquinones, anthrones and dianthrones, most of which occur naturally as glycosides. Their structure and the variety of alternative names given to them have been summarised by Fairbairn and Moss (1970). Their efficacy has been proved many times in clinical trials and their widespread incorporation into laxative medicines (Table 6.1) indicates their well-established safety when used in appropriate circumstances.

The anthracene laxatives exert their effect by passing unchanged into the colon where bacteria hydrolyse the glycoside bond to produce free derivatives which then stimulate directly the myenteric plexus and produce defaecation (Fairbairn and Moss, 1970; Hardcastle and Wilkins, 1970; Godding, 1972). The glycosides are more active than the sugar-free aglycones in their purgative effect so it has been suggested that the glucose molecule protects the anthracene nucleus from oxidation to the less active quinone form during passage through the small bowel whilst also rendering it less readily absorbable by virtue of its large molecular size and greater water solubility (Fairbairn, 1949; Fairbairn and Moss, 1970). Hardcastle and Wilkins (1970) have shown that the glycosides are inactive when introduced into the human colon but after incubation with colonic bacteria stimulate colonic peristalsis which can be blocked by prior application of a local anaesthetic to the mucosa. Although at one time thought to be absorbed (Straub and Triendle, 1937) these compounds are probably not. They are not excreted in the milk of lactating mothers (Werthmann and Krees, 1973).

Direct stimulation of the neuronal plexuses of the colon might be sufficient to account for the laxative effect, but it remains to be seen whether these substances affect colonic electrolyte transport directly and thus have a secretory role of their own. Philips et al (1965) have shown that some anthracene purgatives inhibit sodium absorption in rabbit ileum.

Salines

Magnesium sulphate, hydroxide, carbonate, oxide, citrate, sodium sulphate and phosphate and sodium potassium tartrate are the commonly prescribed and used saline cathartics. It is easy to imagine how they work as all contain poorly absorbed ions which will retain fluid in the intestinal lumen. Their rapid action, within 3 to 6 h of ingestion suggests they affect upper gastrointestinal function mainly. Indeed a 10 g dose of magnesium sulphate increases ileostomy output considerably (Bouchier, Kellock and Manousos, 1963). It is therefore widely assumed that they exert their effect by virtue of their water-retaining property in the gut lumen. Harvey and Read (1975) however have suggested a more imaginative mode of action for these cathartics based on the observation that magnesium sulphate releases the hormone cholecystokinin-pancreozymin (CCK–PZ) from the intestinal mucosa (Harvey et al, 1973). CCK–PZ, or the salt itself, stimulate both small and large bowel motor activity together with small intestinal, pancreatic and biliary secretion thus leading to catharsis by an exaggerated motor and secretory response to normal stimuli. An osmotic effect on small bowel water transport nevertheless remains an additional possibility. Saline cathartics lower faecal pH (Agostini et al, 1972) but not ileal pH (Bouchier et al, 1963) and it is worth remembering that they may also interfere with drug absorption (Mattila, Takki and Jussila, 1974) and alter calcium metabolism (Ray and Rao, 1974).

Phenylmethanes
Phenolphthalein is the best known member of this group which also includes bisacodyl and oxyphenisatin. Although the chemical similarity of the three compounds is far from exact they are all substituted methanes containing one to three phenyl groups and have, for good reasons, been grouped together pharmacologically by various authors. Perhaps because they are easily obtained in a pure form these cathartics have been the subject of a large number of studies. Despite this the precise way in which they act is not clear, although there is nothing to contradict the view that they are in part absorbed from the gut, conjugated in the liver, excreted in the bile and after deconjugation by intestinal bacteria act by stimulating colonic peristalsis (Caldwell and Crane, 1929; Blick, Berardi and Wozasek, 1942; Hardcastle and Mann, 1968; Gooding, 1972). The various stages in their metabolism need further identification and there may well be a secretory component to add to their laxative effect.

There seems little doubt that phenolphthalein is absorbed from the small gut. Between 5 and 20 per cent of an oral dose appears in the urine with peak excretion occurring at 24 h. It is excreted largely in the conjugated form although whether this is mainly a glucuronide or sulphate conjugate seems to be in doubt. Free phenolphthalein may be detected where large doses have been given (Fantus and Dyniewicz, 1938; Pekanmäki and Salmi, 1961). Bile duct ligation experiments and studies in patients with biliary obstruction show that the cathartic effect is reduced or abolished in these circumstances (Steigmann, Barnard and Dyniewicz, 1938; Terada and Machii, 1965). Terada and Machii (1965) have suggested that the conjugate is inactive but requires further metabolism in the colon before producing its effect, a situation analogous with that for the anthracene purgatives. A similar cycle of events has been suggested for bisacodyl (Ferleman and Vogt, 1965), although this preparation also acts directly on the rectum when given as a suppository.

Aside from the ability of the phenylmethanes to stimulate colonic peristalsis they also alter intestinal electrolyte and sugar transport. In both animals and man inhibition of glucose absorption in the proximal small gut has been shown (Hand, Sanford and Smyth, 1966; Adamic and Bihler, 1967; Hart and McColl, 1967, 1968). Tyrosine transport is also inhibited in the rat (Bianchetti and Giachetti, 1972). Perhaps more important is their capacity to impair water and electrolyte absorption or induce secretion in the rat colon (Forth, Rummel and Baldauf, 1966; Ewe, 1972; Forth et al, 1972; Nell et al, 1973a, b). In this context it is interesting to note that the conjugated forms are inactive (Terada and Machii, 1965; Bianchetti and Giachetti, 1972; Forth et al, 1972). A clue to the mechanism whereby these laxatives impair transport processes may lie in the fact that they inhibit sodium–potassium ATPase in rat small gut microsomal preparations (Chignell, 1968). Again the conjugates are inactive in this respect.

Polysaccharides

Better known as the colloid or bulk laxatives this group of substances derived from plants all have one thing in common, namely that they are all polysaccharide polymers which are not broken down by the normal digestive processes of the human upper gastrointestinal tract. These substances enjoyed a great vogue in the 1930s and 1940s as laxatives but subsequently interest in them declined. Today they are once more enjoying a revival of popularity due in part to the allegedly 'natural' way they increase faecal bulk, and also as a consequence of the current debate concerning the value of fibre (under which heading they may be legitimately included) or lack of fibre in our diet. The polysaccharide laxatives may be subdivided into five types (Table 6.3) based

Table 6.3 Revised classification of laxative substances based broadly on their chemical structure and properties

	Class	Example
1.	Anthracene	Senna, aloes, rhubarb, cascara, frangula, danthron
2.	Salts	$MgSO_4$, Na_2SO_4, $Mg(OH)_2$, Na_2HPO_4
3.	Phenylmethanes	Phenolphthalein, bisacodyl, oxyphenisatin
4.	Polysaccharides	i. Cellulose and derivatives ii. Gums—sterculia iii. Mucilages—ispaghula, psyllium iv. Algal—agar, alginates v. Bran
5.	Detergents	Dioctyl sodium sulphosuccinate, bile salts, poloxalkol
6.	Miscellaneous	Lactulose, liquid paraffin, castor oil

on their origin in the plant kingdom and to some extent on their structure. Such a division provides a convenient reminder that different carbohydrate polymers may have distinct properties in the gut.

Cellulose and the more commonly used derivative methyl cellulose (Celevac, Cellucon, Cologel) are unbranched glucose polymers obtained by chemical treatment of plant tissues, particularly wood. In addition to their use as laxatives they are widely incorporated into slimming aids and appetite suppressants.

The plant gums such as those derived from the sterculiaciae family, e.g. sterculia (Inolaxine, Normacol) are sticky exudates obtained from these plants and comprise a complex mixture of highly branched polysaccharide substances. Many once popular gums are little used as laxatives today, e.g. gum arabic, gum acacia, tragacanth, bassora gum.

The mucilages come from a different part of the plant than that of the gums and cellulose. They are found in association with the food reserve carbohydrates of seeds and are obtained by grinding and sieving in a manner similar to flour. Those in current use are obtained from the Plantago family, sp. psyllium (Metamacil, Vi-Siblin) or from Ispaghula (Isogel, Fybogel). They are broadly similar in structure to the gums although tend to have more acidic units.

Algal polysaccharides are so called because they are derived from algae. They include substances such as agar, a sulphated polysaccharide, which is still used in some compound laxative preparations (Agarol), and alginic acid or its salts—alginates, which are little used today in this context.

Bran, the outer layers of the wheat grain obtained by milling, needs no introduction to today's gastroenterologist.

It is widely assumed that the polysaccharide laxatives act by virtue of their ability to retain water in the gut lumen and so promote peristalsis and improve bowel habit. Although this mode of action may be correct none of the many experiments done with these substances has established this, mainly because of the lack, until recently, of appropriate biochemical techniques. In vitro studies demonstrate that these laxatives have undoubted water retaining capacity even against an osmotic gradient. Broadly it would seem that their efficacy in this respect for those tested is of the order, alginates > cellulose derivatives > sterculia sp. > psyllium sp. and agar least (Ivy and Isaacs, 1938; Blythe, Gulesich and Tuthill, 1949; Berger, Ludwig and Wielich, 1953). Water however is not necessarily an appropriate medium for these swelling studies and in fact they almost all swell much less in saline, hydrochloric acid or modified intestinal juice (Gray and Tainter, 1941; Mulinos and Glass, 1953; Ireson and Leslie, 1970).

Their undoubted efficacy in vivo has been shown many times. Whilst direct comparison of experiments is not always possible in general, their in vitro water holding capacity is reflected in their in vivo ability to increase stool bulk with the sterculia gums better than the psyllium mucilages, the cellulose derivatives better than both and the now little used alginates best (Parsons, 1932; Tainter, 1943; Blythe et al, 1949; Berberian, Pauly and Tainter, 1952; Mulinos and Glass, 1953). Most of this work on polysaccharide laxatives was done before 1955 and was well reviewed by Tainter and Buchanan (1954). These studies of the mode of action of polysaccharide laxatives would bear repeating in the light of current thinking about their digestion by colonic bacteria and in addition their possible role in lipid absorption and mineral balance.

Detergents

The property common to bile salts, dioctyl sodium sulphosuccinate (DOSS) and polaxalkol despite their chemical dissimilarity is that they are all detergents. The property of detergency relates to the ability to lower surface tension particularly at an oil–water interface, hence the alternative designation 'surface-active' agents. How, in the light of current knowledge, this relates to their cathartic properties is not clear but when DOSS, for example, was first introduced as a laxative in the 1950s its detergent properties were considered central to its mode of action. DOSS was thought to act solely within the lumen of the bowel, at the surface of colonic contents, to enable penetration of water and so soften the stool. Thus it is sometimes referred to as a 'stool softener'. Whilst DOSS undoubtedly increases the frequency of defaecation in constipated subjects (Cass and Frederick, 1956; Hyland and Foran, 1968) its exact mode of action has not been documented. Recent work has suggested that DOSS, in a manner analogous with bile salts, alters intestinal water and electrolyte transport in human jejunum and colon and rat intestine and therein may lie its cathartic property (Donowitz and Binder, 1975; Saunders, Sillery and Rachmilewitz, 1975). Earlier, Lish (1961) had suggested that DOSS might act by releasing a hormone from the upper gut.

Bile salts have been the subject of intensive research of late particularly into their ability to cause secretion of water and electrolytes in the human gut. Given the right amount, in solution, in the appropriate place in the gut then their cathartic properties seem well established. However, the precise combination of hormonal, motor and secretory effects which lead to the production of an increased faecal weight and frequency by these detergent cathartics remains to be shown. The other physiological properties of bile salts in the gut have quite rightly received much more attention. Bile salts have however been shown to be related to faecal output in patients with limited ileal resections and so their role in regulating faecal weight in normal people deserves further study.

Other cathartics

Of the many other cathartics used from time to time only two deserve further mention, castor oil and lactulose. Those such as liquid paraffin and the plant resins jalap, colocynth and podophyllum are now used with diminishing frequency if at all. Their disadvantages have been outlined by Godding (1972).

Castor oil, although no longer listed in the *BNF* is still used particularly in obstetrics and on occasions when a rapid (2-4 h) effect is required. It has been the subject of several recent investigations as part of an attempt to define the relationship between diarrhoea, the fatty acids and hydroxy fatty acids found in the human gut in steatorrhoea. Castor oil contains the triglyceride of an hydroxy fatty acid, ricinoleic acid (12-OH oleic acid). The triglyceride is hydrolysed in the gut giving free ricinoleic acid which is probably less well absorbed than non-hydroxy fatty acids (Watson and Gordon, 1962; Watson et al, 1963). Ricinoleic acid both impairs water and electrolyte absorption and causes secretion in the jejunum and colon (Ammon and Phillips, 1973; Bright-Asare and Binder, 1973; Ammon, Thomas and Phillips, 1974; Stewart et al, 1975). Other fatty acids do this but the hydroxy fatty acids seem to be especially potent in this respect (Binder, 1973). Ricinoleic acid also alters motor activity in the large bowel either directly (Christensen and Freeman,

1972) or indirectly, possibly through the release of CCK from the jejunal mucosa (Meshkinpour, Dinoso and Lorber, 1974). There are thus several ways in which castor oil might bring about its cathartic effect.

Lactulose, a synthetic disaccharide which is not hydrolysed in the human small intestine, is the only new laxative of recent years. Objective data on its ability to sustain an improvement in bowel habit and increase faecal weight are remarkably few. In two groups of normal subjects studied for purposes other than a direct interest in the laxative effect lactulose did increase faecal weight (Agostini et al, 1972; Bown et al, 1974). An earlier study had shown in constipated geriatric patients that it reduced the need for regular laxatives of other types (Wesselius-de Casparis et al, 1968). Because it is unabsorbed lactulose passes into the large bowel when bacteria metabolise it to short chain fatty acids (SCFA), water, CO_2, H_2 and CH_4. These metabolites, especially lactic acid, are thought to impair colonic water absorption by an osmotic effect and so produce an increased faecal output. Like castor oil, lactulose has attracted a lot of attention for other reasons without its precise mode of action in producing catharsis being defined. Lactulose provides a model for the study of carbohydrate malabsorption, is widely used for the treatment of portasystemic encephalopathy in liver disease, has been used to quantitate hydrogen production in the gut and to measure mouth to caecum transit time. With reference to its possible cathartic effect, however, one fact does seem clear. Lactulose produces acidification of right-sided colonic contents, and to a more variable extent, of the faeces (Agostini et al, 1972; Bown et al, 1974). Faecal pH usually falls to more acid levels when there is the greatest increase in faecal output. Those subjects who show the least effect from lactulose also show least change in faecal pH. The cathartic efficacy of lactulose must therefore be related to the balance between its metabolism to SCFA, their absorption and any resultant changes in colonic absorptive function.

LAXATIVE ABUSE SYNDROME

The laxative abuse syndrome in which a patient takes excessive quantities of laxative in order to simulate ill-health or for other mysterious reasons is a small but problematic facet of the widespread use of laxatives. These patients are sometimes referred to as suffering from a cathartic colon. It may, however, be a little unfair to group all patients who take excessive amounts of laxative under one heading. 'Cathartic colon' should perhaps be reserved for those patients who because of longstanding constipation associated with abdominal discomfort have openly and knowingly consumed greater and greater numbers of laxative tablets until finally they develop a dilated unresponsive colon permanently loaded with faeces. Certainly the management and prognosis of the true 'cathartic colon' patient is better than for laxative abusers. The cathartic colon may be treated successfully by colectomy with ileo-rectal or sigmoid anastomosis (Jones, 1967; Plumley, 1973; Todd, 1973) whilst the covert laxative abuser, who sometimes develops an identical colonic picture is infinitely more difficult to manage and does not welcome any such permanent cure.

The problem of excessive cathartic use was originally recognised from the radiological changes in the colon (Heilbrun, 1943). Since the description by Schwartz and Relman (1953) of the associated metabolic problems it has been reported with increasing frequency. However, only a minority of the 100 or so cases in the literature show the classic features of abdominal discomfort, bowel symptoms, thirst and weakness with hypokalaemia and characteristic radiological and pathological features (see reviews by Sladen, 1972; Cummings, 1974).

CLINICAL FEATURES

This syndrome is almost entirely peculiar to women (only three men are reported) and presents at any age from 20 to 70. The commonest complaints are of a disturbed bowel habit, either diarrhoea or constipation, abdominal pain and discomfort, and weakness (French, Gaddie and Smith, 1956; *British Medical Journal*, 1966; Heizer et al, 1968; Cummings et al, 1974). Bowel symptoms may be completely denied by some patients who go to extraordinary lengths to conceal their diarrhoea by arranging for relatives to dispose of their faeces from the ward and even substituting them with normal stools (Love et al, 1971; Van Rooyen and Ziady, 1972). A history of constipation in childhood is often a significant feature as is some association with the medical profession (Coghill, McAllen and Edwards, 1959; Kramer and Pope, 1964). Other features include nausea and vomiting, weight loss, fever, skin pigmentation (Ramirez and Marieb, 1970; Van Rooyen and Ziady, 1972), finger clubbing which resolves when the laxatives are stopped (Clain et al, 1974; Silk, Gibson and Murray, 1975), bone pain, hypocalaemia, tetany and even osteomalacia (Meulengracht, 1938; Goldfinger, 1969; Frame et al, 1971). A psychiatric disorder is an invariable accompaniment of this syndrome and may be simple depression but more often the disorder is considered to be a variant of anorexia nervosa (Crisp, 1970; Halmi, Brodland and Loney, 1973; Stonehill, 1974). Self-medication with other substances, particularly diuretics, occurs and if accompanied by florid anorexia nervosa the prognosis is particularly poor.

The essence of the syndrome lies in its chronicity with patients repeatedly returning to outpatients and spending months in hospital (and more than one hospital) being investigated for their symptoms. Apart from the metabolic, pathological and radiological features detailed below a variety of other abnormal investigations usually turn up which can be looked upon as 'red-herrings' and only serve to mislead the physician. These include anaemia, a raised ESR, mild steatorrhoea (French et al, 1956; Coghill et al, 1959; Rawson, 1966; Heizer et al, 1968), impaired xylose absorption, gastrointestinal protein loss and impaired glucose tolerance (Heizer et al, 1968; Fleischer et al, 1969;

Frame et al, 1971; Clain et al, 1974). Abnormal pancreatic function is often suspected and there may be spurious hormonal changes (Cummings et al, 1974). Not surprisingly, a majority of these patients come to laparotomy and may even have definitive surgery, but it is a feature of the disease that they relapse soon after even this uncomfortable procedure.

METABOLIC DISTURBANCE

If repeated serum potassium determinations are done over 50 per cent of these patients show hypokalaemia. This is part of a generalised metabolic disturbance which includes weakness, cramps and paralysis, thirst, lassitude, sodium and potassium depletion, increased renin and aldosterone secretion and renal damage (Schwartz and Relman, 1953; Aithchison, 1958; Coghill et al, 1959; Litchfield, 1959; Wolff et al, 1968; Fleischer et al, 1969; Sladen, 1972). Renal damage takes the form of juxtaglomerular hyperplasia, tubular vacuolisation as seen with chronic potassium depletion, arteriolar thickening, focal pyelonephritis and sometimes calculi (Graeff and Schuurs, 1960; Fleischer et al, 1969; Van Rooyer and Ziady, 1972). Aminoaciduria, uraemia and hyperuricaemia may also occur. Other drugs such as analgesics are thought to contribute to the renal damage (Wainscott and Finn, 1974).

The genesis of this metabolic disturbance has been the subject of many investigations, but careful balance studies are fraught with difficulty in such patients. The probable sequence of events starts with sodium and water depletion as a consequence of the diarrhoea. This in turn leads to increased renin and consequently increased aldosterone secretion. Aldosterone causes increased loss of potassium into the urine, gut and most body fluids, and hypokalaemia ensues. Eventually the potassium depletion itself causes renal damage and impairment of renal function with loss of the normal renal compensating mechanisms and therefore further electrolyte losses. This, however, is an over-simplified view not only of the complex relations and feedback control in the renin–angiotensin–aldosterone system but also of the clinical syndrome. For example urine potassium losses may not be increased despite elevated aldosterone secretion levels (Houghton and Pears, 1958; Wolff et al, 1968; Love et al, 1971). Furthermore subjects with chronic diarrhoea from other causes do not develop such metabolic problems (Cummings et al, 1974). The hypokalaemia which dominates the metabolic picture in these subjects is probably of mixed aetiology. Whilst potassium is lost into the gut and initially also in the urine, many patients also vomit and have a highly selective and inadequate dietary intake. In addition some of them take diuretics. Under these circumstances normal homeostatic mechanisms break down and a progressive illness ensues (Aitchison, 1958; Wolff et al, 1968; Love et al, 1971; Fleming et al, 1975).

Fortunately most of this including the renal damage, is reversible once the purgative habit is discontinued. A characteristic feature of the recovery phase is oedema which is probably due to excess sodium retention under the influence of aldosterone. This 're-feeding' type oedema may be combated either by dietary sodium restriction or an aldosterone antagonist such as spironolactone (Graeff and Schuurs, 1960; Heizer et al, 1968; Love et al, 1971; Van Rooyen and Ziady, 1972).

RADIOLOGICAL CHANGES

Chronic cathartic abuse or excess produces a characteristic radiological picture in the bowel (Table 6.4), but it is important to remember that this picture occurs in only a minority of cases probably as few as 1 in 10 (Plum Weber and Sauer, 1960; Cummings et al, 1974). Its absence therefore does not exclude the laxative abuse syndrome. Radiological changes are seen first in the caecum, right colon and terminal ileum, the most characteristic finding being the absence of haustra (Heilbrun, 1943; Heilbrun and Bernstein, 1955). This is associated with a distensible or dilated colon and a generally featureless appearance. The terminal ileum is often involved and appears as a dilated

Table 6.4 Findings at barium enema in laxative abuse and cathartic colon

1. Absent haustra
2. Distensibility of colon
3. Smooth or mosaic mucosal pattern
4. Pseudostrictures
5. Right colon affected more than left
6. Terminal ileum dilated

tube-like structure associated with an incompetent ileocaecal valve (Jewell and Kline, 1954; Lemaitre et al, 1970). The mucosal pattern may be reported as smooth or as having a mottled or mosaic appearance (Heilbrun and Bernstein, 1955). Smooth tapering strictures (pseudostrictures) are seen which characteristically disappear and reappear elsewhere in the colon.

These appearances have been likened to long-standing or 'burnt-out' ulcerative colitis. The cathartic colon may however be distinguished from colitis by the lack of mucosal ulceration, distensibility and predilection for the right side. Rectal changes have not been reported (Marshak and Gershon, 1960; Rawson, 1966). Cathartic abuse and ulcerative colitis may rarely exist together (Coghill et al, 1959).

The inconsistency with which these radiological changes are found could be related to the type of laxative consumed. Where there are x-ray changes the laxative consumed is usually one of the anthracene group or in some early papers a vegetable laxative preparation containing the so-called drastics—jalap, podophyllum and colocynth. Other groups such as the phenylmethanes or polysaccharide cathartics do not seem to be associated with the x-ray changes.

PATHOLOGY

It is something of a disappointment to the physician who thinks he has a florid laxative abuser on his hands to do a sigmoidoscopy and find nothing, or at any rate nothing diagnostic. Although traditionally this syndrome is associated with melanosis coli this is in fact seen in the rectum in only a minority of patients. Nevertheless sigmoidoscopy is an important diagnostic step and may reveal, if not melanosis, a friable inflamed looking mucosa with contact bleeding, resembling colitis. Whatever the appearances, normal or otherwise, a rectal biopsy is essential as this may reveal changes not visible to the naked eye.

In the rectal biopsy a picture first described by Morson (1971) which is characteristic of cathartic abuse may be seen (Table 6.5). This includes infiltration of the mucosa with inflammatory cells, hypertrophy of the muscularis mucosae and possibly melanosis (Clain et al, 1974; Cummings et al, 1974). Unfortunately from the diagnostic viewpoint the rectum is usually least involved in the pathological change as surgical specimens have shown. If the

Table 6.5 Histological and pathological changes in the colon associated with excess laxative consumption

1. Mucosal inflammation
2. Melanosis
3. Hypertrophy of muscularis mucosae
4. Myenteric plexus damage
5. Atrophy of outer muscle layers
6. Proximal colon worse than distal colon

whole colon is examined the proximal part is worst affected showing thinning of the outer muscle layers, loss of haustra and sometimes sacculation (pseudodiverticula). The mucosa may be normal, atrophic or show what Morson and Dawson (1972) describe as a snakeskin or toad's back appearance which would perhaps account for the mosaic-like radiological picture sometimes seen. The muscularis mucosa is thickened, excess adipose tissue may be deposited in the submucosa and melanosis if present affects the right side mainly but stops abruptly at the ileocaecal valve. Smith (1972, 1973) has also described damage to the neurones of the myenteric plexus, which she has reproduced in mice with senna (Smith, 1968).

The inconsistent occurrence of these pathological changes in cathartic abuse may be related to the type of laxative used. Not only has myenteric plexus damage been associated with the anthracene group but so also has melanosis coli (Bockus, Willard and Bank, 1933; Zobel and Susnow, 1935). Melanosis has been experimentally produced in monkeys with cascara (Roden, 1940).

Melanosis coli has excited interest for many years. At the Mayo Clinic it was seen at about 0.8 per cent of sigmoidoscopies (Wittoesch, Jackman and

McDonald, 1958) and is almost exclusively related to the taking of laxatives. Chronic lead or mercury ingestion may lead to black pigmentation in the colon although this is extremely uncommon today (Williams, 1867; Pitt, 1891). The nature of the pigment in melanosis coli is in some doubt but is probably not melanin. It is present in the macrophages and may represent degenerating mitochondria or a complex with an anthracene derivative (Morson and Dawson, 1972; Smith, 1972). Melanosis regresses after the drugs have been discontinued and has usually gone within 12 months (Bockus et al, 1933; Wittoesch et al, 1958). Sigmoidoscopic changes may revert to normal more quickly (Clain et al, 1974). A remarkable case has been described in which melanosis was found not only in the colon of a chronic cascara user but also in the liver and was associated with disturbed liver function (Dubilier and Burkhart, 1974). Four years after stopping the cascara the previously black liver biopsy was normal and the patient well.

DIAGNOSIS (Table 6.6)

The fact that so many of these patients undergo extensive investigation and prolonged inpatient treatment before the precise nature of their illness is established suggests that this syndrome is not readily diagnosed. Like many other less common diseases the diagnosis may be made with a minimum of straightforward investigations but these can only be done once the possibility of laxative abuse has been raised in the clinician's mind. Suspicion should be aroused when confronted by a female patient with indeterminate abdominal symptoms, disturbed bowel function, weakness, tiredness, a poor appetite, perhaps vomiting and a psychiatric disorder. A history of constipation in childhood is often a significant pointer as is some association with the medical profession, i.e. a nurse, medical secretary or medical relative.

Once the possibility of the diagnosis has been raised a sigmoidoscopy and rectal biopsy should be done and a serum potassium. This is followed by a barium enema, at which stage a firm diagnosis can be made in about 30 per cent of cases. Unfortunately the findings are often so non-specific that it is necessary to admit the patient to the ward. This enables a faecal collection to be made to document the diarrhoea and specific chemical tests for laxative ingestion to be made. Fortunately over 70 per cent of the commonly taken laxatives contain either anthracene derivatives or phenylmethanes (Table 6.1), both of which can be detected in the urine and faeces.

Breakdown products of the anthracene group may be detected in the urine using the method described recently by Silk et al (1975) in which the urine is boiled with acid, mixed with carbon tetrachloride, filtered and dilute ammonia added in which a pink colour develops if the patient is taking significant quantities of these laxatives. Testing for the main member of the phenylmethane group, phenolphthalein, is much easier. If an aliquot of urine is made alkaline it will turn pink if this substance is present. This reaction may also occur with some of the anthracene purgatives and so is a useful simple test.

Alkalinisation will, however, detect only free phenolphthalein and as it is conjugated in the liver the test may be improved by first boiling the sample with 2N hydrochloric acid to hydrolyse any conjugates. Free phenolphthalein should be present in the urine if the subject is taking excessive amounts and will be present in only the conjugated form if intake is in the 'normal' range (Fantus and Dyniewicz, 1938; French et al, 1956; Pekanmäki and Salmi, 1961). Faeces may be tested in a similar way for the presence of both phenylmethanes and anthracenes. A specific method for the detection of bisacodyl is also reported (Heizer et al, 1968).

The detection of other laxatives is much more difficult, particularly the salts. Most of these ions are normal body constituents and so some sort of balance study would be required to detect excessive intake. This is clearly outside normal clinical practice. Stools, however, rarely contain much sulphate so a simple test for this such as the addition of barium chloride to an acid extract of faeces might prove useful although this has not been formally studied.

Table 6.6 Diagnosis of laxative abuse

1. Suspect
2. Sigmoidoscopy and rectal biopsy
3. Serum potassium
4. Barium enema
5. Urine and faecal tests for laxatives
6. Search

If there is good evidence to suspect laxative taking then it is generally accepted that the patient's possessions must be searched for them, particularly if they deny taking any such medication. This provides the opportunity to make the diagnosis unequivocal and, by examining any hidden store of purgatives again a few days later, to assess the quantity being taken. Clearly the utmost discretion is needed in the conduct of such an 'investigation'.

MANAGEMENT (Table 6.7)

There are no established guidelines for the management of these patients, nor has anyone reported their long term follow-up in any detail. Having made the diagnosis the clinician is usually faced with the situation of having a patient who is making herself ill with laxatives yet denies taking them. The first problem therefore is whether or not to confront the patient with the facts in the hope that she will see the folly of her ways and be able to return to normality. Many of the reported patients with this syndrome have been faced with the facts and a few have apparently done well (Martensson, 1953; Heizer et al, 1968; Ramirez and Marieb, 1970). This type of confrontation is not by any means always successful and more frequently leads to hostility and denial on the patient's part at first. Some then relent, give up the habit, only to return to it at a later stage. Others admit the problem and continue whilst a further group react badly, discharge themselves from hospital and presumably seek attention elsewhere. Occasionally there may be a frankly psychotic response leading to a suicide attempt (Houghton and Pears, 1958; Rawson, 1966; Cummings et al, 1974). It is because of these bad reactions that the alternative of not confronting the patient should be considered.

In view of the problems associated with telling the patient that she has been discovered and the invariable psychiatric illness present in such patients the advice of a psychiatrist should first be sought. Many of the patients have personality disorders but, in some, problems such as depression may be alleviated and life-threatening situations avoided. Since so few are able to give up the habit completely it is important that they be kept under review and supervised or supported in any way possible.

The problem of laxative abuse is essentially a chronic one and therefore some long-term management policy is useful. At the heart of the matter for the patient is a disordered bowel habit, often starting as constipation, and as such

Table 6.7 Management

1. Seek advice of psychiatrist
2. Discussion with patient?
3. Improve bowel habit
   i. Change to polysaccharide laxative
   ii. Increase dietary fibre intake
4. Monitor and correct electrolyte problems
5. Consider surgery if appropriate
6. Keep under review

may be amenable to treatment. If the patient's confidence can be won then it may be possible to wean her off laxatives likely to damage the large bowel (Smith, 1968, 1972) and substitute other types. Dietary modification may also be possible. Although chronic the syndrome is not entirely benign and every effort should be made to preserve good renal function by avoiding severe electrolyte disturbances. Serum electrolytes can be monitored and potassium supplements given if required. Those who give up the laxatives acutely may require sodium restriction and even diuretics.

The occasional patient may benefit from colectomy although in the disturbed patient this is not a step to undertake lightly. For those who present more of the picture of the cathartic colon it should be considered.

DANGERS OF LAXATIVES

Apart from the peculiar problem of the laxative abuse syndrome already described, laxatives are in general safe therapeutic agents especially in occasional doses. Those reports of their dangers which have appeared usually detail an inappropriate use, or accidental excess of a particular medication. Most of the inherently dangerous, drastic or toxic preparations have now gone from the pharmacopoeia and it is rare to encounter, for example, mercury-containing laxatives, once quite popular as Calomel, bringing about lethal complications (Wands et al, 1974).

Like all drugs, minor sensitivity reactions occur and these have been most frequently reported with phenolphthalein. The commonest form is a skin eruption but hypersensitivity has been blamed in a fatal case of encephalitis which occurred in a child following accidental ingestion of an excessive number of chocolate laxative tablets (Kendall, 1954). Minor skin complaints due to danthron have been reported recently (Bunney and Noble, 1974; Ippen, 1974).

Death due to laxatives is so unusual as to merit a report in the literature. Infants, however, seem to be especially vulnerable to excessive doses of laxative salts. A fatality in a neonate after a magnesium sulphate enema has been reported (Outerbridge, Papageorgiou and Stern, 1973) and hypocalcaemic tetany with coma has occurred both in infants (Levitt, Gessert and Finberg, 1973; Smith, Feldman and Furukawa, 1973) and an adult (Zipser, Bischel and Abrams, 1975) attributable to the high phosphate content of phosphosoda. In all these cases, however, the intake of laxatives greatly exceeded the recommended amount. A fatal outcome does sometimes follow a normal intake of a laxative as occurred with a polysaccharide laxative reported by Souter (1965), but in this case there was severe colonic disease present. One would imagine the polysaccharide laxatives to be relatively safe but the early literature contains a number of reports of problems encountered with them (Tainter and Buchanan, 1954).

Laxatives taken in combination with other medicines may also be a problem. Again the circumstances are unusual but Wainscott and Finn (1974) have suggested that the kidney damage which is associated with analgesics containing phenacetin may only occur when the patient has in addition taken laxatives. In 8 out of 10 of their analgesic nephropathy patients there was a history of concurrent chronic laxative ingestion. The patients were taking between 3 and 30 doses of laxative per week.

Taking combinations of laxatives has led to one of the most prominent arguments about the dangers of laxatives in recent years. This controversy is the probable link between hepatic damage, oxyphenisatin and dioctyl sodium sulphosuccinate (DOSS). The possibility that oxyphenisatin might cause liver damage first came to light several years ago in two reports from Reynolds et al, (1970) and McHardy and Balart (1970) describing jaundice and liver damage in a number of patients taking the laxative Dialose-Plus which contained oxyphenisatin, DOSS and methylcellulose. Several further reports followed (Keeley, Trey and Gottlieb, 1971; Pearson et al, 1971; Willing and Hecker, 1971; Gjone et al, 1972; Goldstein, Lam and Mistilis, 1973) describing a hepatitis-like reaction in the liver with chronic hepatitis and even cirrhosis in some patients. Oxyphenisatin was incriminated as the causal agent. It was then observed that the patients who had developed liver damage whilst taking oxyphenisatin had also been consuming DOSS, a detergent type laxative or 'wetting agent', included in the preparation (Naess, 1970; Godfrey, 1971). The suggestion then was that the detergent enhanced oxyphenisatin absorption and so in some patients produced a reaction in the liver. Subsequent research showed that DOSS did indeed enhance the toxicity of a variety of laxatives (Dobbs, Dawes and Whittle, 1972; Smith, 1972) and also that DOSS itself was absorbed to some extent and was toxic to in vitro liver cell cultures although not to the extent of a DOSS-oxyphenisatin combination (Dujovne and Shoeman, 1972, 1973). However, the final evidence against oxyphenisatin came when patients with hepatic damage who were challenged with the pure substance rapidly developed signs and evidence of further liver damage (Reynolds, Peters and Yamada, 1971; Dietrichson et al, 1974). Oxyphenisatin has now been withdrawn. DOSS remains in wide use as a laxative both alone and in combination with other preparations. The question remains as to what effect these detergent-like substances have on the absorption and metabolism of drugs in general.

SUMMARY AND CONCLUSIONS

Do we really need laxatives or should their use gradually be discontinued? Although there are some dangers associated with them and like most things they are open to abuse by a tiny minority of people, there are not really sufficient grounds for banning them on the basis of safety. But what about the real need for them by the general population? If it is assumed that they are effective mainly in relieving constipation (i.e. are not intended to treat liver, kidney or back disorders, etc) then alternative forms of management for this must be considered. Simple constipation can in all probability be corrected by appropriate dietary changes, such as increasing fibre intake and therefore the use of laxatives for this problem could be reduced. Some more organic causes of constipation cannot be overcome in this way and for these patients laxatives would seem to offer a suitable therapy (Jones, 1972). Their use in hospital practice is well established but should not become routine in any way (Witts, 1937). They are, however, a valuable adjunct to treatment in certain cases of poisoning, infestation with parasites and hepatic coma and in preparation for colonoscopy, bowel surgery and some x-ray procedures. Furthermore the fascinating effect some laxatives have on gastrointestinal salt and water absorption makes them a suitable model for investigation of intestinal transport processes.

Laxatives would seem to have a legitimate place in the pharmacopoeia. Unfortunately some patients will continue to abuse them and so try the diagnostic ability of everyone, and whilst the pressures of our way of life and the suggested inappropriate balance in our diet concentrates people's attention on their bowels, the use of laxatives will remain widespread.

REFERENCES

Adamic, S. & Bihler, I. (1967) Inhibition of intestinal sugar transport by phenolphthalein. *Molecular Pharmacology*, **3**, 188–194.

Agostini, L., Down, P. F., Murison, J. & Wrong, O. M. (1972) Faecal ammonia and pH during lactulose administration in man: comparison with other cathartics. *Gut*, **13**, 859–866.

Aitchison, J. D. (1958) Hypokalaemia following chronic diarrhoea from overdose of cascara and a deficient diet. *Lancet*, **2**, 75–76.

Ammon, H. V. & Phillips, S. F. (1973) Inhibition of colonic water and electrolyte absorption by fatty acids in man. *Gastroenterology*, **65**, 744–749.

Ammon, H. V., Thomas, P. H. & Phillips, S. F. (1974) Effects of oleic and ricinoleic acids on net jejunal water and electrolyte movement. *Journal of Clinical Investigation*, **53**, 374–379.

Berberian, D. A., Pauly, R. J. & Tainter, M. L. (1952) Comparison of a plain methylcellulose with a compound bulk laxative tablet. *Gastroenterology*, **20**, 143–148.

Berger, F. M., Ludwig, B. J. & Wielich, K. H. (1953) Hydrophilic and acid binding properties of alginates. *American Journal of Digestive Diseases*, **20**, 39–42.

Bianchetti, A. & Giachetti, A. (1972) The effect of irritant cathartics on the intestinal transport of tyrosine in rat and guinea-pig. *Archives internationales de Pharmacodynamie et de Thérapie*, **196**, Suppl., 155–157.

Binder, H. J. (1973) Fecal fatty acids—mediators of diarrhea? *Gastroenterology*, **65**, 847–850.

Blick, P., Berardi, J. B. & Wozasek, O. (1942) The mode of action of the laxative action of phenolphthalein. *American Journal of Digestive Diseases*, **9**, 292–297.

Blythe, R. H., Gulesich, J. J. & Tuthill, H. L. (1949) Evaluation of hydrophilic properties of bulk laxatives including the new agent sodium carboxymethyl cellulose. *Journal of the American Pharmaceutical Association*, **39**, 59–64.

Bockus, H. L., Willard, J. H. & Bank, J. (1933) Melanosis coli: the etiologic significance of the anthracene laxatives: a report of 46 cases. *Journal of the American Medical Association*, **101**, 1–6.

Bouchier, I. A. D., Kellock, T. D. & Manousos, O. (1963) The origin of faecal fat in subjects without steatorrhoea. In *Proceedings of the Second World Congress of Gastroenterology*, Munich, 1962, pp. 659–661. Basel and New York: Karger.

Bown, R. L., Gibson, J. A., Sladen, G. E., Hicks, B. & Dawson, A. M. (1974) Effect of lactulose and other laxatives on ileal and colonic pH as measured by a radiotelemetry device. *Gut*, **15**, 999–1004.

Bremner, C. G. (1964) Ano-rectal disease in the South African Banu. *Suid-Afrikaanse Tydskrif vir Chirurgie*, **2**, 119–123.

Bright-Asare, P. & Binder, H. J. (1973) Stimulation of colonic secretion of water and electrolytes by hydroxy fatty acids. *Gastroenterology*, **64**, 81–88.

British Medical Journal (1964) Today's drugs. Laxatives and purgatives, **1**, 1096–1099.

British Medical Journal (1966) A case of purgative addiction, **1**, 1344–1348.

British Medical Journal (1972) Laxative jaundice, **1**, 325.

Bunney, M. H. & Noble, I. M. (1974) Red skin and dorbanex. *British Medical Journal*, **3**, 731.

Caldwell, G. H. & Crane, A. W. (1929) The influence of phenolphthalein on intestinal movements. *Radiology*, **13**, 403–412.

Cass, L. J. & Frederick, W. S. (1956) Doxinate in the treatment of constipation. *American Journal of Gastroenterology*, **26**, 691–698.

Chignell, F. (1968) The effect of phenolphthalein and other purgative drugs on rat intestinal (Na^+–K^+)-adenosine triphosphatase. *Biochemical Pharmacology*, **17**, 1207–1212.

Christensen, J. & Freeman, B. W. (1972) Circular muscle electromyogram in the cat colon: local effect of sodium ricinoleate. *Gastroenterology*, **63**, 1011–1015.

Clain, J., Novis, B. H., Bank, S., Kahn, L. B. & Marks, I. N. (1974) Cathartic colon with unusual histological features. *South African Medical Journal*, **48**, 216–218.

Coghill, N. F., McAllen, P. M. & Edwards, F. (1959) Electrolyte losses associated with the taking of purges investigated with aid of sodium and potassium radioisotopes. *British Medical Journal*, **1**, 14–19.

Connell, A. M., Hilton, C., Irvine, G., Lennard-Jones, J. E. & Misiewicz, J. J. (1965) Variation of bowel habit in two population samples. *British Medical Journal*, **2**, 1095–1099.

Crisp, A. H. (1970) Anorexia nervosa, 'feeding disorder', 'nervous malnutrition' or 'weight phobia'? In *World Review of Nutrition and Dietetics*, ed. Bourne, G. H., Vol. 12, pp. 452–504. London: Pitman.
Cummings, J. H. (1974) Laxative abuse. *Gut*, **15**, 758–766.
Cummings, J. H., Sladen, G. E., James, O. F. W., Sarner, M. & Misiewicz, J. J. (1974) Laxative-induced diarrhoea: a continuing clinical problem. *British Medical Journal*, **1**, 537–541.
Darlington, R. C. (1966) O-T-C laxatives. *Journal of the American Pharmaceutical Association*, N.S. **6**, 470–474.
Department of Health and Social Services. Annual Reports of the Department of Health and Social Security, 1961–1969. London: HMSO.
Department of Health and Social Services. Health and Personal Social Services Statistics for England, 1972, 1973, 1974. London: HMSO.
Dietrichson, O., Juhl, E., Nielson, J. O., Oxlund, J. J. & Christoffersen, P. (1974) The incidence of oxyphenisatin-induced liver damage in chronic non-alcoholic liver disease. A controlled investigation. *Scandinavian Journal of Gastroenterology*, **9**, 473–478.
Dobbs, H. E., Dawes, R. L. F. & Whittle, B. A. (1972) Investigations of toxic interactions of synthetic laxatives with a wetting agent. *Proceedings of the European Society for the Study of Drug Toxicity*, **XIV**, 243–246.
Donowitz, M. & Binder, H. J. (1975) Effect of dioctyl sodium sulfosuccinate on colonic fluid and electrolyte movement. *Gastroenterology*, **69**, 941–950.
Dubilier, L. D. & Burkhart, R. C. (1974) Melanosis coli with liver involvement. *Gastroenterology*, **67**, A.12/789.
Dujovne, C. A. & Shoeman, D. W. (1972) Toxicity of a hepatotoxic laxative preparation in tissue culture and excretion in bile in man. *Clinical Pharmacology and Therapeutics*, **13**, 602–608.
Dujovne, C. H. & Shoeman, D. W. (1973) Surfactant laxatives and hepatotoxicity. *Annals of Internal Medicine*, **79**, 137–138.
Ewe, K. (1972) Effect of laxatives on intestinal water and electrolyte transport. *European Journal of Clinical Investigation*, **2**, 283.
Fairbairn, J. W. (1949) The active constituents of the vegetable purgatives containing anthracene derivatives. I. Glycosides and aglycones. *Journal of Pharmacy and Pharmacology*, **1**, 683–691.
Fairbairn, J. W. & Moss, M. S. R. (1970) The relative purgative activities of 1,8-dihydroxyanthracene derivatives. *Journal of Pharmacy and Pharmacology*, **22**, 584–593.
Fantus, B. & Dyniewicz, J. M. (1938) Phenolphthalein studies. Elimination of phenolphthalein. *Journal of the American Medical Association*, **110**, 796–799.
Ferleman, G. & Vogt, W. (1965) Entacetglierung und Resorption von phenolischen laxantien. *Archiv für experimentelle Pathologie und Pharmakologie*, **250**, 479–487.
Fingl, E. (1970) Cathartics and laxatives. In *The Pharmacological Basis of Therapeutics*, 4th edn, ed. Goodman, L. S. & Gilman, A., pp. 1020–1031. London and New York: Macmillan.
Finn, R. & Wainscott, J. S. (1975) Laxan nephropathy. *Lancet*, **1**, 1202.
Fleischer, N., Brown, H., Graham, D. Y. & Deleña, S. (1969) Chronic laxative-induced hyperaldosteronism and hypercalemia simulating Bartter's syndrome. *Annals of Internal Medicine*, **70**, 791–798.
Fleming, B. J., Genuth, S. M., Gould, A. B. & Kamionkowski, M. D. (1975) Laxative-induced hypokalemia, sodium depletion and hyperreninemia. *Annals of Internal Medicine*, **83**, 60–62.
Forth, W., Rummel, W. & Baldauf, J. (1966) Wasser und Electrolytbewegung am Dunnund Dickdarm unter dem Einfluss von Laxantion ein Beitrag zur Klarung ihres Wirkungmechanismus. *Archiv für experimentelle Pathologie und Pharmakologie*, **254**, 18–32.
Forth, W., Nell, G., Rummel, W. & Andres, H. (1972) The hydragogue and laxative effect of the sulfuric acid ester and the free diphenol of 4,4′-dihydroxydiphenyl-(pyridyl-2)-methane. *Archives of Pharmacology* (N-S), **274**, 46–53.
Frame, B., Guiang, H. L., Frost, H. M. & Reynolds, W. A. (1971) Osteomalacia induced by laxative (phenolphthalein) ingestion. *Archives of Internal Medicine*, **128**, 794–796.
French, J. M., Gaddie, R. & Smith, N. (1956) Diarrhoea due to phenolphthalein. *Lancet*, **1**, 551–553.

Gjone, E., Blomhoff, J. P., Ritland, S., Elgjo, K. & Husby, G. (1972) Laxative-induced chronic liver disease. *Scandinavian Journal of Gastroenterology*, **7**, 395–402.

Godding, E. W. (1972) Therapeutic agents. In *Management of Constipation*, ed. Jones, F. A. & Godding, E. W., pp. 38–76. Oxford: Blackwell.

Godfrey, H. (1971) Dangers of dioctyl sodium sulfosuccinate in mixtures. *Journal of the American Medical Association*, **215**, 643.

Goldfinger, P. (1969) Hypokalemia, metabolic acidosis and hypocalcemic tetany in a patient taking laxatives. *Journal of the Mount Sinai Hospital*, **36**, 113–116.

Goldstein, G. B., Lam, K. C. & Mistilis, S. P. (1973) Drug-induced active chronic hepatitis. *American Journal of Digestive Diseases*, **18**, 177–184.

Graeff, J. de & Schuurs, M. A. M. (1960) Severe potassium depletion caused by the abuse of laxatives. One patient followed for 8 years. *Acta medica scandinavica*, **166**, 407–422.

Gray, H. & Tainter, M. L. (1941) Colloid laxatives available for clinical use. *American Journal of Digestive Diseases*, **8**, 130–139.

Halmi, K., Brodland, G. & Loney, J. (1973) Prognosis in anorexia nervosa. *Annals of Internal Medicine*, **78**, 907–909.

Hand, D. W., Sanford, P. A. & Smyth, D. H. (1966) Polyphenolic compounds and intestinal transfer. *Nature*, **209**, 618.

Hardcastle, J. D. & Mann, C. V. (1968) Study of large bowel peristalsis. *Gut*, **9**, 512–520.

Hardcastle, J. D. & Wilkins, J. L. (1970) The action of sennosides and related compounds on human colon and rectum. *Gut*, **11**, 1038–1042.

Hart, S. L. & McColl, I. (1967) The effect of purgative drugs on the intestinal absorption of glucose. *Journal of Pharmacy and Pharmacology*, **19**, 70–71.

Hart, S. L. & McColl, I. (1968) The effect of the laxative oxyphenisatin on the intestinal absorption of glucose in rat and man. *British Journal of Pharmacology and Chemotherapy*, **32**, 683–686.

Harvey, R. F., Dowsett, L., Hartog, M. & Read, A. E. (1973) A radio-immunoassay for cholecystokinin-pancreozymin. *Lancet*, **2**, 826–828.

Harvey, R. F. & Read, A. E. (1975) Mode of action of the saline purgative. *American Heart Journal*, **89**, 810–812.

Heilbrun, N. (1943) Roentgen evidence suggesting enterocolitis associated with prolonged cathartic abuse. *Radiology*, **41**, 486–491.

Heilbrun, N. & Bernstein, C. (1955) Roentgen abnormalities of the large and small intestine associated with prolonged cathartic ingestion. *Radiology*, **65**, 549–556.

Heizer, W. D., Warshaw, A. L., Waldmann, T. A. & Laster, L. (1968) Protein-losing gastroenteropathy and malabsorption associated with factitious diarrhoea. *Annals of Internal Medicine*, **68**, 839–852.

Houghton, B. J. & Pears, M. A. (1958) Chronic potassium depletion due to purgation with cascara. *British Medical Journal*, **1**, 1328–1330.

Hyland, C. M. & Foran, J. D. (1968) Dioctyl sodium sulphosuccinate as a laxative in the elderly. *Practitioner*, **200**, 698–699.

Ippen, H. (1974) Red skin and dorbanex. *British Medical Journal*, **4**, 345.

Ireson, J. D. & Leslie, G. B. (1970) An in vitro investigation of colloidal bulk-forming laxatives. *The Pharmaceutical Journal*, **205**, 540.

Ivy, A. C. & Isaacs, B. L. (1938) Karaya gum as a mechanical laxative: an experimental study on animals and man. *American Journal of Digestive Diseases*, **5**, 315–321

Jewell, F. C. & Kline, J. R. (1954) The purged colon. *Radiology*, **62**, 368–371.

Jones, F. A. (1967) Cathartic colon. *Proceedings of the Royal Society of Medicine*, **60**, 503–504.

Jones, F. A. (1972) Management of constipation in adults. In *Management of Constipation*, ed. Jones, F. A. & Godding, E. W., pp. 97–131. Oxford: Blackwell.

Keeley, A. F., Trey, C. & Gottlieb, L. S. (1971) Dialose-plus associated jaundice: documentation of abnormal liver function and ultrastructure after challenge. *Gastroenterology*, **60**, 195.

Kendall, A. C. (1954) Fatal case of encephalitis after phenolphthalein ingestion. *British Medical Journal*, **2**, 1461–1462.

Kramer, P. & Pope, C. E. (1964) Factitious diarrhoea induced by phenolphthalein. *Archives of Internal Medicine*, **114**, 634–636.

Lemaitre, G., L'Hermine, C., Decoulx, M., Houcke, M. & Linquette, M. (1970) Aspect radiologique des colites chronique par abus de laxatif. A propos quatre observations. *Journal Belge de Radiologie*, **53**, 339–345.

Levitt, M., Gessert, C. & Finberg, L. (1973) Inorganic phosphate (laxative) poisoning resulting in tetany in an infant. *Journal of Paediatrics*, **82**, 479–481.

Lish, P. M. (1961) Some pharmacological effects of dioctyl sodium sulfosuccinate on the gastrointestinal tract of the rat. *Gastroenterology*, **41**, 580–584.

Litchfield, J. A. (1959) Low potassium syndrome resulting from the use of purgative drugs. *Gastroenterology*, **37**, 483–488.

Love, D. R., Brown, J. J., Fraser, R., Lever, A. F., Robertson, J. I. S., Timbury, G. C., Thomson, S. & Tree, M. (1971) An unusual case of self-induced electrolyte depletion. *Gut*, **12**, 284–290.

Marshak, R. H. & Gerson, A. (1960) Cathartic colon. *American Journal of Digestive Diseases*, **5**, 724–727.

Martensson, J. (1953) Hypopotassaemia with paresis following the abuse of laxatives. *Nordisk Medicin*, **49**, 56–57.

Martindale (1972) *The Extra Pharmacopoeia* 26th edn, ed. Blacow, N. W. Pharmaceutical Press.

Mattilla, M. J., Takki, S. & Jussila, J. (1974) Effect of sodium sulphate and castor oil on drug absorption from the human intestine. *Annals of Clinical Research*, **6**, 19–24.

McConnell, T. H. (1971) Fatal hypocalcemia from phosphate absorption from laxative preparation. *Journal of the American Medical Association*, **216**, 147–148.

McHardy, G. & Balart, L. A. (1970) Jaundice and oxyphenisatin. *Journal of the American Medical Association*, **211**, 83–85.

Meshkinpour, H., Dinoso, V. P., Jr & Lorber, S. H. (1974) Effect of intraduodenal administration of essential amino acids and sodium oleate on motor activity of the sigmoid colon. *Gastro-enterology*, **66**, 373–377.

Meulengracht, E. (1938) Osteomalacia of the spine following the abuse of laxatives. *Lancet*, **235**, 774–776.

MIMS (1975) **17**, pp. 21–24.

Morson, B. C. (1971) Histopathology of cathartic colon. *Gut*, **12**, 867–868.

Morson, B. C. & Dawson, I. M. P. (1972) *Gastrointestinal Pathology*, pp. 587. Oxford: Blackwell.

Mulinos, M. G. & Glass, G. B. J. (1953) Treatment of constipation with new hydrasorbent material derived from kelp. *Gastroenterology*, **24**, 385–393.

Naess, K. (1970) Oxyphenisatin and jaundice. *Journal of the American Medical Association*, **212**, 1961.

Nell, G., Overhoff, H., Forth, W., Kulenkampff, H., Specht, W. & Rummel, W. (1973a) Influx and efflux of sodium in jejunal and colonic segments of rats under the influence of oxyphenisatin. *Archiv für experimentelle Pathologie und Pharmakologie*, **277**, 53–60.

Nell, G., Overhoff, H., Forth, W. & Rummel, W. (1973b) The influence of water gradients and oxyphenisatin on the net transfer of sodium and water in the rat colon. *Archive für experimentelle Pathologie und Pharmakologie*, **277**, 363–372.

Nursing Times (1969) p. 1564.

Outerbridge, E. W., Papageorgiou, A. & Stern, L. (1973) Magnesium sulfate enema in a newborn. Fatal systemic magnesium absorption. *Journal of the American Medical Association*, **224**, 1392–1393.

Parsons, F. B. (1932) Constipation and mechanical laxatives. *Practitioner*, **129**, 70–83.

Pearson, A. J. G., Grainger, J. M., Scheur, P. J. & McIntyre, N. (1971) Jaundice due to oxyphenisatin. *Lancet*, **1**, 994–996.

Pekanmäki, K. & Salmi, H. A. (1961) The glucuronide conjugation of phenolphthalein in man. *Annales medicinae experimentalis et biologiae Fenniae*, **39**, 302–305.

Philips, R. A., Love, A. H. G., Mitchell, T. C. & Neptune, E. M. (1965) Cathartics and the sodium pump. *Nature (Lond.)*, **206**, 1367–1368.

Pitt, G. N. (1891) Colon pigmented black throughout with lead. *Transactions of the Pathological Society of London*, **42**, 109.

Plum, G. E., Weber, H. M. & Sauer, W. G. (1960) Prolonged cathartic abuse resulting in Roentgen evidence suggestive of enterocolitis. *American Journal of Roentgenology, Radium Therapy and Nuclear Medicine*, **83**, 919–925.

Plumley, P. F. (1973) Radical surgery in the treatment of cathartic colon. *Proceedings of the Royal Society of Medicine*, **66**, 243–244.
Ramirez, B. & Marieb, N. J. (1970) Hypokalemic metabolic alkalosis due to Carter's Little Pills. *Connecticut Medicine*, **34**, 169–170.
Rawson, M. D. (1966) Cathartic colon. *Lancet*, **1**, 1121–1124.
Ray, A. K. & Rao, D. B. (1974) Hypercalcemia and malignant disease in the elderly: magnesium sulphate therapy. *Journal of the American Geriatric Society*, **22**, 413–415.
Reynolds, T. B., Lapin, A. C., Peters, R. L. & Yamahiro, H. S. (1970) Puzzling jaundice. *Journal of the American Medical Association*, **211**, 86–90.
Reynolds, T. B., Peters, R. L. & Yamada, S. (1971) Chronic active and lupoid hepatitis caused by a laxative, oxyphenisatin. *New England Journal of Medicine*, **285**, 813–820.
Roden, D. (1940) Melanosis coli. A pathological study: its experimental production in monkeys. *Irish Journal of Medical Sciences*, **6**, 654–674.
Saunders, D. R., Sillery, J. & Rachmilewitz, D. (1975) Effect of dioctyl and sodium sulfosuccinate on structure and function of rodent and human intestine. *Gastroenterology*, **69**, 380–386.
Schwartz, W. B. & Relman, A. S. (1953) Metabolic and renal studies in chronic potassium depletion resulting from overuse of laxatives. *Journal of Clinical Investigation*, **32**, 258–271.
Silk, D. B. A., Gibson, J. A. & Murray, C. R. H. (1975) Reversible finger clubbing in a case of purgative abuse. *Gastroenterology*, **68**, 790–794.
Sladen, G. E. (1972) Effects of chronic purgative abuse. *Proceedings of the Royal Society of Medicine*, **65**, 288–291.
Smith, B. (1968) Effect of irritant purgatives on the myenteric plexus in the man and mouse. *Gut*, **9**, 139–143.
Smith, B. F. (1972) *The Neuropathology of the Alimentary Tract*, pp. 92. London: Edward Arnold.
Smith, B. (1973) Pathologic changes in the colon produced by anthraquinone purgatives. *Diseases of the Colon and Rectum*, **16**, 455–458.
Smith, M. S., Feldman, K. W. & Furukawa, C. T. (1973) Coma in an infant due to hypertonic sodium phosphate medication. *Journal of Pediatrics*, **82**, 481–482.
Souter, W. A. (1965) Bolus obstruction of gut after use of hydrophilic colloid laxatives. *British Medical Journal*, **1**, 166–168.
Steigmann, F., Barnard, R. D. & Dyniewicz, J. M. (1938) Phenolphthalein studies: phenolphthalein in jaundice. *American Journal of Medical Science*, **196**, 673–688.
Stewart, J. J., Gaginella, T. S., Olsen, W. A. & Bass, P. (1975) Inhibitory actions of laxatives on motility and water and electrolyte transport in the gastrointestinal tract. *Journal of Pharmacology and Experimental Therapeutics*, **192**, 458–467.
Stonehill, E. (1974) Laxative-induced diarrhoea. *British Medical Journal*, **2**, 334.
Straub, W. & Triendle, E. (1937) Theaorie der Abfuhrwirkung die Folia Sennas und ihre wirksamen Inhaltsstoffe. *Archiv für experimentelle Pathologie und Pharmakologie*, **185**, 1–19.
Tainter, M. L. (1943) Methyl cellulose as a colloid laxative. *Proceedings of the Society for Experimental Biology in Medicine*, **54**, 77–79.
Tainter, M. L. & Buchanan, O. H. (1954) Quantitative comparisons of colloidal laxatives. *Annals of the New York Academy of Sciences*, **58**, 438–452.
Terada, Y. & Machii, T. (1965) On the mechanism of diarrhoea due to phenolphthalein. *Mie Medical Journal*, **14**, 251–259.
Todd, I. P. (1973) Cathartic colon: surgical aspects. *Proceedings of the Royal Society of Medicine*, **66**, 244–245.
Van Rooyen, R. J. & Ziady, F. (1972) Hypokalemic alkalosis following the abuse of purgatives. Case report. *South African Medical Journal*, **46**, 998–1003.
Wainscott, J. S. & Finn, R. (1974) Possible role of laxatives in analgesic nephropathy. *British Medical Journal*, **4**, 697–698.
Wands, J. R., Weiss, S. W., Yardley, J. H. & Maddrey, W. C. (1974) Chronic inorganic mercury poisoning due to laxative abuse. A clinical and ultrastructural study. *American Journal of Medicine*, **57**, 92–101.
Watson, W. C. & Gordon, R. S. (1962) Studies on the digestion, absorption and metabolism of castor oil. *Biochemical Pharmacology*, **11**, 229–236.

Watson, W. C., Gordon, R. S., Karmen, A. & Jover, A. (1963) The absorption and excretion of castor oil in man. *Journal of Pharmacy and Pharmacology*, **15**, 183–188.

Werthmann, M. W. & Krees, S. V. (1973) Quantitative excretion of senokot in human breast milk. *Medical Annals of the District of Colombia*, **42**, 4–5.

Wesselius-de Casparis, A., Braadbaart, S., Van de Bergh-Bohlken, G. E. & Mimica, M. (1968) Treatment of chronic constipation with lactulose syrup: results of a double-blind study. *Gut*, **9**, 84–86.

Williams, C. T. (1867) Black deposit in the large intestine from the presence of mercury. *Transactions of the Pathological Society of London*, **18**, 111–114.

Willing, R. L. & Hecker, R. (1971) Oxyphenisatin and liver damage. *Australian and New Zealand Journal of Medicine*, **3**, 301–302.

Wittoesch, J. H., Jackman, R. J. & McDonald, J. R. (1958) Melanosis coli: general review and a study of 882 cases. *Diseases of the Colon and Rectum*, **1**, 172–180.

Witts, L. J. (1937) Ritual purgation in modern medicine. *Lancet*, **1**, 427–430.

Wolff, H. P., Vecsei, P., Krück, F., Roscher, S., Brown, J. J., Düsterdieck, G. O., Lever, A. F. & Robertson, J. I. S. (1968) Psychiatric disturbance leading to potassium depletion, sodium depletion, raised plasma renin concentration, and secondary hyperaldosteronism. *Lancet*, **1**, 257–261.

Zipser, R. D., Bischel, M. D. & Abrams, D. E. (1975) Hypocalcemic tetany due to sodium phosphate ingestion in acute renal failure. *Nephron*, **14**, 378–381.

Zobel, A. J. & Susnow, D. A. (1935) Melanosis coli: its clinical significance. *Archives of Surgery*, **30**, 974–979.

7
ALCOHOL AND THE GASTROINTESTINAL TRACT

N. A. G. Mowat   P. W. Brunt

Alcohol is at the same time both a food and a dangerous drug—a pleasure and a poison. The widespread toxic effects of alcohol are now becoming better understood especially its effects upon the gastrointestinal tract which is the site of its absorption, assimilation and metabolism. Alcohol-related disease is becoming a major world health problem. Cirrhosis of the liver, much of it alcohol related, is now the seventh overall commonest cause of death in the USA and continues to show a steady rise (Popper, 1975).

This review attempts to outline some of the recent advances in our understanding of alcohol-induced gastrointestinal injury. No attempt is made to cover the psychosocial aspects of alcoholic disease. There has been much recent work and several excellent reviews on the relation of alcohol to the liver and hence only certain selected aspects are emphasised. By contrast much less has been written on the relation of alcohol to the alimentary tract and pancreas and in these aspects an attempt is made to be more comprehensive.

The term alcohol is used throughout this review to mean *ethanol*. While the congeners and higher alcohols which are present in proprietary beverages in small quantities probably play little role in 'alcohol-related disease' by comparison with ethanol itself, there is little hard evidence available and this subject will not be discussed in this review.

ABSORPTION AND METABOLISM OF ETHANOL

This topic has been well reviewed recently by several authors (Pawan, 1972; Hawkins and Kalant, 1972; Lieber, 1973a, b, 1975a, b; Myerson, 1973; Krebs, 1974). The characteristics of the ethanol molecule explain many of its ubiquitous effects (Table 7.1). After ingestion ethanol is rapidly absorbed from the stomach and proximal jejunum. Halsted, Robles and Mezey (1973a) have shown that immediately after ingestion of a dose of 0.8 g ethanol per kilogram body weight the high concentration of ethanol reached in the jejunum decreases rapidly reaching levels that are in equilibrium with the vascular space by 120 min following ingestion. The absorbed ethanol is distributed throughout the body water and thereafter appears in the breath, urine, spinal fluid and the remainder of the intestine. The appearance and increase of ethanol in the ileum parallels the levels in the vascular space suggesting that ethanol enters the ileum from the vascular space rather than merely travelling the length of the intestine.

Alcohol dehydrogenase (ADH), the principal enzyme catalysing oxidation of ethanol in the liver, has been found in a number of other tissues including the intestine of both rat (Spencer, Brody and Lutters, 1964; Mistilis and Garske, 1969; Carter and Isselbacher, 1971) and man (Spencer et al, 1964). Mezey (1975) has reported ADH activities in the gut of the rat to be highest in the mucosa of the stomach and upper jejunum and low in the ileum. Similar activities of ADH in the mucosa of the upper intestine of the rat have been reported by Spencer et al (1964) Mistilis and Garske (1969) and Carter, Drummey and Isselbacher (1971). Carter et al (1971) calculated the activity of ADH in the intestine to be between half and one and a half times that found in the liver but Mezey (1975) found the activity of ADH of the upper rat intestine is only one-fifth of that in the liver. These discrepancies have resulted from differences in the estimation of liver ADH and almost certainly reflect difficulties of assay methodology.

Table 7.1 Characteristics of the ethanol molecule and its absorption and metabolism

Small molecule with weak properties of dissociation and polarisation
   Freely miscible in water and lipids
   Rapid diffusion through tissues
   Widespread metabolic effects
Oxidation predominantly in liver (very little pulmonary or renal excretion)
No storage mechanisms
No feed-back control of rates of ethanol metabolism
Provides a large caloric load

Intestinal ADH, a zinc-containing enzyme, has been found in the Rhesus monkey to have at least two isoenzymes on agar gel electrophoresis (Von Wartburg and Papenberg, 1966) but further characterisation has not been made. It seems unlikely to be of bacterial origin (Krebs and Perkins, 1970) because it was demonstrated that ethanol can be metabolised to carbon dioxide equally well by rat stomach and small intestinal slices whether these be obtained from germ-free or control animals (Carter and Isselbacher, 1971). Moreover, the rate of metabolism was approximately 68 per cent of that found using liver slices. The biological role of intestinal ADH remains to be elucidated.

Present knowledge suggests that degradation first to acetaldehyde thence to acetate and carbon dioxide and water occurs predominantly in the liver. The first step is catalysed primarily by ADH, and to an unknown extent by a microsomal ethanol oxidising system (MEOS) and by nicotinamide adenine dinucleotide (NAD) phosphate-dependent oxidase/catalase systems. Oxidation of ethanol results in reduction of NAD and NAD phosphate, an alteration in the redox state of the cell and an increasing need to 'export' hydrogen.

Hydrogen equivalents cross the mitochondrial membranes by a complex shuttle system and depress the citric acid cycle. Preferential burning of ethanol as a fuel leads to lipid accumulation. Another effect of the reduction within the hepatocyte is an increase in the lactate–pyruvate ratio, together with hyperlactacidaemia and hyperuricaemia. Finally, 'occupation' and induction of the microsomal oxidising systems will have important repercussions on drug metabolism and this is mirrored by adaptive changes in smooth endoplasmic reticulum visible on electron microscopy (Misra et al, 1971; Tobon and Mezey, 1971; Ishii, Joly and Lieber, 1973). These effects are summarised in Table 7.2. The rate limiting factor is probably availability of NAD rather than enzyme activity.

Table 7.2 Metabolic consequences of ethanol degradation

On mixed function oxidising systems
    Enhancement of ethanol metabolism
    Interference with drug metabolising systems
On hydrogen transport and reduction systems
    Altered redox potential
    Lactate production (lacticacidosis)
    Hyperuricaemia
    Ketosis
On lipid metabolism
    Increased fatty acid synthesis
    Decreased lipid oxidation
    Hepatic triglyceride accumulation
    Hyperlipaemia
On carbohydrate metabolism
    Fall in gluconeogenesis
    Hypoglycaemia

The production of acetaldehyde has interesting consequences and its importance is increasingly being noted (Raskin, 1975). It results in catecholamine release with peripheral vasodilatation and tachycardia. There is inhibition of coenzyme A. Acetaldehyde may also be responsible for diversion of central neuro-amine metabolism and there is some evidence that this effect may be related to the complex development of physical dependence in the alcoholic (Davis and Walsh, 1970; Littleton, 1975).

LIVER

The Spectrum of Alcoholic Liver Injury

Increasing experience with alcoholic liver disease reveals a wide variety of pathological forms ranging from simple hepatomegaly, with mainly electron microscopic changes, to advanced cirrhosis and carcinoma (Rubin, 1973;

Rubin and Lieber, 1975). The nature of the injury in any one individual depends partly on the extent, pattern and length of drinking history (Lelbach, 1975) and partly on unidentified factors relating to intrinsic susceptibility (Brunt, 1971).

Ethanol even in modest quantity consistently produces subcellular changes in the form of increase in the smooth endoplasmic reticulum, probably an 'adaptive' change (Misra et al, 1971) and irregularity and disorganisation of the mitochondria, probably a 'toxic' change (Svoboda and Manning, 1964; Rubin et al, 1972). Sometimes the mitochondria assume giant proportions

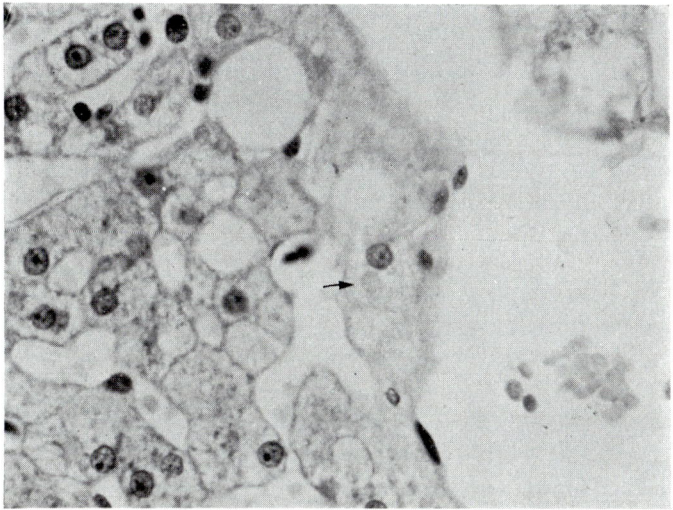

Figure 7.1 Central vein region with adjacent hepatocyte containing intracytoplasmic megamitochondrion (arrowed). Phloxine B ×360. (Courtesy of Dr J. McPhie, Department of Pathology, University of Aberdeen)

(Iseri and Gottlieb, 1971) (Fig. 7.1). They represent the earliest phenomena detectable and there is no convincing evidence that these changes are irreversible.

Alcoholic fatty liver

Hepatic steatosis occurs in a wide variety of conditions including malnutrition, obesity, diabetes mellitus and with many drugs and debilitating diseases. Thus while steatosis is highly characteristic of alcoholic injury (Lieber and Rubin, 1969) it is by no means pathognomonic. The metabolic steps underlying the disorder vary according to the size and duration of the ethanolic load and the amount of dietary fat available (Lieber, Spritz and DeCarli, 1966) and include an increase in fatty acid synthesis and esterification to triglyceride and a decrease in lipoprotein release and fatty acid oxidation. The decreased fatty acid oxidation is probably the dominant mechanism (Isselbacher, Carter and Lui, 1971).

Fat accumulates as fine droplets—circa 50 nm (500 Å)—or as larger intracellular accumulations possibly representing coalescence (Isselbacher et al, 1971; Hartcroft and Porta, 1967). Fat 'cysts' may develop and, with rupture, small fat granulomas may be seen. Clinically, fatty liver is commonly an incidental finding: a large liver in an alcoholic. It is not usually of great significance but occasionally simple steatosis can be massive and may be associated with sudden death from fat embolism or accompanied by deep cholestasis or hepatic failure (Ballard, Bernstein and Farrer, 1961; Popper and Szanto, 1957). The distinction from other forms of alcoholic disease is impossible without liver biopsy although a raised erythrocyte sedimentation rate strongly favours hepatitis or cirrhosis (Brunt et al, 1974).

For the clinician two related questions remain incompletely answered. Is alcohlic steatosis precirrhotic, and what advice should the patient with fatty liver be given?

In experimental animals fatty liver is preventable by lipotropic agents such as choline and by 'super-diets' (Koch, Porta and Hartcroft, 1969); but extrapolation from animals to man is frought with pitfalls (Rogers and Newberne, 1973) and argument persists as to whether human alcoholic steatosis is primarily nutritional or toxic (Hartcroft, 1973; Lieber, 1973a). The weight of opinion favours the latter (Popper and Schaffner, 1974). A survey of the world literature reveals no convincing evidence that steatosis per se leads to cirrhosis (Thaler, 1975). The fatty liver of kwashiorkor is rarely, if ever, superseded by cirrhosis (Cook and Hutt, 1967), although septal fibrosis may occur as with any other cause for hepatic steatosis. Most examples claiming progression of fat to cirrhosis are anecdotal. Cirrhosis occurring after jejunoileal or jejunocolic bypass for obesity (Drenick, Simmons and Murphy, 1970) is currently being quoted as evidence for progression but the cirrhosis may result from some unidentified toxic material absorbed—perhaps lithocholic acid—and be unrelated to the steatosis and 'malnutrition' (Popper and Schaffner, 1974). The strongest evidence against the association is circumstantial but compelling. Fatty change can be produced consistently even in healthy volunteers (Rubin and Lieber, 1968) with relatively modest alcohol intake whereas only a small proportion of very heavy long-standing drinkers develops cirrhosis (Lelbach, 1975) in many of whom biopsy reveals simple steatosis alone.

The conclusion must be that alcoholic steatosis is unaccompanied by any risk of developing cirrhosis. Furthermore cessation of drinking leads to complete resolution of the fatty liver. Sometimes, however, individuals seem to develop hepatitis apparently for the first time after many years of simple steatosis (Galambos, 1972a; Petrie and Brunt, 1976). Factors dictating such a change to hepatitis are unknown hence it is unfortunately not possible to predict a favourable outcome with certainty if ethanol ingestion continues. In our present state of knowledge it is probably wise to advise at least limitation of intake when steatosis is discovered.

Steatonecrosis and hepatitis

Various names have been used for the state of hepatocellular necrosis with ballooning of hepatocytes, expansion of the portal tracts with cellular infiltration, necrosis and sclerosis around the central veins and, characteristically, the striking hyaline inclusions first described by Mallory in 1911. Where fat predominates with occasional foci of necrosis and a relatively mild inflammatory reaction the term *steatonecrosis* seems reasonable. Mallory's hyaline may or may not be present (Christoffersen, Eghoje and Juhl, 1973). With a more florid inflammation a true *alcoholic hepatitis* exists and fat is commonly but not invariably present (Gregory and Levi, 1972). The distinction is somewhat artificial and the crucial point is that, in contrast to steatosis, the presence of necrosis indicates a propensity to progression to cirrhosis. Although the condition is frequently reversible—even the accompanying fibrosis may resolve (Rubin, 1973)—it is of great interest that a few patients progress to cirrhosis even though abstinence is maintained (Galambos, 1972b; Brunt et al, 1974). This has led to an analogy with 'chronic persistent hepatitis' and 'chronic aggressive hepatitis'. A picture resembling the 'chronic aggressive hepatitis' due to other causes, such as hepatitis B, is sometimes seen in alcoholics. The nature of this perpetuation phenomenon is discussed below.

The clinical syndrome of acute alcoholic hepatitis (Beckett, Livingstone and Hill, 1961; Davidson, 1971) is becoming better recognised. The patient usually presents with right upper quadrant pain, progressive sometimes deep jaundice, fever, leucocytosis and a large, tender liver. Distinction from extrahepatic obstruction can be difficult; laparotomy may be fatal. Depression of serum albumin, spider naevi and ascites all suggest primary liver disease rather than extrahepatic obstruction (Reynolds and Edmundson, 1971). Biopsy can be diagnostic and should always be performed if possible but frequently coagulation defects preclude this. Thus the diagnosis may be a considerable clinical challenge, especially if alcohol abuse is denied. In addition portal hypertension with both ascites and bleeding from varices may complicate the picture because central vein compression is a common feature (Reynolds et al, 1969).

Acute alcoholic hepatitis carries a substantial mortality (Hardison and Lee, 1966) particularly if bleeding and coma supervene. This has led to the trial of specific therapy over and above supportive measures—notably prednisolone. The results have been variable and on the whole disappointing, some authors finding improved survival (Helman et al, 1971), others none (Campra et al, 1973) and in some the numbers were too small to reach significance (Porter et al, 1971). One problem is that different authors have evaluated different types and severity of a disease which has a wide range of clinical severity (Green, 1965; Schaffner and Popper, 1970; Reynolds and Edmundson, 1971; Brunt et al, 1974) and an ability to revert completely to normal (Davidson and MacDonald, 1962). Steroids probably should not be used in alcoholic hepatitis and there is no evidence that the drug is of value in alcoholic cirrhosis (Andersen et al, 1969).

Alcoholic hepatitis may become chronic. In addition acute inflammation may complicate an established cirrhosis with a worsening of the prognosis (Rice and Yesner, 1960; Galambos, 1972a; Brunt et al, 1974).

Alcoholic cirrhosis

Traditionally alcoholic cirrhosis has been the finely nodular, fatty, 'hobnail' liver so well described by Laennec. But a coarser, irregular, macronodular or multilobular cirrhosis is becoming increasingly recognised (Popper et al, 1960; Rubin and Lieber, 1975) and probably represents a later stage of the disease when alcohol ingestion may well be less or even have ceased. The risk of hepatoma is allegedly substantially higher in this group—the ironic price of the alcoholic's reform! Broad areas of fibrous scarring are not, however, features of the alcoholic liver and it seems likely that most of the septa in this disease result from new fibre formation rather than from collapse. A further histologically distinct form of cirrhosis has been described as 'incomplete septal cirrhosis' (Popper and Kent, 1975) where the hepatic parenchyma is distorted by discontinuous bands and streaks of fibrous tissue, but nodular regeneration is less marked.

Mallory's Hyaline

For half a century since Mallory of Boston first described the hyaline inclusion characteristic of alcoholic hepatitis (Mallory, 1911) its significance was ill-appreciated; but there has been a resurgence of interest which seems to merit special consideration. Hyaline may well prove to be the Rosetta stone of alcoholic liver disease (Schaffner, 1971).

Hyaline commonly accompanies alcoholic necrosis and is a hallmark of alcoholic hepatitis (Fig. 7.2) where the irregular clear-staining cytoplasmic inclusions are predominantly paranuclear and in centrilobular cells (Gerber et al, 1973). It is not, as was once thought, pathognomonic of ethanolic injury and similar inclusions may be seen in hepatoma, Indian childhood cirrhosis, Wilson's disease and various forms of cholestasis (Keeley, Iseri and Gottlieb, 1972; Roy, Ramalingaswami and Nayak, 1971; Sternlieb, 1975; Ament and Fenster, 1970; French and Davies, 1974). Nevertheless, Gerber and colleagues conclude that '*central* hyaline, with or without cholestasis, in cases with intact lobular architecture is specific for acute alcoholic liver injury . . .' (Gerber et al, 1973). Strikingly similar changes have also been seen following jejuno-ileal bypass (Peters and Reynolds, 1973). Recently, and for the first time, 'alcoholic' hyaline has been produced in experimental animals using griseofulvin (Denk, Gschnait and Wolff, 1975).

Using the electron microscope hyaline is seen as circumscribed masses of electron-dense filaments closely associated with the ribosomes (Kahn, 1973; Wiggers et al, 1973). Three types of hyaline have been recognised (Yokoo et al, 1972):

1. irregular connecting parallel filaments;
2. randomly arranged branching tubular fibrils;
3. non-filamentous granular material.

Its origin remains an enigma although earlier reports that it arose from microsomes or from mitochondria or from lysozomes were incorrect. It is

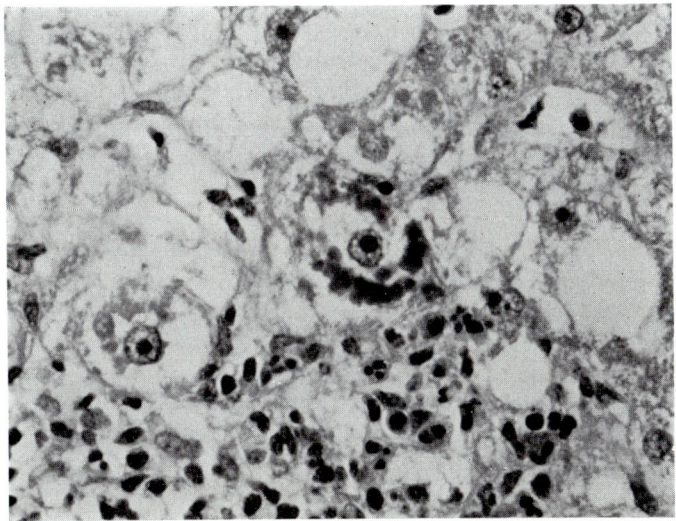

Figure 7.2 Mallory's hyaline in cytoplasm of hepatocytes with associated inflammatory cell infiltrate. Trichrome × 360. (Courtesy of Dr J. McPhie, Department of Pathology, University of Aberdeen)

probably a newly formed protein (Albukerk and Duffy, 1972) possibly derived from ribosomes (French and Davies, 1974) accumulating as a relatively insoluble material either by over-production or lack of clearance.

Hyaline occurs in perhaps 10 to 20 per cent of alcoholic subjects (Christoffersen and Nielson, 1971). Its significance is that it indicates the presence of hepatic necrosis and therefore conveys a poor prognosis (Rice and Yesner, 1960; Kern, Mikkelsen and Turrill, 1969). Leevy believes that it has a positive pathogenetic role and acts as a 'neoantigen' stimulating an immunological reaction (Leevy, Chen and Zetterman, 1975). The significance of its apparent chemotactic action is uncertain (Schaffner and Popper, 1970). The continuing work on its nature and significance will be watched with interest.

Susceptibility and Progression

A fatty liver does not matter; cirrhosis does. In that the term cirrhosis implies the late result of hepatocellular necrosis the essence of the problem is alcoholic hepatitis. There are two basic questions to be answered. Firstly, why are some individuals susceptible and others apparently not? Secondly, what perpetuates the process and drives the disease into irreversibility?

Individual host susceptibility

A major factor in determining the development of hepatitis is clearly the quantity of alcohol drunk. The florid syndrome of alcoholic hepatitis commonly follows a debauch and the histological features of hepatitis rarely occur unless alcohol intake is both high and prolonged (Lelbach, 1975). Many patients will be consuming daily in excess of 160 g (about two-thirds of a bottle of whisky). Pequignot (1961) estimated the risk of developing cirrhosis to be great if more than 160 g are taken while the risk is much less if daily intake falls below 80 g. However, a recent survey in Bouches du Rhone and Ille et Vilaine has caused him to lower the risk margin to 40 g per day (Pequignot and Tuyns, 1975). Experimental evidence in support of these data has finally come now that an animal model for human alcoholic liver disease has been developed (Rubin and Lieber, 1973, 1974). In this study the New York Mount Sinai Group fed alcohol to baboons under carefully controlled circumstances with nutritious diets. When the alcohol was providing 36 per cent of the total calories steatosis, but not hepatitis, developed. However, when it provided 50 per cent of the total calories some animals developed a frank hepatitis similar to the human disease (Lieber, 1975b).

None the less a factor of host susceptibility must still be important to explain why the features of hepatitis are apparently so uncommon compared to the vast numbers of people who drink heavily daily. Hepatitis and cirrhosis are known to occur in only a small proportion of heavy drinkers (Lelbach, 1975). While additional exogenous factors, notably viral hepatitis (Pettigrew et al, 1972), are probably important it is unlikely that these alone can explain all the host individuality observed. There has been much speculation and some research into possible genetic factors determining susceptibility but the results so far have been disappointing and no clear lead has emerged (Brunt, 1971; Lieber, 1975b). Blood group markers are equivocal but some inherited physical characteristics, such as fair skin and brown hair, are associated with cirrhosis and there are undoubtedly some racial predisposing factors involved (Reid et al, 1968). Further work in this field is urgently needed because the identification of those at 'medical' risk from heavy alcohol consumption will be of immense practical importance especially in those parts of the world where the community cost of alcoholic cirrhosis is high (Popper et al, 1969).

Perpetuation and progression

It has been emphasised that alcoholic hepatitis is, in the majority of patients, reversible following reduction of the alcohol intake. Much recent work centres on the mechanisms leading to progression to cirrhosis, and the concept of a 'committed precursor stage' has been advanced (Popper, 1975).

There is some evidence that abnormal immunoreactivity is involved. Levels of IgA are elevated in hepatitis and cirrhosis but not steatosis (Lee, 1965; Steigmann et al, 1974). Abnormal lymphocyte mediated responses have been described by Leevy et al (1975) in hepatitis, comparable to those observed in chronic active hepatitis, but not in steatosis. Further evidence in favour of perpetuation by cell mediated immunity comes from demonstration of liver antigen induced migration inhibition in hepatitis but not in steatosis or cirrhosis (Mihas, Bull and Davidson, 1975). Other workers have shown reductions in circulating T-lymphocytes in aggressive disease, especially hepatitis (Bernstein et al, 1974). The significance of these findings has still to be fully evaluated but the consistent discovery of abnormalities in hepatitis as opposed to other forms of alcoholic liver disease suggests that immunological mechanisms may be involved in perpetuation and progression.

A crucial factor in progression is hepatic collagen metabolism. This is a large subject which has been reviewed recently (Popper and Udenfriend, 1970; Bornstein, 1974; Popper and Kent, 1975; Popper and Becker, 1975). Fibroplasia is stimulated. This may possibly be effected metabolically because hyperlactacidaemia might stimulate collagen synthesis, or else by hepatocyte injury in which there may be the release of 'collagen stimulating factors' (McGee, O'Hare and Patrick, 1973). The process begins by transformation of a precursor cell in the sinusoid, the Ito cell, to a fibroblast. Encirclement of hepatocytes by fibres impairs the cell nutrition and leads to further damage; circumstances are set for the development of a vicious circle. The point of the committed precursor stage is not clear but the development of irreversibility is indicated by a considerable prolongation of the collagen half-life. The development of cirrhosis is heralded by septum formation separating the lobules. Here the linking of the central hyaline sclerosis which is so characteristic of ethanolic damage (Edmondson et al, 1963) with the portal tracts, rather like the bridging in a subacute viral hepatitis, is a fundamental process. At this stage further progression is probable since the septa in cirrhosis produce vascular derangements and intrahepatic shunting followed by yet further compromise of the failing nutritional milieu for the liver cells.

THE MOUTH, PHARNYX AND OESOPHAGUS

Sir Arthur Hurst (1939) reported the incidence of carcinoma of the oesophagus to be four times greater in the alcohol trades than in the general population, whereas in carcinoma of the stomach the difference was much less obvious and there was no difference in carcinoma of the colon. This initial observation has been supported by more recent studies although doubt exists concerning the relative importance of alcohol consumption and cigarette smoking apart from other considerations such as malnutrition.

Kamionkowski and Fleshler (1965) in a study from the United States of patients with carcinoma of the oesophagus reported 73 per cent to be chronic alcoholics; this compared with 19 per cent in a similar group of patients with colonic cancer. Keller (1967) reported an association between cancer of the mouth and pharynx and heavy alcohol consumption independent of the association with cigarette smoking; furthermore this association was more marked when patients had developed alcoholic cirrhosis. Schoenberg, Bailar and Fraumeni (1971) confirmed an epidemiological association between oesophageal cancer and consumption of tobacco and alcohol but also suggested that a third factor, urbanisation, was the most important. Robertson, Harington and Bradshaw (1971) reported that over the previous decade the oesophageal cancer rate in non-white African males in Johannesburg had doubled whilst that in females from the same population had risen five-fold. This dramatic rise in oesophageal cancer rate in non-white South Africans was confirmed by Cook (1971) who suggested a possible association with the consumption of alcoholic drinks made from maize. A more recent South African study (Bradshaw and Schonland, 1974) showed a positive correlation between carcinoma of the oesophagus and the smoking of pipe tobacco but not alcohol consumption. By contrast Pequignot and Tuyns (1975) observed in the Ille et Vilaine study in France that not only was the risk of liver cirrhosis increased above a daily intake of 40 g of ethanol but so also was the risk of development of oesophageal cancer. The precise aetiological relationship between ethanol and carcinoma of the oesophagus remains to be elucidated. Many factors including tobacco smoking, type of alcohol consumed, racial characteristics, geographical location and malnutrition may play a part.

As in other parts of the gut disordered oesophageal motility has been demonstrated (Winship et al, 1968) in patients with chronic alcohol addiction and peripheral neuropathy, characterised by reduced oesophageal peristalsis in the distal oesophagus but preservation of sphincter tone. The clinical relevance of this observation is not yet clear.

STOMACH

Gastric Secretion

Alcohol has a stimulating effect on gastric secretion effecting an increase in acid and gastrin secretion. In addition to the effects of ethanol itself some of the responses may be due to hyperosmolarity. The intravenous administration stimulates gastric secretion even after antrectomy and vagotomy (Woodward, Robertson and Fried, 1957; Daves, Miller and Lemmi, 1965). This gastric secretory response to parenteral alcohol is unchanged following ablation of the pancreas, pituitary, adrenal glands or small intestine, but Weise, Schapiro and

Woodward (1961) reported a decrease in this response in dogs following isolation of the cerebral circulation from the body. This suggested that parenteral alcohol exerts its gastric secretory response via the central nervous system. In part the mechanism whereby ethanol affects the stomach may be its ability, in high concentration, to decrease gastric motility (Schapiro, Cummings and Luckey, 1965). More recently experiments in dogs (Treffot, 1975) have shown that ethanol and meat meals, either alone or in combination, cause a rise in serum gastrin. Chronic ethanol administration causes a higher and better sustained release of gastrin than occurs in non-alcholic control dogs fed with an otherwise identical diet. Chronic ethanol intoxication induces an increased gastrin store and releasing capacity of the gastric antrum. A similar increase occurs with cholecystokinin-pancreozymin (CCK–PZ) in the intestinal mucosa of dogs (Treffot et al, 1976). Chronic ethanol administration has been shown to be a probable stimulant of intrapancreatic ganglia (Tiscornia, Palascinao and Sarles, 1975). Moreover, gastrin release from the antral mucosa is cholinergically mediated through vagal or local reflexes (Grossman, 1967). Thus it may be assumed that chronic ethanol administration exerts its influence on the antral mucosa through either or both of these mechanisms (Maityra, 1963). The enhanced activity of the intramural ganglia on the gastric antrum, as well as those in the pancreas could be the result of a reserpine-like effect of chronic ethanol intoxication (Tiscornia, Palasciano and Sarles, 1976b).

Gastric Mucosal Injury

Following the classical observation of Beaumont (1833) on the acute gastric mucosal changes occurring after St Martin's alcoholic sprees it has been recognised that acute gastritis complicates the administration of alcohol. Gastric haemorrhage is a common complication and seems especially likely to occur following the concomitent ingestion of aspirin with alcohol (Needham et al, 1971; Johnston et al, 1973). These findings may be explained partly by the work of Smith et al (1971) who showed that both aspirin and alcohol increase the permeability of human gastric mucosa to hydrogen ions. The precise mechanism of the gastric mucosal damage is not certain but most studies in man and animals indicate that alcohol interferes with the mucosal barrier (Myerson, 1973) and that this in turn leads to histological changes. The changes produced seem to be dependent on the concentration and amount of alcohol consumed (Williams, 1956; Gillespie and Lucas, 1961; Kawashima and Glass, 1975). Animal studies have shown that stress, especially when following excessive ethanol intake, is a significant factor in the potentiation of acute mucosal injury (Kawashima and Glass, 1975). Despite the observed acute effect of ethanol there is no evidence that *chronic* alcoholism leads to chronic gastritis or gastric atrophy (Palmer, 1954; Wolff, 1970). Indeed, in the study reported by Wolff (1970) patients with histologically normal gastric mucosal biopsies drank *more* alcohol than did those with histological evidence of gastritis! Although ethanol does not produce chronic gastritis Engeset, Lygren and Idsoe (1963) reported an increased incidence of peptic ulceration, particularly gastric ulcers. This may simply reflect the poor nutritional state of many alcoholics rather than a specific effect of ethanol as Mowat, Needham and Brunt (1975) have shown that a significant proportion of patients developing gastric ulcers are already in poor physical condition often with multisystem disease.

The effects of ethanol on the gastric mucosa are reversed by abstinence for a relatively short period of time and most mucosal erosions disappear by 72 h (Kawashima and Glass, 1975). Recently it has been shown that carbenoxolone has no effect in reducing the increased gastric mucosal permeability to hydrogen ions induced by ethanol ingestion (Gordon et al, 1975).

SMALL INTESTINE

Although small bowel malabsorption and pancreatic dysfunction were initially demonstrated in alcoholic patients with cirrhosis of the liver (Baraona et al, 1962; Sun, Albacete and Chen, 1967; Marin, Clark and Senior, 1969) similar abnormalities can occur in chronic alcoholic patients with minimal or undetectable liver disease (Small, Longarini and Zamcheck, 1959; Roggin et al, 1969; Halsted, Criggs and Harris, 1967; Tomasulo, Kater and Iber, 1968; Mezey et al, 1970; Thomson, Baker and Leevy, 1970; Halsted, Robles and Mezey, 1971).

Acute and Chronic Effects of Ethanol in Animals

Experiments have shown that the acute administration of alcohol results in increases in triglyceride (Carter et al, 1971) and cholesterol synthesis (Middleton et al, 1971), an increased triglyceride content of the small intestinal mucosa, and increased lympathic output of triglycerides, cholesterol and phospholipids (Mistilis and Ockner, 1972). Pyrazole partially suppresses the increased triglyceride synthesis and the increased cholesterol synthesis (Carter et al, 1971) is demonstrable only whilst ethanol remains in the intestinal lumen (Middleton et al, 1971). This suggests that the effects of ethanol may be mediated by its metabolism in the intestinal mucosa. Recently Rodgers and O'Brien (1975) examined the effect of acute ethanol treatment of lipid re-esterifying enzymes of the rat and small bowel, and showed that ethanol increases activities of the lipid re-esterifying enzymes in the jejunum. Ileal specific activity of acyl-CoA synthestase is increased. No effect of ethanol on jejunal disaccharidase activity was noted. Ethanol given acutely thus seems to have a specific stimulating effect on intestinal enzymes involved in lipid absorption. It may be that the increased lipid synthesis and output from gastrointestinal lymph may be partly responsible for the hyperlipaemia and fatty liver included by ethanol (Mezey, 1975).

In vitro experiments have shown that ethanol can stimulate adenyl cyclase in both rat and human jejunum (Greene, Herman and Kraemer, 1971). It also causes a decrease in adenosine triphosphate (ATP) levels in the small intestine of rat in vitro and in vivo after both acute and chronic administration (Carter and Isselbacher, 1973). In addition ethanol has an inhibitory effect on sodium, potassium and magnesium-stimulated ATPase activity (Israel, Kalant and Laufer, 1965) which has been shown to be associated with active transport mechanisms (Israel, Salazar and Rosenmann, 1968). These observations may explain why both in vitro and in vivo experiments in the rat have shown that ethanol can inhibit the small intestinal transport of amino acids and glucose (Spencer et al, 1964; Chang, Lewis and Glazko, 1967; Israel et al, 1968).

Krawitt (1973) demonstrated that chronic ethanol ingestion interferes with the ability of the rat duodenum to transport calcium and that this ability existed independently of starvation and of hepatic or pancreatic dysfunction. Further study (Krawitt, 1975) indicated that this effect of ethanol could not be reversed by vitamin D or 25-hydroxycholecalciferol administration. Ethanol ingestion by vitamin D deficient rats did not further suppress transport activity nor interfere with an increase in transport induced by vitamin D. Levels of intestinal calcium-binding activity were not suppressed. Brush-border alkaline phosphatase activity was suppressed by chronic ethanol ingestion and was restored to normal by vitamin D administration. These observations suggest that ethanol interferes with calcium transport by a mechanism at least in part independent of the vitamin D pathway. Changes in alkaline phosphatase and calcium transport although affected by vitamin D may represent independent metabolic consequences (Krawitt, 1975).

In animal morphological changes induced by ethanol have been associated with decreased enzyme activity. Acute administration of ethanol to rats result in haemorrhagic erosions at the tips of the intestinal villi, a decrease in the enzymic activity of lactase and thimidine kinase located principally in the villus and crypt cells respectively, and decreased oxygen consumption (Baraona, Pirola and Lieber, 1974). Chronic administration to rats with an 'adequate' diet causes stunting of the villi, a decrease in the numbers of epithelial cells, and a decrease in the activity of villous enzymes (lactase, sucrase and alkaline phosphatase) but increases in the crypt enzyme thimidine kinase and in the incorporation of thimidine into DNA. Absorption of D-xylose (Broitman et al, 1961) or folic acid (Halsted, Bhanthumnavin and Mezey, in press) is not decreased.

Acute and Chronic Effects of Ethanol in Man

Few studies exist on the effects of ethanol administration on intestinal absorption in man. The direct addition of 2 per cent ethanol to intestinal perfusates inhibits the intestinal uptake of L-methionine (Israel et al, 1969).

Current reports (Halsted et al, 1967; Thomson et al, 1970) suggest that ethanol inhibits the absorption of thiamine and folic acid in only a small proportion of subjects studied. Mezey (1975) has shown that the acute oral administration of a large dose of ethanol (0.8 g/kg body weight) can significantly reduce urinary excretion of D-xylose. It seems that ethanol, in addition to its hyperosmolar effect delaying absorption, also has an inhibitory effect on absorptive capacity. Moreover, the administration of ethanol either orally or intravenously in the above dose alters the motility of the small bowel (Robles et al, 1972). In the jejunum there is inhibition of type I mixing waves that impede the forward progress of intestinal contents, but in the ileum there is enhancement of type III waves which represent a change in tonus of the intestine and are associated with propulsion of intestinal contents. These effects may contribute to 'alcoholic diarrhoea'.

Vitamin B_{12}. Chronic administration of ethanol in subjects taking a nutritious diet result in a decrease of vitamin B_{12} absorption in all patients studied (Lindenbaum and Lieber, 1969). In later studies Lindenbaum and Lieber (1975) have confirmed that B_{12} malabsorption can occur despite a nutritious diet, and that vitamin B_{12} malabsorption is not corrected by giving intrinsic factor or pancreatin. The block of B_{12} absorption presumably occurs at ileal level either by deficient uptake or transport through or out of the ileal cell. It may be dose related. By contrast, some of these patients show surprisingly normal D-xylose and fat absorption. This may be explained by the fact that at the doses of ethanol administered in these absorption studies vitamin B_{12} is absorbed by a specialised active transport mechanism whereas xylose and fatty acids are absorbed by passive diffusion (Lindenbaum and Lieber, 1975). The mechanism for ileal dysfunction in man remains to be established but it is of interest that studies on everted jejunal segments of rats have shown that single doses of ethanol interfere with the active transport of low doses of thiamine but not with passive diffusion at high vitamin concentrations (Hoyumpa et al, 1974). Furthermore, in rats it has been demonstrated that the B_{12} malabsorption occurring with chronic ethanol feeding is associated with both impairment of the ileal uptake step and decreased binding of the vitamin B_{12}-intrinsic factor complex by the villus cell (Lindenbaum et al, 1973).

Folic acid. Chronic ingestion of ethanol causes decreased folate absorption in the relatively few subjects studied (Halsted et al, 1967, 1971). However, among alcoholics abnormalities of intestinal absorption have been found more frequently in patients with a history of poor dietary intake and folate deficiency (Halsted et al, 1967, 1971; Halsted, Robles and Mezey, 1973b). Recovery from malabsorption of folic acid occurs in most patients on institution of a normal diet (Mezey et al, 1970; Halsted et al, 1971). Halsted et al (1973b) showed in alcoholics with very low serum folate levels that the administration of folic acid allowed recovery to occur despite the continuation of a high ethanol intake. In addition the studies of Mezey (1975) suggest that dietary folate deficiency in chronic alcoholics is an important factor in the development of malabsorption and that this occurs before the detection of morphological abnormalities of the intestine detectable by light microscopy.

D-*Xylose*. There is reduced absorption following acute administration of ethanol, but not following chronic administration of even large doses of alcohol (Mezey, 1975). In alcoholics recovery from D-xylose malabsorption rapidly occurs following admission to hospital and institution of a normal diet despite the continuation of alcohol in high dosage.

Fat. Steatorrhoea (faecal fat > 6 g/day) may occur in up to 33 per cent of alcoholics (Mezey, 1975) admitted to hospital and usually disappears when the patient is placed on an adequate diet, whether or not alcohol is continued (Lindenbaum and Lieber, 1975). Where steatorrhoea does persist chronic pancreatitis should be suspected.

Morphology. Although Mezey (1975) reported no light microscopic changes in the mucosa of those studied, Rubin et al (1972) found ultrastructural changes consisting of abnormalities of the mitochondria, endoplasmic reticulum, and Golgi apparatus in chronic alcoholic patients fed ethanol with an adequate diet.

Conclusions

Both ethanol and dietary deficiency play a part in malabsorption found in alcoholics. The acute administration of a single large dose produces histological changes in the mucosa, decreases absorptive capacity and alters intestinal motility. Prolonged ingestion of alcohol, provided it is accompanied by a nutritious diet, results in a demonstrable decrease only of vitamin B_{12} absorption with the absorption of other substances being rarely affected. Since most studies in man have been conducted on highly selected severely ill alcoholics it is not possible to estimate reliably the incidence of alcohol-induced small bowel changes in any general population.

PANCREAS

The most characteristic effect of alcohol on the pancreas is the production of *chronic calcifying pancreatitis*. Although it has been known to occur in alcoholics for nearly 100 years the mechanisms for the pathological changes are incompletely understood.

Since Howard and Jordan (1968) described the features of alcoholic pancreatitis, others (Sarles, Muratore and Sarles, 1961; Sarles et al, 1965; Payan et al, 1972) have confirmed that this disease is characterised by a peculiar group of pathological features usually referred to as chronic calcifying pancreatitis. Similar changes may occur in protein insufficiency during childhood in tropical Africa and Asia; rarely an idiopathic form can occur; an uncommon congenital form also exists and the lesion may be found in association with hyperparathyroidism (Sarles, 1975). The first visible abnormality is the precipitation in ducts and acini of protein plugs formed mainly by the normal pancreatic fluid proteins (Sarles, 1971). Other typical findings are: dilation of ducts and acini forming rounded cavities, the frequent presence of protein plugs or stones in these cavities and intra- and perilobular sclerosis. Half of the patients may have pancreatic cysts or pseudocysts. The course of the illness is one of relapse and remission with oedema and fatty necrosis being commoner than haemorrhagic necrosis. The acute attacks become less frequent as the pancreatic tissue is progressively destroyed (Sarles, 1975). In Europe, South America and probably in North America alcoholism is the main cause of chronic calcifying pancreatitis (Sarles et al, 1965; Sarles, 1973, 1974), most patients will have been drinking a mean quantity of 150 ml of alcohol per day for at least two years. The nature of the alcoholic beverage seems unimportant. Malnutrition has never been proven to play a role in the disease (Sarles, 1975).

Acute Effects of Ethanol on the Pancreas in Animals

In studies of dogs, Menguy et al (1958) and Walton et al (1965) showed that ethanol consumption increases the resistance of the sphincter of Oddi to the flow of bile. Tiscornia et al (1973a) reported that exposure of the duodenal and jejunal mucosae of dogs to ethanol does not cause significant release of secretion of pancreozymin in the waking animal. It has already been noted that Woodward et al (1957) and Treffot et al (1976) demonstrated in dog that contact of ethanol with the antral mucosa increases the release of gastrin which has a direct exciting effect on the pancreatic secretion of protein. In addition the increased gastric secretion of hydrogen ions releases secretin in the duodenum. A direct inhibitory action of ethanol on pancreatic secretion has been observed with inhibition of water, bicarbonate and protein secretion. This inhibition is partly suppressed by the intravenous infusion of atropine and pentolinium and is partially abolished by vagotomy but not by previous administration of reserpine (Tiscornia et al, 1972, 1973b, 1975).

Thus the acute action of ethanol on the dog pancreas is complex, being the sum of mechanisms that simultaneously increase and decrease secretion. The total result is probably a weak stimulation of the gland (Sarles, 1975).

The effects of acute alcohol have been followed in other animals. Studies in rats by Solomon et al (1974) showed that alcohol inhibits water and bicarbonate but not protein secretion and causes a decrease in tissue ATP but has no effect on cyclic AMP content suggesting a direct effect of ethanol on the secretory cell. In the rabbit the sphincter of Oddi pressure also rises significantly following acute alcohol (Sarles and Midejean, 1973).

Histological lesions have never been produced by acute administration of ethanol in either dog or rat (Sarles et al, 1971b).

Acute Effects of Ethanol on the Pancreas in Man

A moderate increase in the tone of the sphincter of Oddi occurs after intraduodenal injection or intravenous infusion of ethanol (Davis and Pirola, 1968; Capitaine and Sarles, 1971) but the increase is less than that which occurs in benign Vaterian stenosis (odditis). This latter causes chronic pancreatitis but never of the calcifying type found in chronic alcoholics (Sarles et al, 1965). Ethanol stimulates a weak pancreatic secretion of water and bicarbonate, but not of proteins. This suggests that when it makes contact with the duodenal mucosa there is release of a small quantity of secretin (Galindo, 1968; Capitaine et al, 1971).

Mott et al (1972) demonstrated that intragastric instillation of 150 ml of 40 per cent (v/v) ethanol gives rise to some inhibition of pancreatic secretion of water and bicarbonate but inhibition of enzyme secretion is much more marked. Maximum inhibition coincided with peak alcohol blood levels at 60 to 75 min after administration of ethanol. Marin, Ward and Fischer (1973) have since confirmed these findings.

Thus in man, as in dogs, pancreatic secretion is only slightly increased following acute ethanol ingestion (Sarles, 1975). There is no evidence that occasional alcohol consumption in people not adapted to its regular use might be a cause of acute pancreatitis. Moreover, there is no proof that the changes induced by the acute effects of alcohol have any part to play in the aetiology of chronic pancreatitis in man.

Chronic Alcoholism and Pancreatic Function in Animals

In dogs adapted to the daily intake of 2 g ethanol per kilogram body weight no significant changes in basal pancreatic secretion was shown (Sarles, 1975). However from the sixth to the fourteenth week of alcohol consumption there is increasing sensitivty of the acinar cells to CCK–PZ infusion; thereafter there is a gradual return to pre-alcoholic levels by the ninth month. On the other hand the response to secretin did not vary during the first eight months. At the twelfth month protein concentration and output during a perfusion with secretin are significantly weaker than before chronic alcohol consumption. Whether this functional decrease is due to the development of chronic pancreatic lesions is not yet reported.

Intraduodenal instillation of 20 ml oleic acid after 14 months of chronic alcoholism leads to a pancreatic secretion of protein six times higher than during the pre-alcoholic period (Sarles, 1975). Water and bicarbonate secretion is only slightly modified. This may be explained by the considerable increase of CCK–PZ release during chronic alcoholism reported by Palasciano et al (1974).

Perhaps the most surprising effect of chronic alcoholism in the dog is the *direct* effect of ethanol on pancreatic secretion (Sarles, 1975). As early as the sixth week the inhibition secondary to an intravenous injection of ethanol

(1.3/kg) begins to decrease. By 40 weeks flow rate increases. By the twelfth month inhibition is no longer observed but there is a marked increase in pancreatic secretion especially in protein output and concentration (Tiscornia, et al, 1976b). The reasons for chronic alcoholism reversing the direct effect of ethanol on the pancreas are not clear.

The consequence of these different effects of chronic ethanol ingestion in the dog is the secretion of a juice with higher concentration of proteins. From the sixth week of intoxication onwards protein precipitations rich in calcium carbonate and identical to human small pancreatic stones are detectable in the pancreatic juice. These protein plugs may sometimes obstruct the ducts. Secretion stops but resumes again abruptly when the plugs are extruded through the pancreatic cannulae (Sarles, 1975).

In the rat spontaneous chronic pancreatitis and spontaneous protein precipitation in pancreatic juice is frequent, but the frequency of this spontaneous disease is significantly increased by the consumption of 20 per cent ethanol over two years (Sarles, 1975). The protein concentration in the pancreatic juice of chronic alcoholic rats is twice as high as that of non-alcoholic controls. Levels of lipase, trypsin, chymotrypsin and amylase are higher in the fasting chronic alcoholic rat than in non-alcoholic controls (Goslin et al, 1965; Sarles, Figarella and Clemente, 1971a). Autoradiographic studies (Jamieson and Palade, 1967) on the intracellular transport of newly synthesised pancreatic proteins in alcoholic rats show that the transit of proteins from the endoplasmic reticulum to the lumen of the acinus is accelerated from the zymogen granules to the lumen. This is possibly under the action of CCK–PZ or acetylcholine. In contrast to protein hypersecretion, protein biosynthetic rates in the alcoholic rat pancreas have been found to be reduced (Sardesai and Orten, 1968; Orrego-Matte et al, 1968; Dagorn et al, 1975) especially in rats fed on high fat diets. This apparent paradox may be partly explained by difficulties in calculating protein biosynthetic rates (Sarles, 1975). Thus although results in regard to biosynthetic rates may be uncertain the pancreatic acinar cell of chronic alcoholic rats is overactive producing a juice rich in protein which precipitates in the ducts.

Chronic Alcoholism and Pancreatic Function in Man

It has been shown (Sarles, 1975) that release of gastrin after ingestion of alcohol is higher in patients with alcoholic calcifying pancreatitis than in controls. In addition, Harvey et al (1973) have shown by radioimmunoassay that CCK–PZ levels are considerably higher in the blood of patients with chronic pancreatic insufficiency than in controls. If the work of Sarles (1975) in dogs is applicable to man the rise in CCK–PZ may be due to a direct effect of chronic alcoholism on CCK–PZ release. An ultrastructural study by Sarles (1975) showed no significant changes in the pancreatic ductal cells, but the acinar cells from patients with chronic calcifying pancreatitis show evidence of hyperfunction with cells that are larger than usual, with larger nuclei, larger nucleoli, an increase in endoplasmic reticulum and Golgi apparatus, and an increase in the numbers of immature zymogen granules. These features are identical to those seen in the animal chronically treated with gastrin or CCK–PZ (Tasso et al, 1973). As in rats the first lesion appears to be the precipitation of normal pancreatic enzymatic proteins in the ducts (Sarles, 1975). These later calcify and possibly form stones; and this change might be influenced by an increased calcium concentration in the pancreatic juice (Goebell et al, 1970; Gullo et al, 1974). The increased calcium concentration is not however specific to the alcoholic but has been shown to occur in acute and chronic pancreatitis of different origin, in pancreatic carcinoma, and in the diabetic pancreas (Goebell et al, 1970). In addition to the increase in calcium concentration the concentration of serum proteins in the pancreatic juice is also increased (Clements et al, 1971) possibly favouring the formation of protein precipitates.

The problem in man is further complicated by the presence in the pancreatic juice of patients with alcoholic chronic calcifying pancreatitis of an unusual high molecular weight protein (mol. wt 78 000) referred to as *lactoferrin* (Colomb et al, 1974; Estevenon, Sarles and Figarella, in press). This is normally found in saliva but not in gastric juice or bile and can occur in the pancreatic juice of up to 5 per cent of normal persons. It is possible that the secretion of lactoferrin predates the morphological changes in the pancreas. It is known that lactoferrin combines with other proteins to form complexes (Heckman, 1971) thereby favouring the precipitation of normal hyperconcentrated proteins. This might explain why few people who take alcohol develop chronic calcifying pancreatitis and might also explain the existence of non-alcoholic forms of chronic calcifying pancreatitis. Recently it has been shown that in patients with chronic alcoholism the trypsin and lipase responses to CCK–PZ are reduced with no significant increase above basal enzyme output, (Minaire et al, 1973; Dimagno, Go and Summerskill, 1973; Dimagno, Malagelada and Go, 1975). Steatorrhoea develops late in chronic alcoholic pancreatitis when lipase outputs in response to CCK–PZ have fallen to less than 10 per cent of normal. All patients with steatorrhoea have enzyme outputs below this level. Creatorrhoea (stool nitrogen greater than 72.5 g/24 h) is related to reduced trypsin outputs because it occurs only when stimulated trypsin outputs are less than 10 per cent of normal maximal trypsin output. It seems there is a gradual and progressive decline of the pancreatic exocrine enzyme output in patients with increasing duration of chronic alcoholism which inevitably leads to steatorrhoea (Dimagno et al, 1975).

Conclusions

As in animals ethanol seems to be harmful to the human pancreas only following prolonged regular consumption. It does so by virtue of increasing pancreatic secretion of proteins without a parallel rise in water and electrolyte secretion. This leads to the eventual precipitation of the hyperconcentrated protein and the formation of protein plugs which subsequently calcify. The presence of lactoferrin may favour this precipitation. The mechanism by which acute effects of ethanol on the pancreas could be linked to chronic pancreatitis is still not understood.

REFERENCES

Albukerk, J. & Duffy, J. L. (1972) Origin of alcoholic hyaline—an electron microscopic study. *Archives of Pathology*, **93**, 510–517.
Ament, M. & Fenster, L. F. (1970) Mallory bodies in chronic cholestasis (Abstract). *Gastroenterology*, **58**, 278.
Andersen, S. B., Balslev, T., Bjorneboe, M., Faber, V., Gjorup, S., Harvald, B., Iversen, K., Jessen, O., Johl, E. & Jorgensen, H. E. (1969) Effect of prednisone on the survival of patients with cirrhosis of the liver. *Lancet*, **1**, 119–121.
Ballard, H., Bernstein, B. & Farrer, J. T. (1961) Fatty liver presenting as obstructive jaundice. *American Journal of Medicine*, **30**, 196–201.
Baraona, E., Orrego, H., Fernández, O., Amenabar, E., Maldonado, E., Tag, F. & Salinas, A. (1962) Absorptive function of the small intestine in liver cirrhosis. *American Journal of Digestive Diseases*, **7**, 318–330.
Baraona, E., Pirola, R. C. & Lieber, C. S. (1974) Small intestinal damage and changes in cell population produced by ethanol ingestion in the rat. *Gastroenterology*, **66**, 226–234.
Beaumont, W. (1833) *Experiments and Observations on the Gastric Juice, and the Physiology of Digestion*, pp. 280. Plattsburgh, New York: J. P. Allen.
Beckett, A. G., Livingstone, A. & Hill, K. R. (1961) Acute alcoholic hepatitis. *British Medical Journal*, **2**, 1113–1119.
Berggren, S. M. & Goldberg, L. (1940) The absorption of ethyl alcohol from the gastrointestinal tract as a diffusion process. *Acta physiologica scandinavica*, **1**, 246–255.
Bernstein, I. M., Webster, K. H., Williams, R. C., Jr & Strickland, R. G. (1974) Reduction in circulating T-lymphocytes in alcoholic liver disease. *Lancet*, **1**, 488–490.
Bornstein, P. (1974) The biosynthesis of collagen. *Annual Review of Biochemistry*, **43**, 567–603.
Bradshaw, E. & Schonland, M. (1974) Smoking, drinking and oesophageal cancer in African males of Johannesburg, South Africa. *British Journal of Cancer*, **30** (2), 157–163.
Broitman, S. A., Small, M. D., Vitale, J. J. & Zamcheck, N. (1961) Intestinal absorption and urinary excretion of xylose in rats fed reduced protein and thyroxine or alcohol. *Gastroenterology*, **41**, 21–28.
Brunt, P. W. (1971) Alcohol and the liver. *Gut*, **12**, 222–229.
Brunt, P. W., Kew, M. C., Scheuer, P. J. & Sherlock, S. (1974) Studies in alcoholic liver disease in Britain. 1. Clinical and pathological patterns related to natural history. *Gut*, **15**, 52–58.
Campra, J. L., Hamlin, E. M., Jr, Kirshbaum, R. J., Olivier, M., Redeker, A. G. & Reynolds, T. B. (1973) Prednisone therapy of acute alcoholic hepatitis: report of a controlled trial. *Annals of Internal Medicine*, **79**, 625–631.
Capitaine, Y. & Sarles, H. (1971) Action de l'éthanol sur le tonus du sphincter d'Oddi chez l'homme. *Biologie gastroenterologie*, **3**, 231–236.
Capitaine, Y., Mott, C. H., Gullo, L. & Sarles, H. (1971) Action de l'éthanol sur la sécrétion pancreatique chez l'homme. *Biologie gastroenterologie*, **3**, 193–198.
Carter, E. A. & Isselbacher, J. K. (1971) The metabolism of ethanol to carbon dioxide by stomach and small intestinal slices. *Proceedings of the Society of Experimental Biology and Medicine*, **138**, 817–819.
Carter, E. A. & Isselbacher, K. J. (1973) Effect of ethanol on intestinal adenosine triphosphate (ATP) content. *Proceedings of the Society of Experimental Biology and Medicine*, **142** 1171–1173.
Carter, E. A., Drummey, G. D. & Isselbacher, K. J. (1971) Ethanol stimulates triglyceride synthesis by the intestine. *Science*, **174**, 1245–1247.

Chang, T., Lewis, J. & Glazko, A. J. (1967) Effect of ethanol and other alcohols on the transport of amino acids and glucose by everted sacs of rat small intestine. *Biochimica et biophysica Acta*, **135**, 1000–1007.

Christoffersen, P. & Nielsen, K. (1971) The frequency of Mallory bodies in liver biopsies from chronic alcoholics. *Acta pathologica et microbiologica scandinavica*, **79**, 274–278.

Christoffersen, P., Eghoje, K. & Juhl, E. (1973) Mallory bodies in liver biopsies from chronic alcoholics. A comparative morphological, biochemical and clinical study of two groups of chronic alcoholics with and without Mallory bodies. *Scandinavian Journal of Gastroenterology*, **8**, 341–346.

Clemente, F., Ribeiro, T., Colomb, E., Figarella, C. & Sarles, H. (1971) Comparaison des protéines de sucs pancréatiques humains normaux et pathologiques. Dosage des protéines sériques et mise en evidence d'une protéine particuliére dans la pancreatitite chronique calcifiante. *Biochimica et biophysica acta*, **251**, 456–466.

Colomb, E., Estevenon, J. P., Figarella, C., Guy, O. & Sarles, H. (1974) Characterisation of an additional protein in pancreatic juice of men with chronic calcifying pancreatitis. Identification of lactoferrin. *Biochimica et biophysica acta*, **342**, 306–312.

Cook, P. (1971) Cancer of the oesophagus in Africa: a summary of the evidence for the frequency of occurrence and a preliminary indication of possible association with the consumption of alcoholic drinks made from maize. *British Journal of Cancer*, **25**, 853–885.

Cook, G. C. & Hutt, M. S. R. (1967) The liver after kwashiorkor. *British Medical Journal*, **3**, 454–457.

Dagorn, J. C., Michel, R., Figarella, C. & Sarles, H. (1975) Effet de l'alcolisme chronique sur la synthège des enzymes pancréatiques chez le rat avant et après stimulation de la sécrétine. *Biologie gastroenterologie* (in press).

Daves, I. A., Miller, J. H. & Lemmi, C. A. E. (1965) Mechanism and inhibition of alcohol-stimulated gastric secretion. *Surgical Forum*, **16**, 305–307.

Davidson, C. S. (1971) Alcoholic hepatitis. *New England Journal of Medicine*, **284**, 1378.

Davidson, C. S. & MacDonald, R. A. (1962) Recovery from active hepatic disease of the alcoholic. *Archives of Internal Medicine*, **110**, 592–595.

Davis, A. E. & Pirola, R. C. (1968) The relationship of alcohol to pancreatic disease. In *Progress in Pancreatology*. Proceedings of the Third Symposium of the European Pancreatic Club, pp. 211–215. Prague, Czechoslovakia: Czechoslovak Medical Press.

Davis, V. E. & Walsh, M. J. (1970) Alcohol, amines and alkaloids: a possible biochemical basis for alcohol addiction. *Science*, **167**, 1005–1007.

Denk, H., Gschnait, F. & Wolff, K. (1975) Hepatocellular hyalin (Mallory bodies) in long-term griseofulvin-treated mice. *Laboratory Investigation*, **32**, 773–776.

Dimagno, E. P., Go, V. L. W. & Summerskill, W. H. J. (1973) Relationship between pancreatic enzyme outputs and malabsorption in severe pancreatic insufficiency. *New England Journal of Medicine*, **228**, 813–815.

Dimagno, E. P., Malagelada, J. R. & Go, V. L. W. (1975) Relationship between alcoholism and pancreatic insufficiency. *Annals of the New York Academy of Sciences*, **252**, 200–207.

Drenick, E. J., Simmons, F. & Murphy, J. F. (1970) Effect on hepatic morphology of treatment of obesity by fasting, reducing diets and small bowel bypass. *New England Journal of Medicine*, **282**, 820–834.

Edmondson, H. A., Peters, R. L., Reynolds, T. B. & Kuzma, O. T. (1963) Sclerosing hyaline necrosis of the liver in the chronic alcoholic: a recognisable clinical syndrome. *Annals of Internal Medicine*, **59**, 646–673.

Engeset, A., Lygren, T. & Idsoe, R. (1963) The incidence of peptic ulcer among alcohol abusers and non-abusers. *Quarterly Journal of Studies on Alcohol*, **24**, 622–626.

Estevenon, J. P., Sarles, H. & Figarella, C. (in press) Abnormal presence of lactoferrin in the duodenal juice of patients suffering from chronic calcifying pancreatitis.

French, S. W. & Davies, P. L. (1974) The Mallory body in the pathogenesis of alcoholic liver disease. In *Biochemical, Epidemiological and Clinical Aspects of the Etiology of Alcoholic Liver Pathology*, ed. Israel, Y.

Galambos, J. T. (1972a) Alcoholic hepatitis—its therapy and prognosis. In *Progress in Liver Disease*, ed. Popper, H. & Schaffner, F., pp. 567–588. Grune & Stratton.

Galambos, J. T. (1972b) Natural history of alcoholic hepatitis. III. Histological changes. *Gastroenterology*, **63**, 1026–1035.

Galindo, F. (1968) Alcoholismo y Pancreatitis. Algunas consideraciones fisiopatogénicas. *Prensa médica argentina*, **55**, 1196.

Gerber, M. A. & Popper, H. (1972) Relation between central canals and portal tracts in alcoholic cirrhosis. *Human Pathology*, **3**, 199–207.

Gerber, M. A., Orr, W., Denk, H., Schaffner, F. & Popper, H. (1973) Hepatocellular hyaline in cholestasis and cirrhosis—its diagnostic significance. *Gastroenterology*, **64**, 89–98.

Gillespie, R. J. G. & Lucas, C. C. (1961) Effect of single intoxicating doses of ethanol on the gastric and intestinal mucosa of rats. *Canadian Journal of Biochemistry and Physiology*, **39**, 237–241.

Goebell, H., Steffen, C. H., Bode, C. H. & Hupe, K. (1970) Calcium ausscheidung im Pankreass aft von Hunden durch Pankreozymin. *Klinische Wochenschrift*, **48**, 755–757.

Gordon, M. S., O'Brien, P., Skillman, J. J. & Silen, W. (1975) The effect of carbenoxolone on changes in canine and human gastric mucosa caused by taurocholate and ethanol. *Surgery*, **77**, 707–714.

Goslin, J., Hong, S. S., Magbe, D. F. & White, T. T. (1965) Relationships between diet, ethyl alcohol consumption and some activities of the exocrine pancreas in rats. *Archives internationales de pharmacodynamie et de therapie*, **157**, 462–469.

Green, J. R. (1965) Subclinical acute liver disease of the alcoholic. *Australasian Annals of Medicine*, **14**, 111–124.

Greene, H. L., Herman, R. H. & Kraemer, S. (1971) Stimulation of jejunal adenyl cyclase by ethanol. *Journal of Laboratory and Clinical Medicine*, **78**, 336–342.

Gregory, D. H. & Levi, D. F. (1972) The clinical-pathologic spectrum of alcoholic hepatitis. *American Journal of Digestive Diseases*, **17**, 479–488.

Grossman, M. I. (1967) Neural and hormonal stimulation of gastric secretion of acid. In *Hand-book of Physiology*, Section 6, Vol. II, p. 935, ed. Code, C. American Physiological Society.

Gullo, L., Sarles, H., Mott, C. D., Tiscornia, O., Pauli, A. M. & Pastor, J. (1974) Pancreatic secretion of calcium in the normal man and in various diseases of the pancreas. *Rendiconti Gastroenterologica*, **6**, 35–44.

Halsted, C. H., Criggs, R. C. & Harris, J. W. (1967) The effect of alcoholism on the absorption of folic acid (^{3}H–PGA) evaluated by plasma levels and urine excretion. *Journal of Laboratory and Clinical Medicine*, **69**, 116–131.

Halsted, C. H., Robles, E. A. & Mezey, E. (1971) Decreased jejunal uptake of labelled folic acid (^{3}H–PGA) in alcoholic patients: roles of alcohol and nutrition. *New England Journal of Medicine*, **285**, 701–706.

Halsted, C. H., Robles, E. A. & Mezey, E. (1973a) Distribution of ethanol in the human gastrointestinal tract. *American Journal of Clinical Nutrition*, **26**, 831–834.

Halsted, C. H., Robles, E. A. & Mezey, E. (1973b) Intestinal malabsorption in folate-deficient alcoholics. *Gastroenterology*, **64**, 526–532.

Halsted, C. H., Bhanthumnavin, K. & Mezey, E. (in press) Jejunal uptake of tritiated folic acid (^{3}H–PGA) in the rat studied by in vivo perfusion.

Hardison, W. G. & Lee, F. I. (1966) Prognosis in acute liver disease of the alcoholic patient. *New England Journal of Medicine*, **275**, 61–66.

Hartcroft, W. S. (1973) The liver—nutritional guardian of the body. In *The Liver*, ed. Gall, E. A. & Mostofi, F. K., pp. 131–149. Baltimore: Williams & Wilkins.

Hartcroft, W. S. & Porta, E. A. (1967) Fatty livers in experimental animals and man: Type A and Type B. *Proceedings of the Canadian Federation Biology Society*, **10**, 46.

Harvey, R. F., Dowsett, L., Hartog, M. & Read, A. E. (1973) A radioimmunoassay for cholestokinin-pancreazymin. *Lancet*, **2**, 826–827.

Hawkins, R. D. & Kalant, H. (1972) The metabolism of ethanol and its metabolic effects. *Pharmacological Reviews*, **24**, 67–157.

Heckman, A. N. (1971) Association of lactoferrin with other proteins, as demonstrated by changes in electrophoretic mobility. *Biochimica et biophysica acta*, **251**, 380–387.

Helman, R. A., Temko, M. H., Nye, S. W., Sylvanus, W. & Fallon, H. J. (1971) Alcholic hepatitis. Natural history and evaluation of prednisolone therapy. *Annals of Internal Medicine*, **74**, 311–321.

Howard, J. M. & Jordan, G. (1968) *Surgical Diseases of the Pancreas*. Philadelphia: Lippincott.

Hoyumpa, A., Middleton, H., Wilson, F. & Schenker, S. (1974) Dual system of thiamine transport: characteristics and effect of ethanol. *Gastroenterology*, **66**, 714.

Hurst, A. (1939) Carcinoma of the oesophagus. *Lancet*, **1**, 621–625.
Iseri, O. A. & Gottlieb, L. S. (1971) Alcoholic hyaline and mega-mitochondria as separate and distinct entities in liver disease associated with alcoholism. *Gastroenterology*, **60**, 1027–1035.
Ishii, H., Joly, J.-G. & Lieber, C. S. (1973) Effect of ethanol on the amount and enzyme activities of hepatic rough and smooth microsomal membranes. *Biochimica et biophysica acta*, **291**, 411–420.
Israel, Y., Kalant, H. & Laufer, I. (1965) Effect of ethanol on the Na, K Mg-stimulated microsomal ATPase activity. *Biochemical Pharmacology*, **14**, 1803–1914.
Israel, Y., Salazar, I. & Rosenmann, E. (1968) Inhibitory effects of alcohol on intestinal amino acid transport in vivo and in vitro. *Journal of Nutrition*, **96**, 499–504.
Israel, Y., Valenzuela, J. E., Salazar, I. & Ugarte, G. (1969) Alcohol and amino acid transport in the human small intestine. *Journal of Nutrition*, **98**, 222–224.
Isselbacher, K. J., Carter, E. A. & Lui, S. (1971) Pathogenesis of the acute alcohol-induced fatty liver in animals. In *Alkohol und Leber*, ed. Gerok, W., Sickinger, K. & Hennekeuser, H. H., pp. 189–200. Stuttgart: Schattauer Verlag.
Jamieson, J. D. & Palade, G. E. (1967) Intracellular transport of secretory proteins in the pancreatic exocrine cell. 1. Role of the peripheral elements of the Golgi complex. *Journal of Cell Biology*, **34**, 577–598.
Johnston, S. J., Jones, P. F., Kyle, J. & Needham, C. D. (1973) Epidemiology and course of gastrointestinal haemorrhage in north-east Scotland. *British Medical Journal*, **3**, 655–660.
Kahn, L. B. (1973) Alcholic hyaline—a review. *South African Medical Journal*, **47**, 1423–1426.
Kamionkowski, M. D. & Fleshler, B. (1965) The role of alcoholic intake in oesophageal carcinoma. *American Journal of Medical Science*, **249**, 696–700.
Kawashima, K. & Glass, G. B. J. (1975) Alcohol injury to gastric mucosa in mice and its potentiation by stress. *American Journal of Digestive Diseases*, **20** (2), 162–172.
Keeley, A. F., Iseri, O. A. & Gottlieb, L. S. (1972) Ultrastructure of hyaline cytoplasmic inclusions in a human hepatoma: relationship to Mallory's alcoholic hyalin. *Gastroenterology*, **62**, 280–293.
Keller, A. Z. (1967) Cirrhosis of the liver, alcoholism and heavy smoking associated with cancer of the mouth and pharnyx. *Cancer*, **20**, 1015–1022.
Kern, W. H., Mikkelsen, W. P. & Turrill, F. L. (1969) The significance of hyaline necrosis in liver biopsies. *Surgery, Gynecology and Obstetrics*, **129**, 749–754.
Koch, O. R., Porta, E. A. & Hartcroft, W. S. (1969) A new experimental approach in the study of chronic alcoholism, No. 5, 'Superdiet'. *Laboratory Investigation*, **19**, 298.
Krawitt, E. L. (1973) Ethanol inhibits calcium transport in rats. *Nature*, **243**, 88–89.
Krawitt, E. L. (1975) Effects of ethanol ingestion on duodenal calcium transport. *Journal of Laboratory and Clinical Medicine*, **85** (4), 665–671.
Krebs, H. A. (1974) The metabolism of ethanol. In *Topics in Gastroenterology*—2, ed. Truelove, S. C. & Trowell, J., pp. 283–291. London: Blackwell.
Krebs, H. A. & Perkins, J. R. (1970) The physiological role of liver alcohol dehydrogenase. *Biochemical Journal*, **118**, 635–644.
Lee, F. I. (1965) Immunoglobulins in viral hepatitis and active alcoholic liver disease. *Lancet*, **2**, 1043–1046.
Leevy, C. M., Chen, T. & Zetterman, R. (1975) Alcoholic hepatitis, cirrhosis and immunologic reactivity. *Annals of the New York Academy of Sciences*, **252**, 106–115.
Lieber, C. S. (1973a) Liver adaptation and injury in alcoholism. *New England Journal of Medicine*, **288**, 356–362.
Lieber, C. S. (1973b) Hepatic and metabolic effects of alcohol (1966–1973). *Gastroenterology*, **65**, 821–846.
Lieber, C. S. (1975a) Interference of ethanol in hepatic cellular metabolism. *Annals of the New York Academy of Sciences*, **252**, 24–50.
Lieber, C. S. (1975b) Hepatitis, cirrhosis and their inter-relationships. *Annals of the New York Academy of Sciences*, **252**, 63–83.
Lieber, C. S. & Rubin, E. (1969) Alcoholic fatty liver. *New England Journal of Medicine*, **280**, 705–708.
Lieber, C. S., Spritz, N. & DeCarli, L. M. (1969) Fatty liver produced by dietary deficiencies: its pathogenesis and potentiation by ethanol. *Journal of Lipid Research*, **10**, 398–405.

Lelbach, W. K. (1966, 1967) Leberschäden bei chronischem Alkoholisms. *Acta hepatosplenologica*, **13**, 321–349; **14**, 9–39.

Lelbach, W. K. (1975) Cirrhosis in the alcoholic and its relation to the volume of alcohol abuse. *Annals of the New York Academy of Sciences*, **252**, 85–105.

Lindenbaum, J. & Lieber, C. S. (1969) Alcohol induced malabsorption of vitamin B_{12} in man. *Nature*, **224**, 806.

Lindenbaum, J. & Lieber, C. S. (1975) Effects of chronic ethanol administration on intestinal absorption in man in the absence of nutritional deficiency. *Annals of the New York Academy of Sciences*, **252**, 228–234.

Lindenbaum, J., Shea, N., Saha, J. R. & Lieber, C. S. (1973) Mechanism of alcohol-induced malabsorption of vitamin B_{12}. *Gastroenterology*, **64**, 762.

Littleton, J. M. (1975) The experimental approach to alcoholism. *British Journal of Addiction* **70**, 99–122.

Maityra, B. B. (1963) Influence of ethanol on gastric secretion. *Annals of Biochemistry and Experimental Medicine*, **23**, 539–549.

Mallory, F. B. (1911) Cirrhosis of the liver—five different types of lesions from which in may arise. *Bulletin of the Johns Hopkins Hospital*, **22**, 69–75.

Marin, G. A., Clark, M. L. & Senior, J. R. (1969) Studies of malabsorption occurring in patients with Laënnec's cirrhosis. *Gastroenterology*, **56**, 727–736.

Marin, G. A., Ward, N. L. & Fischer, R. (1973) Effect of ethanol on pancreatic and biliary secretions in humans. *American Journal of Digestive Diseases*, **18**, 825–833.

McGee, J. O'D., O'Hare, R. P. & Patrick, R. S. (1973) Stimulation by factors released from injured liver. *Nature (New Biology)*, **243**, 121–123.

Menguy, R. B., Hallenbeck, G. A., Bollman, J. L. & Grindlay, J. H. (1958) Intraductal pressures and sphincteric resistance in canine pancreatic biliary ducts after various stimuli. *Surgery, Gynecology and Obstetrics*, **106**, 306.

Mezey, E. (1975) Intestinal function on chronic alcoholism. *Annals of the New York Academy of Sciences*, **252**, 215–227.

Mezey, E., Jow, E., Slavin, R. E. & Tabon, F. (1970) Pancreatic function and intestinal absorption in chronic alcoholism. *Gastroenterology*, **59**, 657–664.

Middleton, W. R. J., Carter, E. A., Drummey, G. D. & Isselbacher, K. J. (1971) Effect of oral ethanol administration on intestinal cholesterogenesis in the rat. *Gastroenterology*, **60**, 880–887.

Mihas, A. A., Bull, D. M. & Davidson, C. S. (1975) Cell mediated immunity to liver in patients with alcoholic hepatitis. *Lancet*, **1**, 951–953.

Minaire, Y., Descos, L., Daly, J. P., Bererd, M. B. & Lambert, R. (1973) The inter-relationships of pancreatic enzymes in health and disease under cholecystokinin stimulation. *Digestion*, **9**, 8–20.

Misra, P. S., Lefèvre, A., Ishii, H., Rubin, E. & Lieber, C. S. (1971) Increase of ethanol, meprobamate and pentobarbital metabolism after chronic ethanol administration in man and rats. *American Journal of Medicine*, **51**, 346–351.

Mistilis, S. P. & Garske, A. (1969) Induction of alcohol dehydrogenase in liver and gastrointestinal tract. *Australasian Annals of Medicine*, **18**, 227–231.

Mistilis, S. P. & Ockner, R. K. (1972) Effects of ethanol on endogenous lipid and lipoprotein metabolism in small intestine. *Journal of Laboratory and Clinical Medicine*, **80**, 34–46.

Mott, C. D., Sarles, H., Tiscornia, O. & Gullo, L. (1972) Inhibitory action of alcohol on human exocrine pancreatic secretion. *American Journal of Digestive Diseases*, **17**, 902–910.

Mowat, N. A. G., Needham, C. D. & Brunt, P. W. (1975) The natural history of gastric ulcer in a community: a four-year study. *Quarterly Journal of Medicine*, N.S. **XLIV** (173) 45–56.

Myerson, R. M. (1973) Metabolic aspects of alcohol and their biological significance. *Medical Clinics of North America*, **57**, 925–940.

Needham, C. D., Kyle, J., Jones, P. F., Johnston, S. J. & Kerridge, D. F. (1971) Aspirin and alcohol in gastrointestinal haemorrhage. *Gut*, **12**, 819–821.

Orrego-Matte, H., Navia, E., Feres, A. & Costamaillere, L. (1968) Ethanol ingestion and incorporation of ^{32}P into phospholipids of pancreas in the rat. *Gastroenterology*, **56**, 280–285.

Palasciano, G., Tiscornia, O., Hage, G. & Sarles, H. (1974) Chronic alcoholism and endogenous CCK-PZ. *Biomédecine*, **21**, 94–97.

Palmer, E. D. (1954) Gastritis: a revaluation. *Medicine*, **33**, 199–290.
Pawan, G. L. S. (1972) Metabolism of alcohol (ethanol) in man. *Proceedings of the Nutrition Society*, **31**, 83–89.
Payan, H., Sarles, H., Demirdjian, M., Gautier, A. P., Cros, R. C. & Burbec, J. P. (1972) Study of the histological features of chronic pancreatitis by corresponding analysis. Identification of chronic calcifying pancreatitis as an entity. *Review of European and Clinical Biology*, **17**, 663–670.
Pequignot, G. (1961) Die rolle des Alkohols bei der Ätiologie von Leberzirrhosen in Frankreich. *Münchener medizinische Wochenshrift*, **103**, 1464–1468.
Pequignot, G. & Tuyns, A. (1975) Rations d'alcool déclarées et resques pathologiques. In *Symposium Franco-Britannique sur L'alcoolisme* (to be published).
Peters, R. L. & Reynolds, T. B. (1973) Hepatic changes simulating alcoholic liver disease, post ileo-jejunal bypass (Abstract). *Gastroenterology*, **65**, 364.
Petrie, M. X. E. & Brunt, P. (1976) Studies in alcoholic liver disease in Britain. II. Liver disease in north-east Scotland (in preparation).
Pettigrew, M. N., Govdie, R. B., Russell, R. I. & Chaudhuri, A. K. R. (1972) Evidence for a role of hepatitis virus B in chronic alcoholic liver disease. *Lancet*, **2**, 724–725.
Popper, H. (1975) Cirrhosis. *Clinics in Gastroenterology*, **4**, 225–226.
Popper, H. & Becker, K., ed. (1975) *Collagen Metabolism and the Liver*. New York: Stratton Intercontinental.
Popper, H. & Kent, G. (1975) Fibrosis in chronic liver disease. *Clinics in Gastroenterology*, **4**, 315–332.
Popper, H. & Schaffner, F. (1974) Steatosis–Mallory's hyaline–cirrhosis. *Gastroenterology*, **67**, 185–188.
Popper, H. & Szanto, P. B. (1957) Fatty liver with hepatic failure in alcoholics. *Journal of the Mount Sinai Hospital*, **24**, 1121–1131.
Popper, H. & Udenfriend, S. (1970) Hepatic fibrosis. *American Journal of Medicine*, **49**, 707–721.
Popper, H., Rubin, E., Krus, S. & Schaffner, F. (1960) Post-necrotic cirrhosis in alcoholics. *Gastroenterology*, **39**, 669–686.
Popper, H., Davidson, C. S., Leevy, C. M. & Schaffner, F. (1969) The social impact of liver disease. *New England Journal of Medicine*, **281**, 1455–1458.
Porter, H. P., Simon, F. R., Pope, C. E., Volwiler, W. & Fenster, L. F. (1971) Corticosteroid therapy in severe alcoholic hepatitis. *New England Journal of Medicine*, **284**, 1350–1355.
Raskin, N. H. (1975) Alcoholism or acetaldehydism? *New England Journal of Medicine*, **292**, 422–423.
Reid, N. C. R. W., Brunt, P. W., Bias, W. B., Maddrey, W. C., Alonso, B. A. & Iber, F. L. (1968) Genetic characteristics and cirrhosis: a controlled study of 200 patients. *British Medical Journal*, **2**, 463–465.
Reynolds, T. B. & Edmundson, H. A. (1971) Alcoholic hepatitis. *Annals of Internal Medicine*, **74**, 440–442.
Reynolds, T. B., Hidemura, R., Michel, H. & Peters, R. (1969) Portal hypertension without cirrhosis in alcoholic liver disease. *Annals of Internal Medicine*, **70**, 497–506.
Rice, J. D., Jr & Yesner, R. (1960) The prognostic significance of so-called Mallory bodies in portal cirrhosis. *Archives of Internal Medicine*, **105**, 99–104.
Robertson, M. A., Harington, J. S. & Bradshaw, E. (1971) The cancer pattern in Africans at Baragwanath Hospital, Johannesburg. *British Journal of Cancer*, **25**, 377–384.
Robles, E. A., Mezey, E., Halsted, C. H. & Schuster, M. (1972) Effect of ethanol on intestinal motility in man (Abstract). *Gastroenterology*, **67**, 799.
Rodgers, J. G. & O'Brien, R. J. (1975) The effect of acute ethanol treatment on lipid re-esterifying enzymes of the rat small bowel. *American Journal of Digestive Diseases*, **20**, 354–358.
Rogers, A. E. & Newberne, P. M. (1973) Animal models of human disease. Alcoholic or nutrition fatty liver and cirrhosis. *American Journal of Pathology*, **73**, 817–820.
Roggin, G. M., Iber, F. L., Kater, R. M. H. & Tobon, F. (1969) Malabsorption in the chronic alcoholic. *Johns Hopkins Medical Journal*, **125**, 321–330.
Roy, S., Ramalingaswami, V. & Nayak, N. D. (1971) An ultrastructural study of the liver in Indian childhood cirrhosis with particular reference to the structure of alcoholic hyaline. *Gut*, **12**, 693–701.

Rubin, E. (1973) The spectrum of alcoholic liver injury. In *The Liver*, ed. Gall, E. A. & Mostofi, F. K., pp. 199–217. Baltimore: Williams & Wilkins.
Rubin, E. & Lieber, C. S. (1968) Alcohol induced hepatic injury in non-alcoholic volunteers. *New England Journal of Medicine*, **278**, 869–876.
Rubin, E. & Lieber, C. S. (1973) Experimental alcoholic hepatitis: a new primate model. *Science*, **182**, 712–713.
Rubin, E. & Lieber, C. S. (1974) Fatty liver, alcoholic hepatitis and cirrhosis produced by alcohol in primates. *New England Journal of Medicine*, **290**, 128–135.
Rubin, E. & Lieber, C. S. (1975) Relation of alcoholic liver injury to cirrhosis. *Clinics in Gastroenterology*, **4**, 247–272.
Rubin, E., Beattie, D. S., Toth, A. & Lieber, C. S. (1972) Structural and functional effects of ethanol on hepatic mitochondria. *Federation Proceedings*, **31**, 131–140.
Rubin, E., Rybak, B. J., Lindenbaum, J., Gerson, C. D., Walker, G. & Lieber, C. S. (1972) Ultrastructural changes in the small intestine induced by ethanol. *Gastroenterology*, **63**, 801–814.
Sardesai, V. M. & Orten, J. M. (1968) Effect of prolonged alcohol consumption in rats on pancreatic protein synthesis. *Journal of Nutrition*, **96**, 241–246.
Sarles, H. (1971) Alcoholism and pancreatitis. *Scandinavian Journal of Gastroenterology*, **6**, 193–198.
Sarles, H. (1973) An international survey on nutrition and pancreatitis. *Digestion*, **9**, 389–403.
Sarles, H. (1974) Chronic calcifying pancreatitis. Chronic alcoholic pancreatitis. *Gastroenterology* (Progress Report), **66**.
Sarles, H. (1975) Alcohol and the pancreas. *New York Academy of Sciences*, **252**, 171–182.
Sarles, J. C. & Midejean, A. (1973) Electromyographic study of the action of alcohol upon the sphincter of Oddi. *Digestion*, **9**, 93–94.
Sarles, H., Muratore, R. & Sarles, J. C. (1961) Étude anatomique des pancréatites de l'adulte. *Semaine des hôpitaux de Paris*, **37**, 1507–1522.
Sarles, H., Sarles, J. C., Bamatte, R., Muratore, R., Gaini, M., Guien, C., Pastor, J. & Leroy, F. (1965) Observations on 205 confirmed cases of acute pancreatitis, recurring pancreatitis and chronic pancreatitis. *Gut*, **6**, 545–559.
Sarles, H., Figarella, C. & Clemente, F. (1971a) The interactions of ethanol, dietary lipids and proteins on the rat pancreas. 1. Pancreatic enzymes. *Digestion*, **4**, 13–22.
Sarles, H., Lebreuil, G., Tasso, F., Figarella, C., Clemente, F., Devaux, M. A., Fagonde, B. & Payan, H. (1971b) A comparison of alcoholic pancreatitis in rat and man. *Gut*, **12**, 377–388.
Schaffner, F. (1971) Electron microscopy of acute alcoholic hepatitis. In *Alcohol and the Liver*, ed. Gerok, W., Sickinger, K. & Hennekauser, H. H., pp. 273–279. Stuttgart: Schattauer.
Schaffner, F. & Popper, H. (1970) Alcoholic hepatitis in the spectrum of ethanol-induced liver injury. *Scandinavian Journal of Gastroenterology*, Suppl., **7**, 69.
Schapiro, H., Cummings, A. J. & Luckey, S. (1965) Dissociation between gastric secretion and motility. *American Journal of Digestive Diseases*, **10**, 751–757.
Schoenberg, B. S., Bailar, J. C. & Fraumeni, J. F. (1971) Certain mortality patterns of oesophageal cancer in the United States. *Journal of the National Cancer Institute*, **46**, 63.
Small, M., Longarini, A. & Zamchek, N. (1959) Disturbances of digestive physiology following acute drinking episodes in 'skid-row' alcoholics. *American Journal of Medicine*, **27**, 575–585.
Smith, B. M., Skillman, J. J., Edwards, B. G. & Silen, W. (1971) Permeability of the human gastric mucosa. Alteration by acetyl salicylic acid and ethanol. *New England Journal of Medicine*, **285**, 716–721.
Solomon, N., Solomon, T. E., Jacobson, E. D. & Shanbour, L. L. (1974) Direct effects of alcohol on in vivo and in vitro exocrine pancreatic secretion and metabolism. *American Journal of Digestive Diseases*, **19**, 253–260.
Spencer, R. P., Brody, K. R. & Lutters, B. M. (1964) Some effects of ethanol on the gastrointestinal tract. *American Journal of Digestive Diseases*, **9**, 599–604.
Steigmann, F., Dourderekas, D., Shobassy, N., Vittal, S. B. V., Szanto, P. B., Ainis, H., Khin, U. & Telischi, M. (1974) Humoral response in patients with liver disease. *American Journal of Gastroenterology*, **61**, 349–355.
Sternlieb, I. (1975) The development of cirrhosis in Wilson's disease. *Clinics in Gastroenterology*, **4**, 367–379.

Sun, D. C. H., Albacete, R. A. & Chen, J. K. (1967) Malabsorption studies in cirrhosis of the liver. *Archives of Internal Medicine*, **119**, 567–572.
Svoboda, D. J. & Manning, R. T. (1964) Chronic alcoholism with fatty metamorphosis of the liver: mitochondrial alterations in hepatic cells. *American Journal of Pathology*, **44**, 645–662.
Tasso, F., Stemmelin, N., Clop, J., Cros, R. C., Durbec, J. P. & Sarles, H. (1973) Comparative morphometric study of the human pancreas in its normal state and in primary chronic calcifying pancreatitis. *Biomédecine*, **18**, 134–144.
Thaler, H. (1975) Relation of steatosis to cirrhosis. *Clinics in Gastroenterology*, **4**, 273–280.
Thomson, A. L., Baker, H. & Leevy, C. M. (1970) Patterns of ^{35}S-thiamine hydrochloride absorption in the malnourished alcoholic patient. *Journal of Laboratory and Clinical Medicine*, **76**, 34–35.
Tiscornia, O. M., Gullo, L., Sarles, H., Devaux, M. A., Michel, G. & Grimaud, R. (1972) The inhibition of canine exocrine pancreatic secretion by intravenous alcohol. *Gastroenterology*, **62**, 866.
Tiscornia, O. M., Gullo, L., Sarles, H., Devaux, M. A., Michel, G. & Grimaud, R. (1973a) The inhibition of canine exocrine pancreatic secretion by intravenous ethanol. *Digestion*, **9**, 231–240.
Tiscornia, O. M., Hage, G., Palasciano, G., Brasca, A., Devaux, M. A. & Sarles, H. (1973b) The effects of pentolinium and vagotomy on the inhibition of canine exocine pancreatic secretion by intravenous ethanol. *Biomédecine*, **18**, 159–163.
Tiscornia, O. M., Palasciano, G. & Sarles, H. (1975) Atropine and exocrine pancreatic secretion in alcohol fed dogs. *American Journal of Gastroenterology*, **63**, 33–36.
Tiscornia, O. M., Palasciano, G., Dzieniszewski, J. & Sarles, H. (1976a) Simultaneous changes in pancreatic and gastric secretion induced by acute intravenous ethanol infusion. Effects of atropine and reserpine (to be published).
Tiscornia, O. M., Palasciano, G. & Sarles, H. (1976b) Canine exocrine pancreatic secretory changes induced by acute and chronic ethanol administration. *American Journal of Gastroenterology* (in press).
Tobon, F. & Mezey, E. (1971) Effect of ethanol administration on hepatic ethanol and drug-metabolising enzymes and on rates of ethanol degradation. *Journal of Laboratory and Clinical Medicine*, **77**, 110–121.
Tomasulo, P. A., Kater, R. M. U. & Iber, F. L. (1968) Impairment of thiamine absorption in alcoholism. *American Journal of Clinical Nutrition*, **21**, 1340–1344.
Treffot, M. J. (1975) Chronic alcoholism and endogenous gastrin. *American Journal of Gastroenterology*, **63** (1), 29, 32.
Treffot, M. J., Tiscornia, O. M., Palasciano, G., Hage, G. & Sarles, H. (1976) Chronic alcoholism and endogenous gastrin. *American Journal of Gastroenterology* (in press).
Von Wartburg, J. P. & Papenberg, J. (1966) Alcohol dehydrogenase and ethanol metabolism. *Psychosomatic Medicine*, **28** (11), 405–413.
Walton, B. E., Shapiro, H., Yeung, T. & Woodward, E. R. (1965) Effect of alcohol on pancreatic duct pressure. *American Journal of Surgery*, **31**, 142–144.
Weise, R. E., Schapiro, H. & Woodward, E. R. (1961) Effect of parenteral alcohol on gastric secretion. *Surgical Forum*, **12**, 281–282.
Wiggers, K. D., French, S. W., French, B. A. & Carr, B. N. (1973) The ultrastructure of Mallory body filaments. *Laboratory Investigation*, **29**, 652–658.
Williams, A. W. (1956) Effects of alcohol on gastric mucosa. *British Medical Journal*, **1**, 256 259.
Winship, D. H., Calflisch, C. R., Zboralske, F. F., & Hogan, W. J. (1968) Deterioration of oesophageal peristalsis in patients with alcoholic neuropathy. *Gastroenterology*, **55**, 173–178.
Wolff, G. (1970) Does alcohol cause chronic gastritis? *Gastroenterology*, **5**, 289–291.
Woodward, E. R., Robertson, C. & Fried, W. (1957) Further studies on the isolated gastric antrum. *Gastroenterology*, **32**, 868–877.
Woodward, E. R., Robertson, C., Ruttenberg, H. D. & Shapiro, H. (1957) Alcohol as a gastric secretory stimulant. *Gastroenterology*, **32**, 727–737.
Yokoo, H., Minick, O. T., Batti, F. & Kent, G. (1972) Morphologic variants of alcoholic hyalin. *American Journal of Pathology*, **69**, 25–40.

8
ENDOSCOPIC CANNULATION OF THE PAPILLA OF VATER
Clinical and Research Developments
Peter B. Cotton

The historical aspects and technical basis of endoscopic cannulation of the papilla of Vater have been reviewed in detail elsewhere (Cotton, 1972). This contribution attempts to assess the clinical relevance of endoscopic retrograde cholangio-pancreatography (ERCP) alongside other diagnostic techniques, and explores the new developments such as endoscopic sphincterotomy and analysis of pure secretions.

TECHNIQUE AND HAZARDS

Basic instrumentation has scarcely changed since the initial introduction of specialised lateral-viewing duodenoscopes (Oi, 1970; Ogoshi, Tobita and Hara, 1970). Cannulation is also possible with slightly larger lateral-viewing endoscopes and with instruments with a swing-lens system. Developments in endoscopy have in one sense made cannulation more difficult. Contrary to earlier practice, most doctors now start endoscopy with forward-viewing instruments, which are not suitable for cannulation. The use of a lateral-viewing system requires reorientation. Attempts at cannulation are doomed to failure if not preceded by some months of personal familiarisation with a suitable instrument, and with the duodenal loop. At this stage, the beginner can expect to achieve papillary cannulation in about half of the first 30 to 40 patients; ideally these attempts should be made in the presence of an expert. All examiners with experience of over 200 to 300 patients report technical success rates of around 90 per cent for entering the pancreatic duct and slightly less for the bile duct. A few attempts fail because of poor patient toleration or instrument breakdown. Gross disease or operative distortion of the stomach or duodenum may render deep duodenoscopy impossible. Using standard instruments, cannulation is difficult in patients under the age of 10 years. The Billroth II partial gastrectomy often provides an exceptional challenge, which may be overcome with a forward-viewing instrument. Previous sphincter surgery may prevent cannulation if stenosis has occurred, and also if scarring from the surgical duodenotomy has significantly reduced the duodenal lumen. In the absence of these factors, the experienced examiner will always be able to see the papilla, and to pass a cannula into its apex. Occasionally, repeated insertions of the cannula from different angles fails to allow opacification of the relevant duct, even after ensuring sphincter relaxation with drugs such as glucagon. This failure may be due to disease within or beneath the papilla. When cannulation fails, gastroduodenoscopy alone can provide diagnostic information in patients with biliary or pancreatic problems.

Complications have been rare but occasionally serious. Endoscopy itself carries a small risk of medication reactions and perforation. The two hazards peculiar to ERCP are acute pancreatitis and the introduction of infection into stagnant systems, producing cholangitis and infection of pseudocysts. Febrile reactions, cholangitis and overt septicaemia have only been seen in the presence of biliary stasis particularly in patients already suffering from recurrent cholangitis. Whilst the overall incidence of such complications is less than 2 per cent (Cremer and Engelholm, 1973), a figure of 20 per cent has been reported in patients with biliary disease (Liguory et al, 1974). Oi (1974) encountered 14 deaths from cholangitis in a survey of over 7000 procedures. Nebel et al (1975) reviewed North American experience of 3884 examinations; there were 25 patients with cholangitis and two deaths. It is likely that symptoms of cholangitis arise from the dissemination of bacteria already present in a stagnant system, but the introduction of infection cannot be excluded. There are no data to validate the routine use of parenteral or intraductal antibiotics. When we demonstrate biliary stasis we commence parenteral antibiotics (usually gentamicin and ampicillin) and recommend definitive surgery within 48 h.

A transient rise in serum amylase and lipase occurs in most patients following pancreatography. We found no evidence that the prophylactic administration of aprotinin (Trasylol) reduced the rise of amylase, but glucagon is effective (Silvis and Vennes, 1975). Clinically overt acute pancreatitis is rare. In the North American survey, there were 51 patients (1.2 per cent) with two deaths (Nebel et al, 1975). However, the Erlangen group reported a higher figure of 7.4 per cent in 569 patients, with three deaths (Ruppin et al, 1974). We have seen five pancreatic complications in over 700 examinations, all of them occurring in patients already suffering from recurrent episodes of pancreatitis; three had pseudocysts. These patients are at greater risk (Seifert et al, 1974) even when the cyst itself is not opacified.

CLINICAL RELEVANCE OF DIAGNOSTIC ERCP

ERCP is technically complex and serious complications can occur. Does it provide any advantage over alternative techniques in any given clinical context? These will be discussed in turn.

Jaundice

In many patients the diagnosis of extrahepatic obstructive jaundice can be made without difficulty. There may be a typical history of biliary pain and fever, or an insidious onset with a palpable gallbladder. Grey-scale ultrasonography permits the inclusion of other patients into this category by demonstrating dilated intrahepatic ducts (Taylor et al, 1974). In such patients the radiological practice varies. Many surgeons proceed direct to laparotomy and perform any radiological investigations on the operating table. Others prefer to undertake preoperative cholangiography. This can be performed via the liver (transhepatic cholangiogram), or the papilla. When there is already a commitment to surgery, transhepatic cholangiography would seem the most appropriate technique, particularly since the introduction of the fine-bore needle (Okuda et al, 1974; Conn, 1975; Elias et al, 1975).

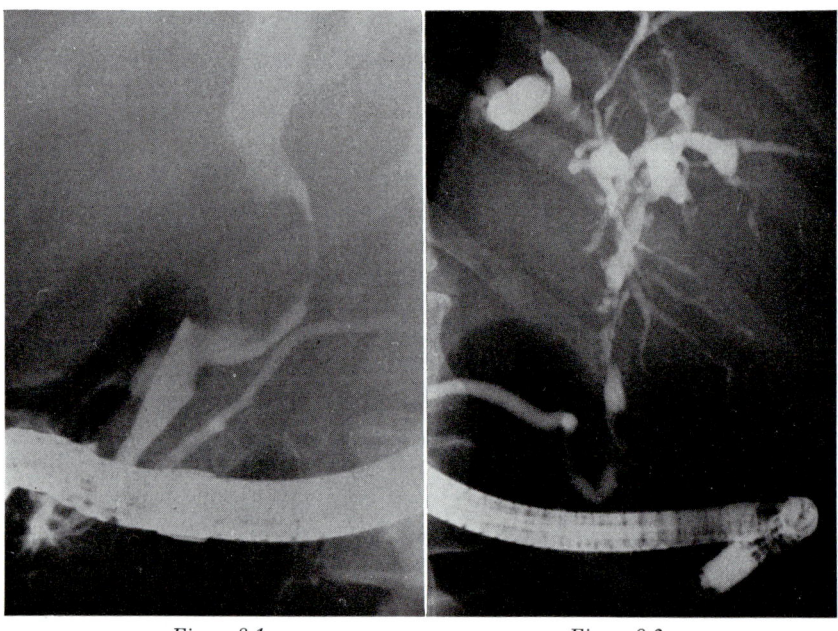

Figure 8.1   Figure 8.2

Figure 8.1 Obstructive jaundice. Carcinoma of gallbladder involving common bile duct
Figure 8.2 Advanced sclerosing cholangitis in a patient with ulcerative colitis. (Image reversed, patient lying prone during examination)

However, the situation is different in patients where the distinction between intra- and extrahepatic obstruction remains in doubt. The likelihood of entering non-obstructed ducts via the transhepatic route is small; there remains a risk of biliary leakage or bleeding in patients where surgery is not primarily required. In patients with difficult jaundice it is no longer necessary to procrastinate and keep the patient under observation, for retrograde cholangiography along with the associated gastroduodenoscopy can provide a precise diagnosis in a high percentage of patients (Blumgart, Salmon and Cotton, 1974; Cremer and Engelholm, 1973). The clinical dilemma is immediately defused whether the ducts are shown to be normal or obstructed. Where an abnormality is seen its cause is usually clear (Fig. 8.1). Calculi rarely provide complete obstruction and usually move up the duct during contrast injection. The distinction between cholangiocarcinoma and sclerosing cholangitis (Fig. 8.2) may occasionally prove difficult. Intraductal cytology and even biopsy can be helpful. We emphasise the small but definite risk of post-ERCP cholangitis where biliary stasis is demonstrated. These patients require surgical relief at an early stage.

Problems Following Biliary Surgery

Many patients continue to have symptoms following cholecystectomy (Johnston, 1975; Bodvall, 1973; Way, Admirand and Dunphy, 1972) and some are incapacitated by recurrent pain. Even in the absence of jaundice

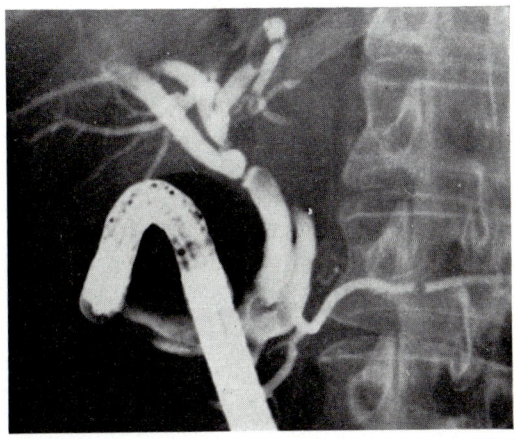

Figure 8.3 Recurrent pain and jaundice following cholecystectomy. ERCP shows a stricture of the common hepatic duct and left intrahepatic duct. There is a long cystic duct remnant, and calculi are present within it and the common bile duct

intravenous cholangiograms may fail to provide diagnostic radiographs and in these patients, retrograde cholangiography has proved to be a major advance. High quality studies can demonstrate once and for all whether there is a stricture (Fig. 8.3), a stone, or no abnormality. In the latter situation endoscopy and ERCP have the added advantage of contributing to the investigation of gastric, duodenal and pancreatic disease. The adequacy and function of any previous sphincter surgery can be assessed. Papillary manometry and endoscopic sphincterotomy will be discussed later.

Known Recurrent Pancreatitis

Whilst such patients can be classified into those with relapsing chronic and relapsing acute disease the clinical problem is the same. It concerns the need to eliminate aetiological factors such as gallstones, to assess the state of the duct systems and to define any role for surgery (Cotton and Beales, 1974). There is no indication for pancreatography in patients with a calcified pancreas except when symptoms are sufficient to warrant consideration of surgery. We have demonstrated a major duct lesion on pancreatography in almost half of a group of 63 patients with recurrent episodes of acute pancreatitis (Table 8.1). A number of these patients had pseudocysts which had not been suspected on prior clinical examination or barium studies. Ultrasonography should be performed prior to ERCP using a sensitive technique (Fig. 8.4). If symptoms are sufficient to warrant surgical intervention, endoscopic pancreatography may be useful immediately prior to operation (Figs. 8.5, 8.6). The evolution of smaller pseudocysts can be followed by serial ultrasonography.

Table 8.1 Results of ERCP in patients with relapsing acute pancreatitis

No pancreatogram obtained	7
Normal duct system	20
Minor abnormalities	8
Major duct lesions	28
Generalised	6
Localised	
Cysts	6 ⎫
Block	5 ⎬ 22
Stenosis	11 ⎭
Gallstones detected	5(+1)
Total patients	63

Previously undetected gallstones were found in five patients. In one other, retrograde cholangiography appeared normal, but surgery demonstrated stones in the gallbladder.

Follow-up of the patients detailed in Table 8.1 remains incomplete, and is too short to allow definite conclusions concerning the value of surgery based on the pancreatogram findings. However, the prognosis for patients with a normal or virtually normal duct system is certainly good if the initial cause for the pancreatitis is established and eliminated. Endoscopic pancreatography should reduce the inappropriate usage of exploratory laparotomy and of sphincter surgery in recurrent pancreatitis. In some patients ERCP may provide unexpected findings such as duodenal ulcers and gallstones (Table 8.1) even when standard x-rays have proved negative. Endoscopic pancreatography has a role in the assessment of patients after pancreatic surgery, in particular to establish the patency of any duct diversion procedure.

Abdominal Pain: Could it be Pancreatic?

The precise diagnostic contribution to pancreatic disease of endoscopic pancreatography remains in doubt. It has to be considered alongside the proliferating alternative techniques including function tests, arteriography and scanning (using isotopes, ultrasound, or EMI computer-assisted tomography). The analysis of pure pancreatic secretion may also have diagnostic application. A good test should be applicable to hospitals of all sizes since obscure abominal pain is a common condition.

Perhaps the most accurate test for pancreatic disease is a careful clinical history. In our experience pancreatography rarely provides a diagnosis of chronic pancreatic disease in the absence of suggestive symptoms or biochemical alterations. Pancreatography is an accurate method for diagnosing pancreatic cancer at the stage at which patients usually present for investiga-

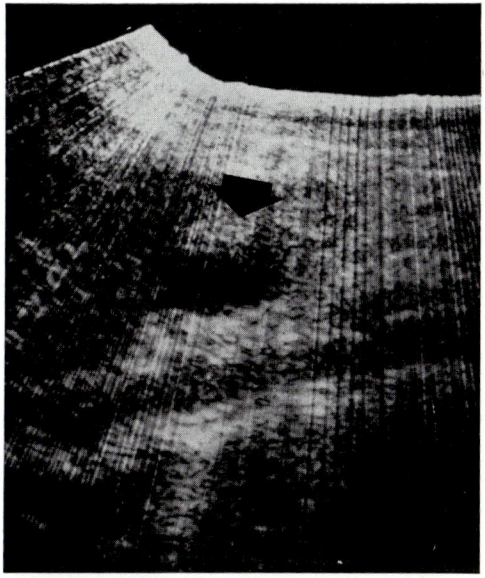

Figure 8.4 Sagittal ultrasound scan of the abdomen showing a pseudocyst (arrowed) lying anteriorly to the great vessels

tion (Stadelman et al, 1974). Although cannulation may fail to provide a pancreatogram in some 20 per cent of such patients, this failure is immediately obvious and in some it is possible to obtain diagnostic histology or cytology from the papillary area (Hatfield et al, 1975). The most frequent radiological findings are those of complete obstruction or stenosis (Fig. 8.7) (Classen et al, 1975). In some cases the distinction between chronic pancreatitis and cancer cannot be made on the radiographs alone and reliance must be placed on cytology or indeed the clinical history. Carcinoma and pancreatitis may occasionally coexist. Very few curable pancreatic cancers have been detected by pancreatography and endocrine adenomas are not seen with this technique. The diagnosis of smaller lesions requires detailed interpretation of branch duct patterns of which the normal variations are not yet documented (Cotton,

G

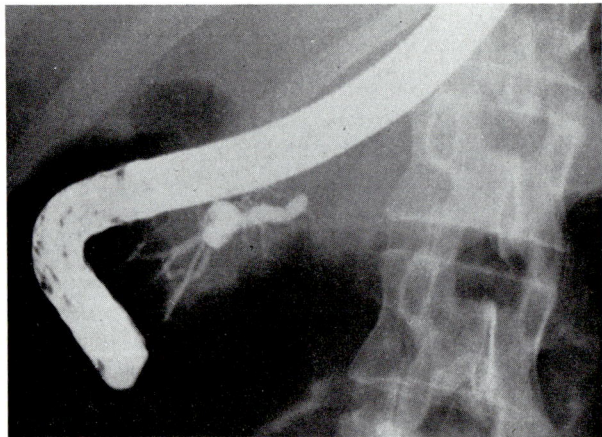

Figure 8.5 Complete obstruction of the pancreatic duct at the junction of the head and body. Traumatic pancreatitis causing a pseudocyst, as demonstrated by ultrasound in Figure 8.4

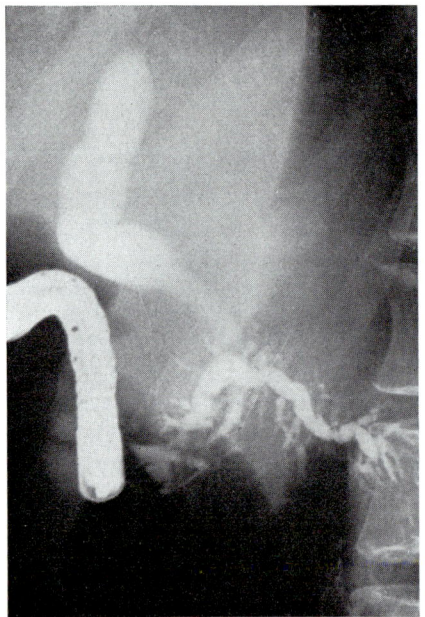

Figure 8.6 Chronic pancreatitis. Dilated pancreatic duct and branch ducts. Oedema of the pancreatic head causing distortion and narrowing of the retropancreatic portion of the bile duct, with dilatation above

1974). Most investigators avoid too extensive opacification of the smallest branches and parenchyma for fear of precipitating pancreatitis.

The abnormalities of established chronic pancreatitis are obvious (Fig. 8.8) but minor changes are more difficult to interpret (Fig. 8.9) (Kasugai et al, 1972). Recurrent pancreatitis occurs quite frequently in the presence of a normal main pancreatic duct system (Table 8.1) (Cotton and Beales, 1974). A good quality normal endoscopic pancreatogram virtually excludes cancer but does not exclude pancreatitis as a cause of recurrent pain.

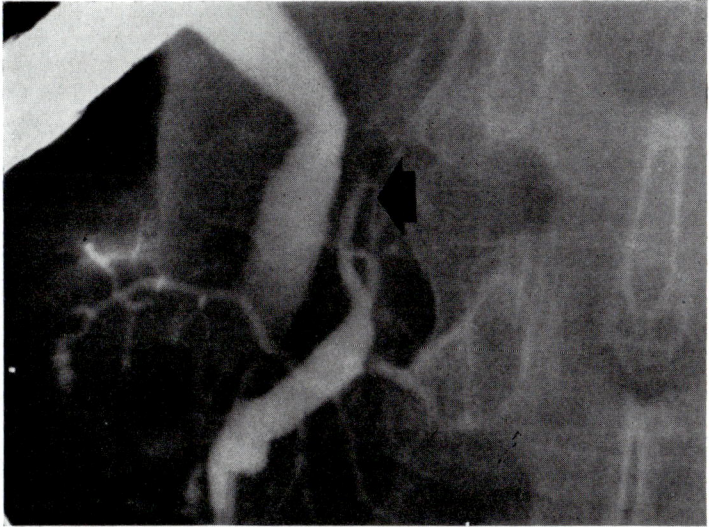

Figure 8.7 Cancer of the pancreatic head causing a 'rat-tail' stenosis and obstruction of the pancreatic duct (arrowed), and distortion of the bile duct

Comparison with Alternative Diagnostic Techniques

Imaging techniques are clinically attractive since they are non-invasive and virtually free of hazard. Isotope pancreatic scanning has proved somewhat disappointing. False positive scans (i.e. the pancreas is incorrectly labelled as abnormal) are sufficiently common to raise doubt about the significance of an abnormal scan (Baron, 1975), but the unequivocally normal scan may be helpful. In a recent British study (Spencer et al, 1974) none of the 110 patients with a normal scan was subsequently judged to have pancreatic disease. Scanning provided an effective screening test. Other results have not been so impressive. False normal scans have been found in 1 to 20 per cent of series (Charlesworth, Testa and Watson, 1970; Braganza, et al, 1973). In the largest report, 110 of 728 patients with a normal pancreatic image were subsequently found to have pancreatic disease (Miale, Rodriguez and Gill, 1972). Cotton et al (1975) compared endoscopic pancreatography with pancreatic scanning, in 62 patients. Four patients with normal gamma camera scans were found to have chronic pancreatic disease (two cancer, two chronic pancreatitis). Pancreatography had been positive in two, normal in one, and a failure in the fourth. The degree of observer variation in the reporting of pancreatic scan images was disturbing. Three experienced observers looked at each of the scans on three separate occasions. Answering the question as to whether or not the scan image was normal, the observers were unanimous in their individual reports in only 47, 66 and 73 per cent of cases. The observer variation in interpretation of pancreatograms is currently under study.

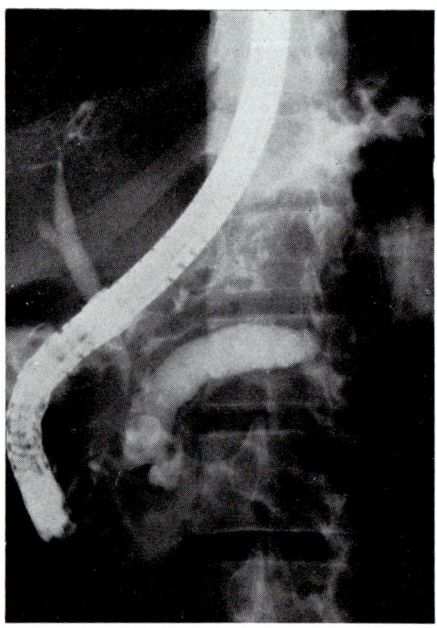

Figure 8.8 Chronic pancreatitis. Gross dilatation of the duct in the head and body. There is obstruction to the duct in the tail, and calculi within the duct at the head.

Pancreatic isotope scanning has been available long enough for clinicians to make their own pragmatic judgements. In most centres this judgement is not complementary and many departments have discontinued the technique for routine clinical purposes.

Ultrasonography has recently advanced with the development of more sophisticated apparatus particularly the grey-scale attachment. Whilst it was originally recommended only for the detection and analysis of cystic structures (Fig. 8.4) more extensive claims are now being made (Taylor et al, 1974; Weill et al, 1975; Sahel and Pietri, 1975; Walls et al, 1975). Current results of ultrasonography are highly dependent upon the enthusiasm and skill of the investigator in obtaining and interpreting the images and also sometimes in the adaptation and development of equipment. An overall assessment is impossible but the potential can be judged from a few examples. Engelhart (1975) demonstrated a tumour on ultrasound scan in 37 out of 39 patients confirmed by operation or autopsy. Weill et al (1975) showed the lesion in 38 out of 43 pancreatic cancers. In 162 patients with pancreatic disease, these authors gave only 13 false negative and 12 false positive reports. There were 4 false positive reports amongst 58 patients judged to have a normal pancreas. Sahel and Pietri (1975) compared pancreatography and ultrasonography in the diagnosis of 67 patients. Both techniques were correct in around 90 per cent of cases in the diagnosis of pancreatic cancer and the normal pancreas. In combination the accuracy was virtually complete. They recommend ultrasonography as the primary diagnostic investigation. Our own preliminary assessment of ultra-

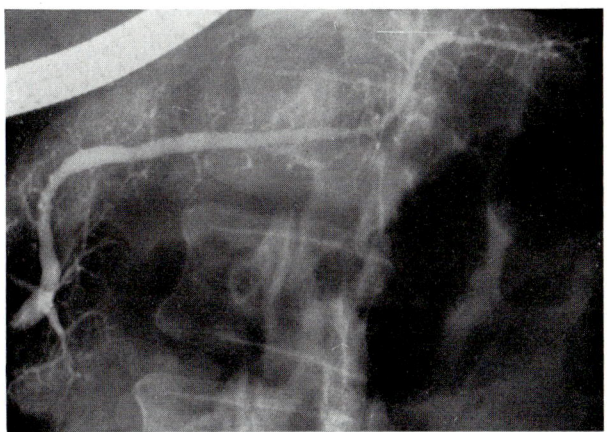

Figure 8.9 Minor abnormalities of the branch ducts consistent with an early stage of chronic pancreatitis

sonography is less impressive and we restrict its use to the search for cysts in patients with recurrent pancreatitis. However, the technique must continue to develop and may well have a much wider clinical role in the future. The potential for EMI computer-assisted tomography is perhaps even greater.

Arteriography has been widely used in the diagnosis of pancreatic disease particularly in continental Europe and North America. In expert hands the diagnosis and operability of cancer can be established in around 90 per cent of patients particularly when superselective techniques are used (Rösch and Holman, 1975). Kramann (1975) used arteriography and pancreatography in 23 patients with advanced chronic pancreatitis. The results were normal in two and three cases respectively but the abnormalities on pancreatography were more often gross.

Pancreatic function studies. Pancreatography and function studies measure different parameters and their direct comparison is artificial. However, in practice it is necessary to decide which technique should be used first in the diagnosis or exclusion of chronic pancreatic disease. Cancer is a space-occupying condition where anatomical diagnostic techniques such as pancreatography and imaging would seem most appropriate, until superseded by serology (Banwo, Versey and Hobbs, 1974). By contrast, pancreatitis is primarily a parenchymal disease with secondary effects on the duct system; functional changes might be detectable prior to anatomical abnormalities.

Are function tests sensitive enough at this stage in the disease? They are virtually always abnormal in patients with well-established chronic pancreatitis and compare favourably when a late diagnostic end-point such as pancreatic calcification or surgical histology is being used. Dreiling (1975) claims a 90 per cent diagnostic accuracy for the secretin test. His group has correlated function studies and pancreatography in 24 patients with histologically proven chronic pancreatitis (Waye, Adler and Dreiling, 1975). Both tests were abnormal in 13 patients: in 7 the function test was abnormal and pancreatography normal. In 4 the reverse was true. In none of the patients were both

Table 8.2 Results of ERCP and a secretin function test in patients with chronic and relapsing acute pancreatitis

	Normal	Abnormal	No result
ERCP	8	10	6
Secretin	7	15	2

tests normal. In our own comparison (Cotton et al, 1975), 24 patients with a final diagnosis of chronic or relapsing pancreatitis underwent both pancreatography and a secretin study. Table 8.2 shows that both tests were often normal, at least in the early stages of the disease. The apparent advantage over the secretin test was negated by the significant number of abnormal secretin results obtained in patients subsequently judged to have no pancreatic disease. Salmon et al (1975) performed a secretin test, a Lundh test and pancreatography in 48 patients with recurrent pancreatitis. When the pancreatogram changes were severe, the secretin test was abnormal in 12 out of 13 patients. When the changes were minimal, as described by Kasugai et al (1972), the secretin test was abnormal in only four whereas the Lundh test was abnormal in 10 patients. Dobrilla et al (1975) compared the results of a secretin/pancreozymin test with pancreatography in 17 patients with proven chronic pancreatitis. The function test was normal in one patient and pancreatography normal in two.

When faced with the patient with pain which is as yet undiagnosed there remains a large range of possible investigative techniques. EMI scanning and ultrasonography have still to prove themselves and the contribution of isotope scanning is questionable. Function tests are not easy for the patient but provide good discrimination in expert hands.

Endoscopic pancreatography is complex and expensive, but is becoming more widely used as a result of the increasing experience with fibreoptic endoscopes. ERCP has certain advantages in the patient with undiagnosed abdominal pain. It should be possible to exclude peptic ulcer disease en route to the papilla, and a normal pancreatogram virtually excludes symptomatic cancer. When the pancreatogram shows abnormalities of pancreatitis it provides the anatomical map required in any discussion of surgical intervention. When it is normal a diagnosis of pancreatitis must rest on function studies, but the normal pancreatogram excludes the necessity for exploratory surgery.

All the techniques of pancreatic diagnosis presently depend upon considerable technical and interpretive expertise. This means that the conclusions from one centre are by no means universally applicable. In an individual hospital the most useful technique is that which is available.

RECENT DEVELOPMENTS

Collection of Pure Pancreatic Juice and Bile

Most data on human pancreatic secretion have been derived from collection and analysis of duodenal aspirates which are inevitably contaminated by bile and intestinal secretions. The recovery of duodenal juice is incomplete, an error which can be partially corrected by the use of non-absorbable markers (Lagerlof, Schultz and Holmer, 1967). Work on pure uncontaminated pancreatic secretion in man has been restricted until recently to the study of a few patients with pancreatic fistulae, and some in whom a catheter has been left in the pancreatic duct at the time of surgery (Elmslie, White and Magee, 1964). Direct endoscopic cannulation of the bile duct and pancreatic duct provides an opportunity to collect pure secretions uncontaminated by other fluids (Cotton et al, 1974; Cotton and Heap, 1975). Bile can be recovered by gentle aspiration, but the collection of pancreatic juice requires a stimulus such as secretin.

Cytology

Cytodiagnosis is of clinical relevance where x-rays of the bile duct and pancreatic duct show a stricture or obstruction of uncertain cause. The interpretation of cholangiograms is usually straightforward, although the distinction between sclerosing cholangitis and carcinoma may sometimes be difficult. Witte and Riegg (1973) have reported a study of bile duct cytology.

Collection of pure secretions for cytology is more often relevant for pancreatic diagnosis where the radiographic distinction between chronic pancreatitis and carcinoma can be difficult. Our own results have been disappointing; using cytology only when the diagnosis is in doubt, malignant cells have been detected in less than 50 per cent of cases subsequently shown to have cancer. When employed in every patient the results may be improved (Kozu, 1973; Endo et al, 1974). Hatfield et al (1975) found the main value of cytology to be in patients where pancreatography failed to opacify the duct due to cancer involving the head. In no patient has cytology proved positive in the presence of a normal pancreatogram.

Juice can be obtained immediately after pancreatography for diagnostic cytology. The cannula is left in the duct, and a bolus injection of secretin is given intravenously. The admixture with contrast material does not appear to affect cytodiagnosis. Juice collection should not precede pancreatography since this will necessitate contrast injection against the flow; this provokes pain and may be dangerous.

Biochemistry

Contrast materials, anticholinergic agents and the pancreatic stimulus of ERCP itself will affect the biochemical analysis and results in pure pancreatic juice. Formal biochemical studies should be performed as a separate procedure from pancreatography, using little or no sedation and no antiperistaltic agents. Since collection is the only aim the procedure need not take place in the x-ray department.

The catheter used for pure juice collection should be primed with normal saline or water which can be marked with a dye to identify catheter deadspace. Air bubbles should be excluded. We have found it convenient and effective to collect juice by simple syphonage at a level about 60 cm below the patient. There is no true basal flow. The standard duodenoscope cannula has a single end hole which may impact against the duct wall and result in intermittent flow. This may be avoided by using a catheter with several lateral holes if deep cannulation is achieved. Even then some pancreatic juice may escape around the cannula, and the collection will be incomplete particularly where there is a patent accessory papilla. A balloon-tipped catheter would reduce this loss and allow conclusions concerning the output of pancreatic juice constitutents as well as concentrations. However, the safety of such catheters has not been established. The need for a balloon inflation lumen reduces the collection lumen to a size where the resistance to flow is impressive. Even using the standard length and diameter cannulation catheter the pressure required to achieve a flow of 5 ml/min exceeds 30 mmHg (Laurence et al, 1976). With a longer catheter and a narrower lumen the pressure characteristics suggest that it may be unsafe to obstruct the pancreatic duct with a balloon.

Pancreatic juice beings to flow briskly following a stimulus. Many different stimuli have been used during traditional duodenal drainage function tests, with an emphasis on large doses such as 1 unit/kg of secretin or pancreozymin given by bolus injection or intravenous infusion. Given at the time of ERCP this range of stimulus produces a rapid flow of pure juice except in patients with major pancreatic disease. We have been interested to discover the pancreatic response to much smaller doses and those which provide more physiological blood levels (Fig. 8.10). There are differences in volume response as between patients with a normal or abnormal pancreas (Cotton et al, 1974; Cremer, Jacobs and Deltenre, 1975; Gregg and Sharma, 1975), but the differences in bicarbonate concentrations are much less than those expected from duodenal drainage studies.

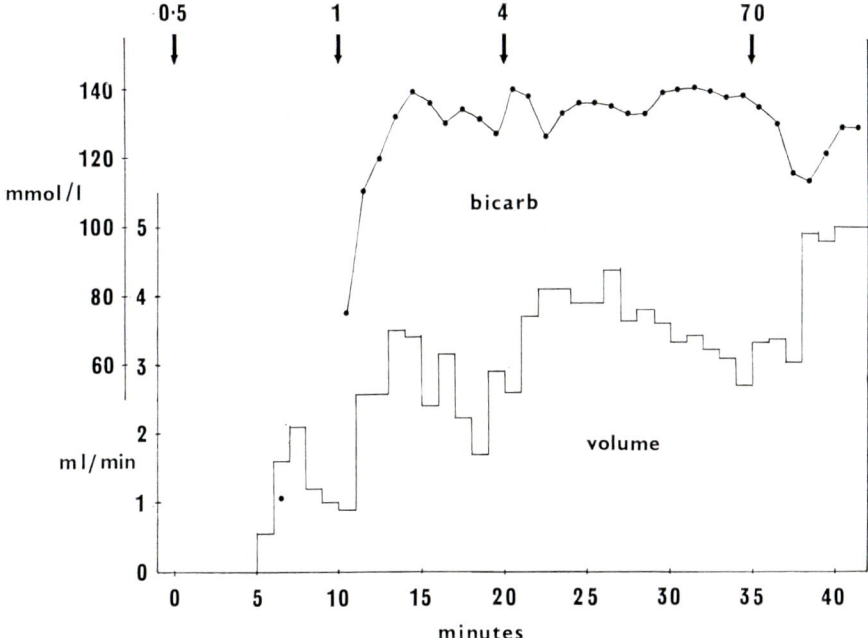

Figure 8.10 Pure pancreatic juice response to bolus injections of GIH secretin (0.5, 1, 4, 70 units). Minute by minute collections demonstrate a brisk volume response even to small doses, and a maximum bicarbonate concentration following the single unit stimulus. There is a fall in bicarbonate concentration following the 70 unit bolus

The lowest maximum bicarbonate concentration we have yet experienced in a patient with chronic pancreatitis is 99 mmol/litre. The total protein excretion closely reflects the output of pancreatic enzymes (Robberecht et al, 1975). Detailed comparisons of enzyme concentrations and outputs are not yet available from pure juice studies but we anticipate that qualitative differences may well be of more interest than quantitative ones. Detailed electrophoretic analysis of pure juice proteins (Keller and Allan, 1967) could yield exciting data. It may even be possible to find specific abnormalities of diagnostic relevance such as lactoferrin (Colomb et al, 1974). Kawanishi, Sell and Pollard (1975) found high pure juice levels of carcinoembryonic antigen in patients with cancer. There was some overlap with chronic pancreatitis but all normal patients had low levels. Calcification is a classical marker of pancreatitis; pure juice studies should allow detailed analysis of calcium dynamics and protein interrelationships.

Uncontaminated bile can also be collected for biochemical studies. We have established a technique for leaving a balloon-tipped catheter in the bile duct in man with withdrawal of the endoscope (Shapiro and Cotton, 1975). This provides a new avenue for studies on hepatic metabolism of clinical relevance in the context of gallstones and their diagnosis.

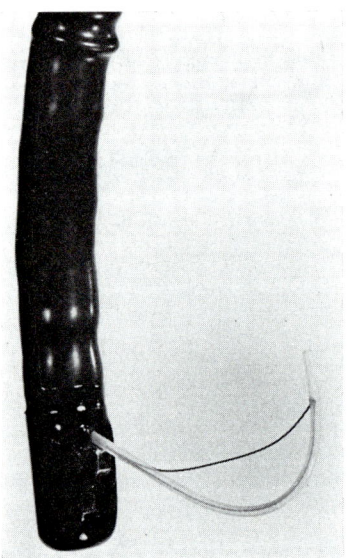

Figure 8.11 Endoscopic sphincterotomy. Tip of experimental duodenoscope, with catheter and diathermy wire exposed

Endoscopic sphincterotomy

Surgical interference with the sphincter of Oddi has had a long but somewhat controversial history. Neither the indications nor the results have always been clear. In selected patients the early results of endoscopic diathermy sphincterotomy have been impressive and certain techniques and indications are now established (Kawai et al, 1974; Koch, 1975; Classen and Safrany, 1975). The prime indication has been for the removal of retained common bile duct stones in elderly and frail patients who have already undergone cholecystectomy. There are many such patients in whom surgical re-exploration is not without hazard or failure.

Endoscopic sphincterotomy is performed using the standard cannulating duodenoscope or a slightly larger insulated instrument. Following endoscopic cholangiography and confirmation of the need for sphincterotomy the standard catheter is replaced by one incorporating a diathermy wire (Fig. 8.11).

Under careful visual and fluoroscopic control, the catheter and wire are placed within the sphincter so that the wire is projecting towards the duodenal lumen. Diathermy is then applied to produce a sphincterotomy along a length of about 1 cm. It is difficult at the time to be certain of the size of sphincterotomy performed. This can be measured by using balloon-tipped catheters (Laurence et al, 1975), a procedure probably best delayed for a week or so following the initial sphincterotomy. At this time endoscopic cholangiography is repeated; in many cases the stone or stones will have passed spontaneously and can be

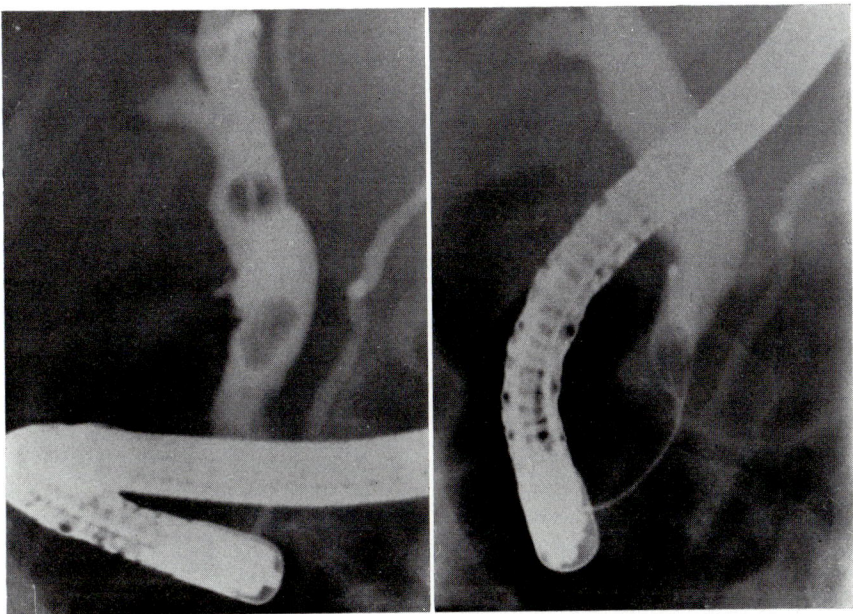

Figure 8.12   *Figure 8.13*

Figure 8.12 Gallstone extraction. Balloon catheter inflated in the bile duct above a calculus
Figure 8.13 Gallstone extraction. Calculus trapped in a dormia basket in the process of extraction through the papilla

found in the faeces. If the stones are still present they can usually be removed using balloon catheters or a dormia-type basket. (Figs. 8.12, 8.13). The size of the sphincterotomy must be tailored to the size of stone present on cholangiography. Our results of this procedure have been encouraging; the sphincterotomy is virtually always successful and complications have been few. Classen and Safrany (1975) achieved sphincterotomy in 50 out of 59 attempts. Where gallstone removal was the aim this was achieved in 33 out of 39 patients. There were no serious complications. Rosch (1975) reviewed the procedure in 130 patients from Germany. There were four episodes of haemorrhage, one of pancreatitis and four of perforation, with two deaths.

Since the majority of patients were selected because of their poor operative risk this complication rate is remarkably low. Endoscopic sphincterotomy has been performed in a few patients with papillary stenosis and in some very elderly and frail patients with jaundice due to common bile duct stones who were unfit for cholecystectomy. There have been isolated reports of sphincterotomy as a palliative procedure in patients with jaundice due to carcinoma in the papillary region.

Endoscopic sphincterotomy is a new technique and the long-term results have yet to be established. Follow-up examinations at one year show that subsequent stenosis is very unusual. Whilst the procedure was introduced for patients unfit for further surgery its relative ease and safety may well lead to more widespread use.

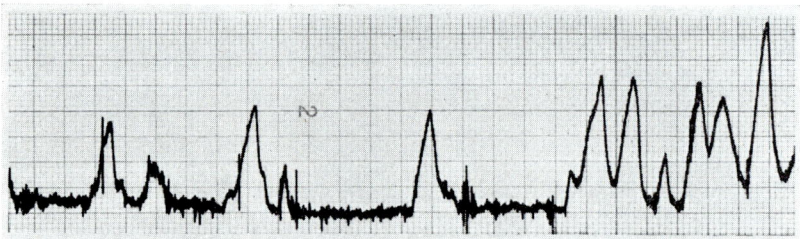

Figure 8.14 Measurement of pressure in the sphincter of Oddi using a side-hole constantly perfused catheter during duodenoscopy. Full trace deflection 100 mmHg. The catheter was initially pulled through the sphincter, giving three consistent readings for sphincter pressure of approximately 40 mmHg. The catheter was then left in the sphincter zone and increasing spontaneous contractions measured following mechanical stimulation of the papilla

Papillary manometry

Some patients continue to complain of severe episodes of pain following cholecystectomy in the absence of any major structural biliary abnormality. The pain can often be reproduced by over-distension of the biliary tree during cholangiography, reinforcing the belief that it may be due to inefficient biliary emptying caused by a disturbance of the sphincter mechanism. Endoscopic cannulation of the papilla allows manometry of the sphincter in the conscious patient using a constantly perfused side-hole catheter system. Pressure profiles are recorded in the resting state and after the use of various drugs (Fig. 8.14). Nebel (1975) has published data for normal sphincter pressures but in individual patients the peaks are somewhat variable. It is possible to demonstrate that previous sphincterotomy or sphincteroplasty has been effective but the detection of the high pressure sphincter is more difficult. Cannulation may fail with intense spasm or stenosis. When there is high pressure (like the patient's symptoms) it may be intermittent and an isolated reading may be of little relevance. We have so far encountered two patients with recurrent pain following cholecystecomy where the sphincter pressure exceeded 50 mmHg in the absence of bile duct dilatation. Both patients have had good short-term results after sphincteroplasty.

Pancreaticoscopy and choledochoscopy

Operative choledochoscopy is well established in some centres. Classen, Schwemmle and Demling (1972) have described operative pancreaticoscopy using a fibrebronchoscope. There have now been reports of per-oral pancreaticoscopy and cholangioscopy, using experimental fine fibrescopes passed through the operating channel of a larger instrument (Nakamura et al, 1974). These small instruments are fragile and provide images of poor quality; the technique is unlikely to attain clinical relevance.

CONCLUSION

The clinical role of endoscopic papillary cannulation is being defined more clearly. In careful hands it has a high yield in the diagnosis of pancreatic cancer and in the management of recurrent pancreatitis. It can provide an early and precise diagnosis in patients with jaundice and is particularly helpful in the investigation of patients with symptoms following biliary surgery. Endoscopic sphincterotomy is an advance in the treatment of certain patients with retained common duct stones. The role of ERCP in the diagnosis of chronic pancreatitis is still being defined and must await further large series of comparisons with other anatomical and functional techniques. The ability to collect pure secretions opens a new avenue for clinical and physiological research.

ACKNOWLEDGEMENTS

I wish to acknowledge invaluable assistance with various aspects of this work given generously by colleagues in radiology (Dr M. Chapman and Dr J. S. M. Beales), surgery (Professor L. LeQuesne and Professor M. Hobsley), biochemistry (Dr A. Miller, Miss J. Townson, Miss S. Tough) and medicine (Dr A. Reuben, Dr T. Heap, Dr R. Stern, Dr M. Denyer). We have been generously supported by the Special Trustees of the Middlesex Hospital, and by the Wellcome Trust.

REFERENCES

Banwo, O., Versey, J. & Hobbs, J. E. (1974) New oncofetal antigen for the pancreas. *Lancet*, **1**, 643–645.

Baron, J. H. (1975) Pancreatic function tests. In *Topics in Gastroenterology*, Vol. 3, Ch. 9. Oxford: Blackwells.

Blumgart, L. H., Salmon, P. R. & Cotton, P. B. (1974) Endoscopy and retrograde choledochopancreatography (ERCP) in the diagnosis of the jaundiced patient. *Surgery, Gynecology and Obstetrics*, **138**, 565–570.

Bodvall, B. (1973) The postcholecystectomy syndromes. In *Clinics in Gastroenterology*, Vol. 2, Diseases of the Biliary Tract, ed. Bouchier, I. A. D., Ch. 6, London: W. B. Saunders.

Braganza, J., Critchley, M., Howat, H. T., Testa, H. J. & Torrance, H. B. (1973) An evaluation of ^{75}Se Selenomethionine scanning as a test of pancreatic function compared with the secretin/pancreozymin test. *Gut*, **14**, 383–389.

Charlesworth, D., Testa, H. J. & Watson, A. (1969) Radioisotope scanning of the pancreas and spleen. *Journal of the Royal College of Surgeons, Edinburgh*, **14**, 115–156.

Classen, M., Anacker, H., Stadelmann, O., Seifert, E. & von Fritsch, E. (1975) The diagnosis of tumours of the papilla of Vater and of the pancreas by endoscopic-radiologic cholangio-pancreaticography (ERCP). In *Efficiency and Limits of Radiologic Examination of the Pancreas*, ed. Anacker, H., pp. 203–209. Stuttgart: Georg Thieme.

Classen, M. & Safrany, L. (1975) Endoscopic papillotomy and removal of gall stones. *British Medical Journal*, **4**, 371–374.

Classen, M., Schwemmle, K. & Demling, L. (1972) Endoscopy of the pancreatic duct. *Endoscopy*, **4**, 221–224.

Colomb, E., Estevenon, J. B., Figarella, C., Guy, O. & Sarles, H. (1974) Characterisation of an additional protein in pancreatic juice of men with chronic calcifying pancreatitis. Identification to lactoferrin. *Biochimica biophysica Acta*, **342**, 306–312.

Conn, H. O. (1975) Liver biopsy in extrahepatic biliary obstruction and in other contraindicated disorders. *Gastroenterology*, **68**, 817–821.

Cotton, P. B. (1972) Cannulation of the papilla of Vater by endoscopy and retrograde cholangio-pancreatography (ERCP). *Gut*, **13**, 1014–1025.

Cotton, P. B. (1974) The normal endoscopic pancreatogram. *Endoscopy*, **6**, 65–70.

Cotton, P. B. & Beales, J. S. M. (1974) Endoscopic pancreatography in management of relapsing acute pancreatitis. *British Medical Journal*, **1**, 608–611.

Cotton, P. B., Cremer, M., Robberecht, P. & Christophe, J. (1974) Biochemical studies of pure pancreatic juice obtained by duodenoscopic cannulation of the pancreatic duct in conscious patients. *Gut*, **15**, 838.

Cotton, P. B. & Heap, T. R. (1975) The analysis of pancreatic juice. *British Journal of Hospital Medicine*, **14**, 659–666.

Cotton, P. B., Ponder, B. A. J., Beales, J. S. M. & Croft, D. N. (1975) Pancreatic diagnosis: comparison of endoscopic pancreatography (ERCP), isotope scanning, and secretin tests in 62 patients. *Gut*, **16**, 405.

Cremer, M. & Engelholm, L. (1973) La cholangio-wirsungographie endoscopique dans la diagnostic des icteres obstructifs. *Acta gastro-enterologica belgica*, **36**, 642–675.

Cremer, M., Jacobs, W. & Deltenre, M. (1975) Study of pure human pancreatic secretion. Comparison of the results obtained by perfusion and after a bolus injection of secretin. *8th Symposium, European Pancreatic Club*, Toulouse.

Dobrilla, A., Fratten, A., Valentini, M., Vantini, I., Kavalini, G., Angelini, G. Mirachian, R. & Mora, R. (1975) Diagnosis of chronic pancreatitis. Comparison between endoscopic pancreatography and secretin pancreozymin test. *8th Symposium European Pancreatic Club*, Toulouse.

Dreiling, D. A. (1975) Pancreatic secretory testing in 1974. *Gut*, **16**, 653–657.

Elias, E., Hamlin, A. N., Jane, S., Long, R., Summerfield, J. A., Dick, R. & Sherlock, S. (1975) A randomised trial of percutaneous transhepatic cholangiography versus endoscopic retrograde cholangiography for bile duct visualisation in cholestasis. *Gut*, **16**, 831.

Elmslie, R. G., White, T. T. & Magee, D. F. (1964) Observation on pancreatic function in eight patients with controlled pancreatic fistulas. *Annals of Surgery*, **160**, 937–948.

Endo, Y., Morii, T., Tamura, H. & Okuda, S. (1974) Cytodiagnosis of pancreatic malignant tumours by aspiration under direct vision using a duodenal fibrescope. *Gastroenterology*, **67**, 944–951.

Engelhart, G. J. (1975) Diagnosis with ultrasound in the region of the pancreas. In *Efficiency and Limits of Radiologic Examination of the Pancreas*, ed. Anacker, H., pp. 245–253. Stuttgart: Georg Thieme.

Gregg, J. A. & Sharma, M. M. (1975) The effect of secretin on pancreatic juice flow rates during endoscopic cannulation of the main pancreatic duct. *Gastroenterology*, **68**, 905.

Hatfield, A. R. W., Smithies, A., Wilkins, R. & Levi, A. J. (1975) Endoscopic retrograde cholangio-pancreatography (ERCP) and pure pancreatic juice cytology: a combined diagnostic approach in pancreatic disease. *Gut*, **16**, 405.

Johnston, A. G. (1975) Cholecystectomy and gallstone dyspepsia. *Annals of the Royal College of Surgeons, England*, **56**, 69–80.

Kasugai, T., Kuno, N., Kizu, M., Kobayashi, S. & Hattori, K. (1972) Endoscopic pancreato-cholangiography. II. The pathological endoscopic pancreato-cholangiogram. *Gastroenterology*, **63**, 227–234.

Kawanishi, H., Sell, J. E. & Pollard, H. M. (1975) Combined endoscopic pancreatic fluid collection and retrograde pancreatography. *Gastroenterology*, **68**, 4, 1033.

Kawai, K., Akasaka, Y., Murakami, K., Tada, M., Kohli, Y. & Nakajima, M. (1974) Endoscopic sphincterotomy of the ampulla of Vater. *Gastrointestinal Endoscopy*, **20**, 148.

Keller, P. J. & Allan, B. J. (1967) The protein composition of human pancreatic juice. *Journal of Biological Chemistry*, **242**, 281–287.

Koch, H. (1975) Endoscopic papillotomy. *Endoscopy*, **7**, 89–93.

Kozu, T. (1973) Duodenoscopic collection of intraductal pure pancreatic juice and its application to the cytodiagnosis. In *Endoscopy of the Small Intestine with Retrograde Pancreatocholangiography*, ed. Demling, L. & Classen, M., pp. 70–74. Stuttgart: Georg Thieme.

Kramann, B. (1975) A comparative study on duodenoscopic pancreaticography, arteriography and barium meal examination in the diagnosis of chronic pancreatitis. In *Efficiency and Limits of Radiologic Examination of the Pancreas*, ed. Anacker, H., pp. 209–214. Stuttgart: Georg Thieme.

Lagerlof, H. O., Schultz, H. B. & Holmer, S. (1967) A secretin test with high doses of secretin and correlation for incomplete recovery of duodenal juice. *Gastroenterology*, **52**, 67–77.

Laurence, B., Cotton, P. B., Shapiro, H. & Heap, T. R. (1976) Balloon catheters in the biliary and pancreatic ducts. *Gut* **17**, 78.

Liguory, C., Goueron, H., Chavy, A., Coffin, J. C. & Huguier, M. (1974) Endoscopic retrograde cholangio-pancreatography. *British Journal of Surgery*, **61**, 359.

Miale, A., Rodriguez, Antounis, A. & Gill, W. M. (1972) *Seminars in Nuclear Medicine*, pp. 201–219.

Nakamura, M., Takasaka, T., Toki, F., Kozu, T., Hamano, K., Takada, T., Hayna, F. & Takemoto, T. (1974) The research of transduodenal pancreaticoscopy. *3rd World Congress of Gastrointestinal Endoscopy*, Mexico.

Nebel, O. T. (1974) Endoscopic manometry: a new technique for the physiologic study of the human sphincter of Oddi. *Gastroenterology*, **56**, 818.

Nebel, O. T., Silvis, S. E., Rogers, G., Sugawa, C. & Mandelstam, P. (1975) Complications associated with endoscopic retrograde cholangio-pancreatography. Results of the 1974 ASGE surgery. *Gastrointestinal Endoscopy*, **22**, 34–36.

Ogoshi, K., Tobita, Y. & Hara, Y. (1970) Endoscopic observation of the duodenum and pancreato-choledochography using duodenal fibrescope under direct vision. *Gastroenterological Endoscopy* (*Tokyo*), **12**, (1), 83.

Oi, I. (1970) Fibre duodenoscopy and endoscopic pancreato-cholangiography. *Gastrointestinal Endoscopy*, **17**, 59.

Oi, I. (1974) Complications of duodenoscopy. *3rd World Congress of Gastrointestinal Endoscopy*, Mexico.

Okuda, K., Tamkawa, K., Emura, T. et al (1974) Non-surgical percutaneous transhepatic cholangiography—diagnostic significance in medical problems of the liver. *American Journal of Digestive Disease*, **19**, 21–36.

Robberecht, P., Cremer, M., Vandermers, A., Vandermers-Piret, M-C., Cotton, P. B., de Neef, P. & Christophe, J. (1975) Pancreatic secretion of total protein and of three hydrolases collected in healthy subjects via duodenoscopic cannulation. Effects of secretin, pancreozymin and caerulein. *Gastroenterology*, **69**, 374–379.

Rösch, J. & Holman, D. C. (1975) Superselective arteriography of the pancreas. In *Efficiency and Limits of Radiologic Examination of the Pancreas*, ed. Anacker, H., pp. 159–167. Stuttgart: Georg Thieme.

Rosch, W. (1975) Workshop: operative endoscopy, *Endoscopy*, **7**, 157–160.

Ruppin, H., Amon, R., Etti, W., Classen, M. & Demling, L. (1974) Acute pancreatitis after endoscopic/radiological pancreaticography (ERP). *Endoscopy*, **6**, 94–98.

Sahel, J. & Pietri, H. (1975) Endoscopic wirsungography and ultrasonography. 2. Complementary examinations in pancreatology. *8th Symposium European Pancreatic Club*, Toulouse.

Salmon, P. R., Baddeley, H., Machada, G., Lobear, T., Rees-Davies, E. & Trapnell, J. (1975) Endoscopic pancreatography, scintigraphy and exocrine function in pancreatitis: a comparative study, *Gut*, **16**, 830–831.

Seifert, E., St Stender, H., Safrany, L., Lesch, P., Luska, G. & Misaki, F. (1974) X-ray findings of pancreatic cysts diagnosed by endoscopic pancreato-cholangiography. *Endoscopy*, **6**, 77–83.

Shapiro, H. A. & Cotton, P. B. (1975) Leaving a balloon-tip catheter in the bile duct at duodenoscopy. *Lancet*, **1**, 13–14.

Silvis, S. E. & Vennes, J. A. (1975) The role of glucagon in endoscopic cholangio-pancreatography. *Gastrointestinal Endoscopy*, **21**, 162–164.

Spencer, A. M., Patel, M. P., Smitz, B. J. & Williams, J. D. F. (1974) Pancreatic scanning as a diagnostic tool in the district general hospital. *British Medical Journal*, **4**, 153–156.

Stadelman, O., Safrany, L., Leuffle, A., Barnar, L., Midere, S. E., Papp, J., Kalfe, C. & Sobbe, A. (1974) Endoscopic retrograde cholangio-pancreatography in the diagnosis of pancreatic cancer. *Endoscopy*, **6**, 84–94.

Taylor, K. J. W., Carpenter, D. A. & McCready, V. R. (1974) Ultrasound and scintigraphy in the differential diagnosis of obstructive jaundice. *Journal of Clinical Ultrasound*, **2**, 105–116.

Walls, W. J., Gonzalez, G., Martin, N. L. & Templeton, A. W. (1975) B-Scan ultrasound evaluation of the pancreas. *Radiology*, **114**, 127–134.

Way, L. W., Admirand, W. H. & Dunphy, J. E. (1972) Management of choledocholithiasis. *Annals of Surgery*, **176**, 347–357.

Waye, J. D., Adler, M. & Dreiling, D. A. (1975) The pancreas. A correlation of function structure and histopathology. *Gastroenterology*, **68**, 1010.

Weill, F., Kraehenbuhl, J. R., Becker, J. C., Gillett, M. & Bourgoyne, A. (1975) Echo tomography of the pancreas: a critical and comparative study. In *Efficiency and Limits of Radiologic Examination of the Pancreas*, ed. Anacker, H., pp. 253–263. Stuttgart: Georg Thieme.

Witte, S. & Riegg, H. (1973) Cytological findings in the bile after endoscopic cannulation of the papilla of Vater. In *Endoscopy of the Small Intestine with Retrograde Pancreatocholangiography*, International Workshop at Erlangen, 1972, ed. Demling, L. & Classen, M., pp. 94–98. Stuttgart: Georg Thieme.

9
CLINICAL ASPECTS OF BILE ACID METABOLISM

K. W. Heaton

WHAT DOES A GASTROENTEROLOGIST NEED TO KNOW ABOUT NORMAL BILE ACID METABOLISM?

Steroid chemistry and detergent physics are not everybody's bedside reading and to most people bile acid (bile salt) metabolism is dauntingly complex. It is easy to see why. Even the so-called trivial names are long and clumsy, such as glycochenodeoxycholate. The synthesis of conjugated bile acids from cholesterol has at least 16 steps and, in the faeces, there are over 30 bacterial metabolites of bile acids. However, bile acid metabolism need not be complicated. Only two or three synthetic steps are clinically important (being rate-limiting or being the first committed step along the pathway to one or other of the two primary bile acids), while the great majority of bacterial metabolites can be ignored, having no known physiological or clinical role.

Everything that matters happens in the enterohepatic circulation (Fig. 9.1). This is a very efficient recycling system. It ensures that about 20 g of bile acid pour into the duodenum each day at the trivial cost of only 500 mg lost in the faeces. Lost bile acid is replaced by newly synthesised material and this daily synthesis of 500 mg or 1 mmol[1] represents nearly half the body's disposal arrangements for cholesterol. It could be perilous to reduce it. In hypercholesterolaemia (type IIa hyperlipidaemia) there is reduced synthesis of bile acids. Most diseases in which bile acids are implicated are disorders of the enterohepatic circulation.

When a meal is eaten and the gallbladder contracts, the 2 to 3 g (4–6 mmol) pool of conjugated bile salt enters the duodenum through the relaxed sphincter of Oddi. In the upper small bowel, bile salts are present in a concentration of 5 to 40 mmol/litre, which is well above the critical level necessary for micellar aggregates to form. The chief function of bile salts is to disperse into micellar solution the almost insoluble products of fat digestion, long-chain fatty acids and their 2-monoglycerides. Micelles are capable of taking up and so dissolving the other important dietary lipids, including cholesterol, carotene, retinol (vitamin A), tocopherols (vitamin E) and vitamin K. They may be regarded as miniature lipid transporters, ferrying packets of lipid repeatedly to the absorptive membrane of the microvilli. For the absorption of cholesterol and fat-soluble vitamins micellar solubilisation is essential, but it is merely an accelerator of fatty acid and monoglyceride absorption. At least half the normal dietary load of fat can be absorbed when bile salts are completely absent from the intestine. There are other ways in which bile acids aid fat absorption. They help to emulsify fat before it is split by pancreatic lipase, they lower the pH optimum of lipase, and in some way activate it, and they seem to stimulate the resynthesis of triglyceride in the intestinal mucosa. There are no important differences in the capacity of the different bile acids to perform these functions,

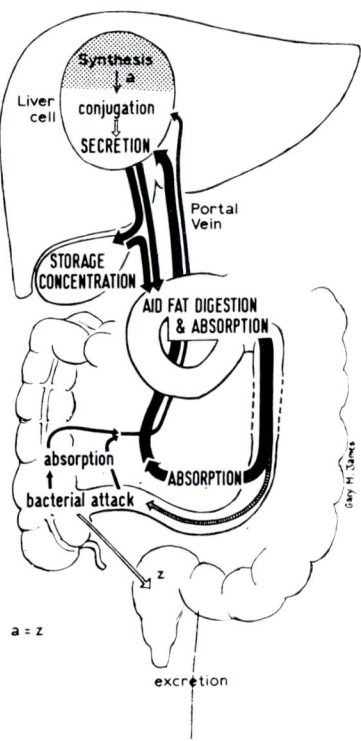

Figure 9.1 The main events in the enterohepatic circulation

and it is puzzling that mammals bothered to evolve two different primary bile acids.

In the synthesis of cholic and chenodeoxycholic acids the crucial step is the first one, the 7α-hydroxylation of cholesterol. This is the rate-limiting step, on which is exercised negative feedback control. The enzyme concerned, 7α-hydroxylase, is inhibited by reabsorbed bile salts returning to the liver in the portal vein. When feedback inhibition is increased, for example by the infusion of bile salts, the activity of 7α-hydroxylase decreases within a few hours. This enzyme determines the *amount* of bile salt to be produced, but the

[1] Where possible values are expressed in SI units; otherwise metric units are used.

type depends on the activity of another enzyme, 12α-hydroxylase. The insertion of a 12α-hydroxyl group commits the liver to produce cholic acid (3α,7α,12α-trihydroxycholanic acid), whereas failure to do so leads to chenodeoxycholic acid (3α,7α-dihydroxycholanic acid). This enzyme is inhibited by thyroid hormone and seems to be low in activity in cirrhotic livers. Hence, there is a relative deficiency of cholic acid in hyperthyroidism and in cirrhosis.

There must also be a rate limiting step somewhere in the pathway leading exclusively to chenodeoxycholic acid (CDC), since the synthesis of this bile acid, but not of cholic acid, can be inhibited by feeding small amounts of deoxycholic acid (Pomare and Low-Beer, 1975).

Deoxycholic acid (DC) (3α,12α-dihydroxycholanic acid) is the third of the three main bile acids in human bile, the relative proportions being about 40 per cent cholate, 40 per cent CDC and 20 per cent DC. Its presence in bile is the result of two events in the colon—removal of the 7α-hydroxyl group from cholate by anaerobic bacteria, and absorption of this degraded or secondary bile acid by passive diffusion. One or both of these events is inhibited by dietary fibre (Pomare and Heaton, 1973c). Patients with ileostomies have little if any deoxycholate in their faeces or their bile.

Human bile also contains minute quantities of a fourth bile salt, lithocholate (3α-hydroxycholanic acid). This is analogous to DC, since it is produced in the colon by 7α-dehydroxylation of CDC. However, because it has only one hydroxyl group, it has low polarity and water-solubility. Most of it is excreted. The absorbed fraction is transformed in the liver which esterifies the weakly polar 3α-hydroxyl group into a much more polar sulphate group. This sulphation probably represents a detoxification. It certainly prevents accumulation as, in the sulphated form, lithocholate is less easily absorbed from the small intestine (Cowen et al, 1975b). The main bile salts in human faeces are deoxycholate, lithocholate and isolithocholate (the 3β isomer of lithocholate).

The other main bacterial modification undergone by bile salts is deconjugation, in which anaerobic organisms hydrolyse the amide bond between the steroid nucleus and the glycine or taurine sidechain. This reaction, which occurs to a variable extent in the healthy ileum as well as the colon, does not prejudice the chances of a bile salt molecule being absorbed, unless it is a prelude to dehydroxylation. Deconjugation has attracted much attention from clinicians because it is a marker of the exposure of bile salts to intestinal bacteria (see section on the Breath Test).

Intestinal reabsorption of bile salts is 96 to 97 per cent efficient. It takes place mainly in the terminal ileum, whose mucosa possesses an active transport system specific for bile salts. This system is less efficient with unconjugated (free) than with conjugated bile acids, but this is offset by the fact that free bile acids are less polar and so more freely diffusible. They are absorbed by passive non-ionic diffusion at all levels of the intestine. The jejunum is particularly permeable to bile acids. It is theoretically capable of absorbing all the glycine-conjugated dihydroxy bile salts, which are the least polar of the conjugates

(Krag and Phillips, 1974). However, in real life it does not seem to do this (Low-Beer et al, 1974). This may be because, after a meal, bile acids are normally present in the jejunum in mixed micelles containing dietary and biliary lipids, which may well reduce passive uptake. During fasting, when bile acid secretion is occurring slowly but constantly due to 'incontinence' of the sphincter of Vater, reabsorption may well be mainly jejunal. This could explain why fasting serum contains five times more conjugates of chenodeoxycholic than of cholic acid (Erb, Schreiber and Walczak, 1972), the latter being less easily diffusible.

Reabsorbed bile acids are carried to the liver in the portal vein, loosely bound to albumin. The liver takes up bile acids with amazing avidity, as much as 92 per cent being cleared on a single passage. The half-life of intravenously injected bile salt is only 2 to 3 min (Cowen et al, 1975c). Unconjugated bile acids are immediately conjugated in proportion to the prevailing ratio of glycine to taurine conjugates in bile (G/T ratio). The normal G/T ratio lies between 1 and 6, and can vary considerably from week to week in normal individuals.

For a fuller account of bile salt metabolism and for references up to 1972, the reader is referred to Heaton (1972), and for an advanced but less up to date treatise to Nair and Kritchevsky (1971).

ARE SERUM BILE ACID MEASUREMENTS PRACTICAL AND USEFUL IN CLINICAL PRACTICE?

The fact that, in hepatobiliary diseases, it is routine to measure serum bile pigments and not serum bile acids is paradoxical. Altered bilirubin metabolism has no important ill-effects except in the neonate, whereas altered bile acid metabolism is responsible for both the lipid malabsorption and the pruritus of these conditions, and it may even tend to perpetuate the disease. Moreover, raised serum bile acid levels are probably a more sensitive indicator of liver dysfunction than raised serum bilirubin, or indeed than other routine liver function tests (Demers and Hepner, 1975; Frosch and Wagener, 1967; Korman et al, 1973). Why then is serum bile acid not a routine measurement? The reason is technical. Available methods for measuring total serum bile acids are simply much more time consuming than those for bilirubin. Moreover, it has not been shown that the management of patients would be improved if a more sensitive liver function test was available. It could be argued that needless anxiety would be raised, at least in non-specialist minds, by the 'discovery' that liver function remains abnormal for longer than expected after an attack of hepatitis or an episode of cholestasis.

Nevertheless, gastroenterologists wishing to study their patients more closely may wish to have their serum total bile salts estimated. Enzymatic assay using the 3α-steroid dehydrogenase is within the capacity of a routine biochemistry laboratory, but the low levels found in normal subjects are measurable only if the assay is combined with fluorimetry (Murphy, Billing and Baron, 1970; Panveliwalla et al, 1970). In hepatic dysfunction or portasystemic shunting of blood, the serum bile acid level is substantially higher after a meal than in the fasting state. This is presumably due to impaired hepatic uptake of the bolus of bile salt which rests in the gallbladder during fasting. In testing for these conditions, therefore, it should be most informative to measure bile acid levels 1 to 2 h after a meal. In a study of 26 patients with various liver diseases, the only test which was abnormal in all cases was the 2 h postprandial serum bile acid level (Kaplowitz, Kok and Javitt, 1973). The fasting serum bile acid level was abnormal in only 62 per cent. For comparison, the frequency of abnormality in the routine liver function tests was as follows: BSP retention 82 per cent, alkaline phosphatase 74 per cent, 5'-nucleotidase 58 per cent, SGOT 58 per cent, SGPT 41 per cent, bilirubin 35 per cent. These authors advocated the use of the 2 h postprandial bile acid concentration as a screening test for liver disease. It should be noted that their estimations involved the use of gas chromatography.

In the past, a great deal of effort has been spent on analysing the relative amounts of the individual bile acids in the blood of patients with hepatobiliary disease (Makino, Nakagawa and Mashimo, 1969; Carey 1970; Neale et al, 1971). These have revealed certain characteristic patterns in cirrhosis and cholestasis. However, there is so much overlap between different groups of patients that these analyses are of little clinical value. Moreover, they involve time-consuming extractions and complex chromatographic techniques. Should radioimmunoassay of bile salts become widely available the picture could change (Demers and Hepner, 1975). However, this method is by no means free of technical problems, and a separate assay system is needed for each class of bile acids.

At a more theoretical level, the Mayo Clinic group has recently discovered that serum bile acid measurement can provide a window on to events in the enterohepatic circulation. Using the sensitive radioimmunoassay for cholylglycine which they had developed (Simmonds et al, 1973) they found that serum bile acids rose significantly after meals in normal subjects, that this rise was less in ileectomy subjects with bile acid malabsorption, and that in cholecystectomy subjects who have a constantly circulating bile acid pool the fasting level was high but there was little increase with meals (LaRusso et al, 1974). All this implies that, with a normal liver and biliary tract, the main determinant of the serum bile acid level is the rate of intestinal absorption of bile salts. This opens the possibility that states of bile acid malabsorption could be diagnosed by the finding of an abnormally low postprandial serum level.

An interesting and so far unexplained finding is that patients with the stagnant loop syndrome have high serum levels of unconjugated bile acids (Lewis et al, 1969). The most plausible explanation is increased absorption of deconjugated bile acids which are bound more tightly to plasma albumin than are conjugated bile acids. There is certainly no other evidence of liver dysfunction.

It seems certain that analysis of serum bile acids will continue to be a valuable research technique, but it is less likely that it will become routine in clinical practice in the foreseeable future.

WHAT HAPPENS TO BILE ACID METABOLISM IN HEPATOBILIARY DISEASE?

Cholestasis is the ultimate insult to bile acid metabolism. Deprived of all access to the enterohepatic circulation, bile acids are compelled to wander uselessly, and irritatingly, round the body. Serum bile acid concentrations are from 4 to 60 times the normal level, that is 15 to 285 μmol/litre (Neale et al, 1971). Presumably bile acid synthesis is depressed, though there are no data available on this, nor on bile acid pool sizes. However, it was recently found that the activity of the enzyme controlling bile acid synthesis, 7α-hydroxylase, was only 22 per cent of normal in the livers of five patients with biliary obstruction (Salen et al, 1975).

In complete biliary obstruction the main pathway of bile salt excretion is probably the urinary tract, and in six subjects this accounted for 32.6 μmol/24 h (Makino et al, 1975). This is much less than the normal daily turnover of bile salts (about 1000 μmol/24 h), but it far exceeds their normal urinary excretion (<1 μmol/24 h). This increased urinary loss is associated with and made possible by the sulphation of hydroxyl groups in the liver. Sulphated bile acids are more water soluble than their parent substances, and their renal clearance is 20 to 200 times greater (Stiehl, Earnest and Admirand, 1975). Sulphation occurs minimally in health and seems to be a protective response of the obstructed liver, designed to promote renal excretion of bile acids and to prevent toxicity from accumulation of bile acids within the liver cell (Stiehl, 1974). Sulphation is both more necessary and more complete with the mono- and dihydroxy bile acids than with cholate. Nevertheless, in prolonged cholestasis, the liver concentration of unsulphated CDC can reach levels at which detergent damage occurs (Greim et al, 1972). Dihydroxy bile acids are particularly prone to damage the microsomal cytochrome P-450 system (Denk, Greim and Hutterer, 1971), which is important in the metabolism of drugs, steroid hormones and cholesterol, as well as of bile acids themselves. Accumulation of unsulphated CDC in liver cells could explain why cholestasis is sometimes very persistent. It may also explain some of its metabolic effects.

The cholestatic liver is prone to synthesise curious bile acids. This was first shown in infants with biliary atresia, but it now appears that all infants with cholestasis have in their urine an unsaturated, monohydroxy bile acid (3β-hydroxy-5-cholenoic acid; Norman and Strandvik, 1973). It has also been reported, together with lithocholic acid, in five adults with extrahepatic biliary obstruction and five with viral hepatitis (Back, 1972). This is intriguing because in animals infusing monohydroxy bile acids can cause cholestasis (Javitt and Emerman, 1968). Other exotic bile acids which have been found in the urine of cholestatic patients include a primitive 27 carbon acid normally found in toads and crocodiles (trihydroxycoprostanic acid; Eyssen et al, 1972) and a bile acid which is native to the pig (hyocholic acid; van Berge Henegouwen et al, 1975).

Phenobarbitone, which induces microsomal enzymes, is of therapeutic value in intrahepatic cholestasis, relieving pruritus and reducing serum bile acids (Admirand and Bauer, 1971; Stiehl, Thaler and Admirand, 1972). This is probably because it stimulates the secretion of bile, since it is known to increase the fraction of bile flow which is independent of bile salt secretion (Gumucio et al, 1973). Unfortunately, this effect of phenobarbitone cannot be used to distinguish between intrahepatic and extrahepatic cholestasis, as it can have the same effect in extrahepatic obstruction (Metreau et al, 1975).

The pruritus of cholestasis is probably caused by the retention of bile acids in the skin, since itching patients have high concentrations of bile acids on their skin and the levels tend to fall to normal on the same day as pruritus is relieved (Schoenfield, 1969). Evidence that bile acids can actually cause pruritus has recently been provided by Kirby, Heaton and Burton (1974). When applied to blister bases in a concentration of 1 mmol/litre, all three major bile acids and their conjugates caused itching, the most effective being unconjugated chenodeoxycholate.

In *cirrhosis* bile salt metabolism is disturbed in almost every possible way. Nearly all reported studies have been performed on patients with alcoholic cirrhosis in the United States. The total bile acid pool is little more than half its normal size, mainly due to a marked lack of cholic acid (Vlahcevic et al, 1971) which in turn is the result of reduced synthesis. The latter is present even in patients with clinically mild disease, but with advanced cirrhosis synthesis declines to a mere 68 mg/d (normal 333 ± 149) (McCormick et al, 1973). Curiously, CDC synthesis is affected much less, which suggests that there is a specific deficiency of the enzyme 12α-hydroxylase (Vlahcevic et al, 1972b). The small cholic acid pool is turned over at only half the normal rate, probably because in the colon of cirrhotic patients there is far less dehydroxylation of cholic acid than normal (Yoshida et al, 1975). The reason for this is unknown, but as a result the bile of a cirrhotic patient contains remarkably little deoxycholate or even none at all (Mehta et al, 1974).

The uptake of bile acids by the cirrhotic liver is impaired (Blum and Spritz, 1966; Williams and Senior, 1971). Consequently serum bile acid levels are elevated, though seldom to the same extent as in cholestasis. It has repeatedly been shown that there is a relative excess of dihydroxy bile acids and of taurine conjugates in the blood (Makino et al, 1969; Carey, 1970; Neale et al, 1971). More recently, it has been found that the urine contains increased amounts of sulphated bile acids (Makino et al, 1975; Stiehl et al, 1975).

Cirrhotic patients secrete large amounts of dilute bile (Turnberg and

Grahame, 1970; Lenthall, Reynolds and Donovan, 1970). In English non-alcoholic patients, the duodenal concentration of bile salts during digestion is low if there is steatorrhoea, and this was thought to be the major factor in the malabsorption of cirrhosis (Badley et al, 1970). In alcoholic patients, duodenal bile salt levels seem to be similar whether steatorrhoea is present or not, and the main factor in causing malabsorption is pancreatic exocrine deficiency (Gourgoutis, 1975; Williams and Senior, 1971).

When patients with *chronic active hepatitis* were studied after undergoing full clinical and biochemical remission, some were found to retain high fasting serum bile acid levels, as measured by radioimmunoassay (Korman et al, 1973). On follow-up, these patients were particularly prone to relapse. Moreover, all patients who relapsed had rising serum bile acids several weeks before other tests including SGOT became abnormal. Similarly, the onset of viral hepatitis was detected by the postprandial bile acid concentration in all of five children who had been inoculated with the hepatitis B virus, even though four remained anicteric (Hofmann, Korman, and Krugman, 1974).

An even more sensitive test for detecting occult hepatitis is the cholyglycine tolerance test, in which a dose of 5 μmol/kg body weight is given intravenously and serum cholyl conjugates are measured by radioimmunoassay at zero time and after 10 min (Korman et al, 1975). Eleven patients were studied who had biopsy-proven chronic liver disease but normal conventional liver function tests. Cholylglycine tolerance was impaired in nine of the eleven, whereas fasting serum cholylglycine was increased in only three out of ten (LaRusso et al, 1975). It is perhaps salutary to note that a very similar test was advocated by Josephson in 1941. Then, as now, the chief obstacle to its widespread use was the technical difficulty of measuring cholic acid in blood. This problem could be circumvented if the bile acid tolerance test was performed using a tracer dose of ^{14}C-labelled cholylglycine or cholic acid and measuring the radio-activity of plasma drawn 10 min later. It would be of interest to compare this test with the 2 h postprandial serum bile acid concentration.

WHATEVER HAPPENED TO LITHOCHOLATE?

A few years ago, lithocholate was strongly suspected of being involved in the pathogenesis of chronic liver disease (Carey et al, 1966) and of perpetuating if not causing cholestasis (Schaffner and Popper, 1969). Fear of lithocholate-induced liver injury resulted in chenodeoxycholate therapy for gallstones being introduced with great caution. These anxieties sprang from the fact that, experimentally, this poorly soluble monohydroxy bile salt is extremely toxic. Injected intramuscularly into volunteers in doses of only 6 mg, lithocholic acid or its glycine conjugate cause within 12 h a high fever, with intense malaise, headache and nausea, followed by a marked and prolonged local inflammatory reaction (Palmer, Glickman and Kappas, 1962). The average American carries about 100 mg lithocholate in his enterohepatic circulation (Cowen et al,

1975a). When fed to animals and birds of many species, lithocholate injures the liver (for references see Heaton, 1972). In low doses, it causes mainly bile duct changes, ductular proliferation and hyperplasia. The rabbit liver is particularly sensitive, being damaged when the diet contains only 0.25 per cent lithocholate. In even smaller amounts, lithocholate or its conjugates induce cholestasis, with no damage visible except electron microscopic evidence of injury to bile canaliculi (Fisher and Miyai, 1971).

In spite of all this, recent years have seen a growing conviction that lithocholate is quite harmless after all, or at least that it is singularly absent from the scenes of crimes it had been suspected of committing. Thus high hepatic levels of lithocholate have been sought but not found in patients with cholestasis (Greim et al, 1972) and with liver injury following jejuno-ileal shunting for obesity (Sherr et al, 1974). Patients with ulcerative colitis have normal levels of lithocholate in their portal blood and also in their peripheral blood when they have liver disease (Siegel et al, 1975). In patients fed chenodeoxycholic acid for the treatment of gallstones, up to 30 per cent of the bile salts in fasting gallbladder bile are lithocholates (Danzinger et al, 1973), and serum levels of lithocholate are raised, and yet in 270 patient-years of CDC treatment no case of clinically significant hepatotoxicity has been discovered (Allan et al, 1975; Iser et al, 1975).

If lithocholate is, after all, benign this is probably because it is not allowed to circulate in unmodified form. When radioactive lithocholate is injected intravenously, it is rapidly and completely cleared into the bile, where, after but a single passage through the liver, 100 per cent is conjugated and 60 per cent is sulphated at the 3α-hydroxyl group (Palmer, 1967; Cowen et al, 1975a). Sulphation is particularly important as it renders lithocholate much more soluble in water and therefore probably less prone to bind to tissue proteins. For this reason or not, sulphated lithocholate is much less toxic to the isolated perfused rat liver than is the parent substance (Fisher and Miyai, 1971). Sulphation also promotes the excretion of lithocholate in the faeces (Cowen et al, 1975b). It does this by making the molecule more polar and so less easily reabsorbed by passive diffusion (Low-Beer, Tyor and Lack, 1969). In short, sulphation is an ingenious and effective detoxication system. It continues to operate in the obstructed liver, when it prevents accumulation by allowing free excretion of lithocholate into the urine (Stiehl, 1974; Makino et al, 1975).

WHAT IS THE PLACE AND VALUE OF THE BREATH TEST?

The radioactive glycocholate or cholylglycine breath test was the first test involving bile acids to become widely used in clinical practice. This is because, in the modest words of its inventor, it is 'extremely simple and moderately useful' (Hofmann and Thomas, 1973). The test was introduced in 1971 as a means of detecting excessive bile acid deconjugation. The principle is as follows: when glycine conjugated bile acids, which normally make up about three-quarters of the total in bile, are deconjugated in the intestine, the liberated glycine is either metabolised by anaerobic bacteria or absorbed and metabolised by the body. In either case, the end products include CO_2, most of which is excreted in the breath. When the glycine is labelled with ^{14}C, radioactive CO_2 is expired at a rate proportional to the rate of bile salt deconjugation. In health, the majority of the bile salt pool is absorbed intact from the ileum, but it has been estimated from isotopic studies that 15 to 20 per cent is deconjugated before it is absorbed (Hepner, Hofmann and Thomas, 1972). The rate of deconjugation is markedly increased: (a) if bacteria have access to the circulating bile salt pool more proximally in the intestine than normal, and (b) if a larger than normal fraction of the bile salt pool descends into the bacteria-rich colon, that is if there is dysfunction of the terminal ileum and so malabsorption of bile salts. Thus the main causes of a positive breath test are bacterial overgrowth in the small intestine, and ileal disease or resection, or a combination of both situations (see also Chapter 4).

The test is simple, non-invasive and without significant radiation hazard. The result should be available within 48 h. After an overnight fast, the patient is given a liquid test meal containing a 5 μCi dose of cholylglycine (glycocholic acid), labelled in the carboxyl atom of the glycine moiety. This material is obtainable from the Radiochemical Centre at Amersham. It should be mixed with 50 mg unlabelled bile acid as carrier. At hourly intervals for 4 or 5 h, the patient blows into a solution of a CO_2 trapping agent, Hyamine hydroxide, which contains an acid-base indicator. This changes colour when 1 ml of Hyamine has taken up 1 mmol of CO_2. The radioactivity that has been expired in 1 mmol of CO_2 is measured in a liquid scintillation counter to obtain the specific activity of the CO_2.

The results can be expressed in different ways but preferably as the percentage of the administered dose expired per hour, or per 5 h. This figure is arrived at by dividing the specific activity data by the dose of radioactivity administered, to obtain percentage of dose per mmol CO_2, and then multiplying by the estimated CO_2 production of the patient (conveniently assumed to be 9 mmol/kg h^{-1}).

False positive results are rare, but have occurred in severe constipation (Hofmann and Thomas, 1973). Mildly abnormal results have been reported in primary biliary cirrhosis and are unexplained (James, Agnew and Bouchier, 1973). Negative results are obtained in diarrhoea of colonic origin, in coeliac disease and in pancreatic steatorrhoea. Positive results are consistently obtained in patients with steatorrhoea due to the *stagnant loop syndrome*, as for example after Billroth II gastrectomy, or with jejunal diverticulosis, gastrocolic fistula or systemic sclerosis. In a study of 13 patients with small bowel diverticula, only three of whom had steatorrhoea, seven had an abnormal breath test and, in these, jejunal aspirates contained greater numbers of bacteria than in the six with a normal breath test (Parkin et al, 1972). Five of the seven with a positive test had high numbers of bacteroides or clostridia, which actively deconjugate bile acids. Six of the seven had a high ratio of glycine to taurine conjugates, which is a finding common to situations where the liver has an excessive amount of bile acid conjugation to perform (Heaton, 1972). In the study of Parkin et al (1972), there was poor correlation between the breath test and the presence of unconjugated bile acids in a jejunal aspirate, but this could have been due to abnormal deconjugation below the aspiration site. More disturbingly, one of the three patients with steatorrhoea had a normal breath test. Studies are needed on a much larger series of patients with small bowel bacterial overgrowth to assess the frequency of false negative results and to determine their cause.

It is in *ileal disorders* that the breath test has been most widely used and evaluated, perhaps because the pathophysiological state is easier to quantify than with bacterial overgrowth. If ileum has been resected, the abnormality should be proportional to the length of bowel resected. However, the terminal quarter of the small intestine must be counted more important in bile acid absorption than the third quarter, since active transport sites for bile acid absorption are concentrated in this area (Lack and Weiner, 1961). Bile acid malabsorption follows the resection of as little as 40 cm of terminal ileum and is severe when 60 cm are lost (Hofmann and Poley, 1972), but there is no direct relationship between length of resection and severity of bile acid malabsorption. There is also no correlation between either of these parameters and the amount of $^{14}CO_2$ expired in the breath test (Fromm, Thomas and Hofmann, 1973). Unfortunately, up to 20 per cent of patients with proven bile acid malabsorption have normal breath tests (Fromm et al, 1973; Pedersen, Arnfred and Hess Thaysen, 1973). This has been blamed on rapid transit through the colon, with failure of bacteria to detach the labelled glycine or to convert it to $^{14}CO_2$ or both. Nevertheless, the breath test is probably more sensitive than the Schilling test in detecting ileal dysfunction (Fromm et al, 1973). The two tests can be performed simultaneously, since radioactivity from one does not interfere with measurements of radioactivity from the other (see also Chapter 4).

In the commonest ileal disease, Crohn's disease, a positive breath test is often hard to interpret, because both bile acid malabsorption and bacterial overgrowth can be present. It was originally proposed that these be distinguished by measuring the faecal radioactivity as well, since an increase in this is diagnostic of bile acid malabsorption and does not occur with bacterial overgrowth (Fromm and Hofmann, 1971). However, this requires different and quite specialised technology and negates the great virtue of the breath test, its simplicity. Giving antibiotics and repeating the test is unhelpful, since this may reduce bacterial deconjugation in the colon as well as the small intestine.

To overcome these limitations, two modifications of the breath test have been suggested. Hepner (1975a) has proposed a prolonged test, with collection of breath samples at 2, 4, 6, 8, 12, 18 and 24 h, followed by calculation of the percentage of the total 24 h expired radioactivity which is excreted in the first 12 h. In control subjects, including some with diarrhoea, 39 ± 13 (s.d.) per cent of the 24 h breath $^{14}CO_2$ was expired in the first 12 h. Patients with ileitis or ileal resection expired their $^{14}CO_2$ more rapidly, so that in the first 12 h 78 ± 9 per cent had been excreted. Only 1 of 19 patients with ileal dysfunction overlapped with the controls, whereas half of them overlapped on comparing the rate of $^{14}CO_2$ excretion in the first 2 h. Unfortunately, the extra length of the test makes it much less suitable for clinical practice. A quite different approach has been proposed by Hirschowitz et al (1975). They have added ^{99}Tc-labelled sulphur colloid to the meal containing the ^{14}C-cholylglycine and scanned the abdomen hourly to determine the location of the meal when breath $^{14}CO_2$ is at its peak. In this way they claim to be able to decide if deconjugation is occurring chiefly in the small intestine or in the colon. Again, unfortunately, the simplicity of the test is sacrificed and extra technology introduced. However, in suitably equipped departments this modification could be attractive, provided of course that the claims made are substantiated.

Unfortunately, unoperated cases of ileal Crohn's disease are very prone to give negative breath tests. In one study, a positive result was obtained in only 1 out of 10 such patients (Lenz, 1975). This was in spite of the fact that the disease was judged to be active in four patients and that six of them had bile acid malabsorption documented by increased ^{14}C in the stools. This disappointing finding indicates that, in clinical practice, the breath test is of no value as a screening test for ileal disease unless it is combined with measurements of faecal radioactivity.

An interesting application of the breath test is to the detection of *cholangitis*. James et al (1973) studied six patients and found $^{14}CO_2$ excretion to be markedly increased in three and slightly increased in two of them.

The breath test is an attractive tool for *research*. Newman et al (1973) applied it to 17 randomly selected patients who had received pelvic radiotherapy for gynaecological malignant disease. All but one had an abnormal breath test. This was interpreted as evidence of radiation injury to the terminal ileum and was thought to explain the fact that most of the patients had noticed a permanent change in bowel habit after radiotherapy. Increased bile salt degradation by intestinal bacteria occurs after cholecystectomy (Pomare and Heaton, 1973a; Hepner et al, 1974) and this can be detected by the 24 h breath test (Hepner, 1975a). For research workers, it is a happy fact that $^{14}CO_2$ excretion after ^{14}C-cholylglycine correlates very closely with the more direct but far more laborious measurement of cholylglycine deconjugation—the daily fractional turnover of the glycine moiety (Hepner et al, 1972).

WHAT IS THE ROLE OF BILE ACIDS IN THE STAGNANT LOOP SYNDROME?

It is many years since this question was first raised (Dawson and Isselbacher, 1960), but a definite answer is still not possible. Two different mechanisms have been proposed. Both start from the premise that, whenever there is malabsorption due to bacterial contamination of the small intestine, there is extensive deconjugation of bile salts in the upper reaches of the small bowel. Much evidence supports this belief. Patients and experimental animals with the stagnant loop syndrome have repeatedly been shown to have abnormal amounts of free bile acids in their jejunal aspirates (Donaldson, 1970; Tabaqchali, 1970) and patients regularly have positive ^{14}C-cholylglycine breath tests. When careful bacteriological techniques are used, the main bacteria found in jejunal aspirates are anaerobes, especially bacteroides, capable of deconjugating bile salts (Drasar and Shiner, 1969) and, when intestinal contents are aspirated at different levels, there is usually a relationship between the presence of bacteroides and of free bile acids (Gorbach and Tabaqchali, 1969). The evidence is not absolutely consistent, since the occasional patient has a negative breath test (Parkin et al, 1972) or complete bile acid deconjugation without steatorrhoea (Hamilton et al, 1970). Strongly positive breath tests are often found in the absence of malabsorption (Fromm and Hofmann, 1971; Parkin et al, 1972). However, when eight patients with malabsorption and stagnant loops (four proximal, four distal) were studied after administration of radioactive taurocholate, all showed isotopic evidence of increased deconjugation, whereas taurocholate metabolism was normal in three subjects who had proximal diverticula and no malabsorption (Arnesjö et al, 1974). There was also increased dehydroxylation.

The main source of disagreement is whether steatorrhoea is caused by the toxicity of free dihydroxy bile acids or by reduced concentrations of conjugated bile acids, that is by detergent deficiency.

The detergent deficiency hypothesis arose from the finding by Tabaqchali, Hatzioannou and Booth (1968) of concentrations below 5 mmol/litre of conjugated bile salts in the upper jejunum of six patients and the reduction of faecal fat in one patient by feeding taurocholate. These studies are hard to interpret because they were performed on fasting subjects. However, low postprandial levels of conjugated bile salts, 3.4 mmol/litre compared with 7.4 in controls, have been reported (Northfield, 1973). Total bile salt concentration can be misleadingly normal, because it includes the sediment of intestinal aspirates and this contains precipitated free bile acids, whose solubility is low at the relatively low pH of the upper small bowel. In dogs with experimental blind loops, the small bowel after a fatty meal contains markedly subnormal levels of micellar lipid (Kim et al, 1966).

Detergent deficiency may not, however, be the whole explanation of the steatorrhoea of the stagnant loop syndrome. Contrary to previous beliefs, the small bowel mucosa is often abnormal both morphologically and functionally in patients with bacterial overgrowth. When multiple jejunal biopsies are examined, definite if patchy abnormalities can be seen on light microscopy (Paulley, 1969; Ament et al, 1972) while electron microscopy shows far more extensive damage to absorptive cells; intriguingly, many normal-looking cells can be seen to have difficulty in absorbing fat (Ament et al, 1972). Similarly, rats with experimental blind loops have patchy ultrastructural changes in the contaminated small intestine (Gracey, Papadimitriou and Bower, 1974) and reduced enzymatic activity both in the brush border and in intracellular organelles (Gracey, Thomas and Houghton, 1975; Toskes et al, 1975).

Are these changes due to the toxic effects of free dihydroxy bile acids? Evidence in man is limited. When three healthy subjects underwent overnight infusion of the jejunum with deoxycholate 1 or 2 mmol/litre, there was no ultrastructural damage detectable but, after a test meal, there was evidence of impaired fat absorption, namely a marked decrease in the number of fat particles in the apical areas of absorptive cells (Shimoda, O'Brien and Saunders, 1974). There was also a delay in transport of chylomicrons out of the cells into the intercellular spaces. The same changes were seen in patients with the stagnant loop syndrome. They could represent an inhibitory effect of unconjugated bile salts on re-esterification of fatty acids by the jejunal mucosa, since this has been demonstrated in vitro with deoxycholate (Dawson and Isselbacher, 1960; Dietschy, 1967). Failure to produce more severe changes may have been due to the short duration of the experiment or to the protective action of conjugated bile salt micelles. When deoxycholate is fed daily to rats for three or four days, quite severe absorptive cell damage is evident under the electron, but not light microscope (Gracey et al, 1973). This includes blunting and actual loss of microvilli, mitochondrial swelling and fragmentation of rough endoplasmic reticulum—changes very similar to those seen in rats with experimental blind loops. In both situations too, there is inhibition of both brush border and intracellular enzymes (Giannella, Rout and Toskes, 1974; Gracey, Houghton and Thomas, 1975).

It is quite possible, therefore, that mucosal damage by deconjugated bile acids explains at least some of the malabsorption of the stagnant loop syndrome. This is not ruled out by the reduction in steatorrhoea produced by feeding conjugated bile salts, since the extra micelles may solubilise free bile acids and so keep them from the mucosa.

The watery diarrhoea so troublesome in some patients with this syndrome may also be caused by free bile acids.

The fate of bile salts themselves has received remarkably little attention. It has for long been assumed that deconjugated bile acids are freely absorbed by passive diffusion throughout the small bowel, so that there is no excessive loss of bile acids from the body. This belief was strengthened by the finding of normal faecal radioactivity in patients undergoing the ^{14}C-cholylglycine breath test (Fromm and Hofmann, 1971; Pedersen et al, 1973). However, recently Arnesjö et al (1974) reported that, in four out of eight patients with the stagnant loop syndrome, labelled taurocholate disappeared from the bile so fast that its half-life could not be measured. In the other four patients, in whom kinetic data could be collected, the half-life was shortened and the pool size reduced. All this suggests that there was malabsorption of bile salts. However, the data need to be confirmed after administration of labelled free cholate and chenodeoxycholate.

In clinical practice, how far should one go in the investigation of patients thought to have the stagnant loop syndrome? Since bile salt deconjugation seems to be the sine qua non of this disorder, it is obviously desirable to demonstrate its presence. This is most easily done by the breath test. A negative result makes bacterial overgrowth very unlikely. However, positive results are obtained in some patients with bacterial overgrowth, but without malabsorption, so in a given patient an abnormal breath test can only be interpreted in the light of his faecal fat excretion. According to Northfield, Drasar and Wright (1973), the test which correlates best with steatorrhoea is analysis of a postprandial upper jejunal aspirate for deconjugated bile acids, using thin layer chromatography. Free bile acids were found in eight out of nine patients with malabsorption, but in none out of six patients with an anatomical stagnant loop that was not causing steatorrhoea. Poor discrimination was found with bacterial culture of the aspirate, and with the Schilling test. A different experience was reported by Egger and Kessler (1973). Of 38 patients with the stagnant loop syndrome, less than 60 per cent had free bile acids in their upper intestinal aspirates. These workers therefore developed an ingenious and relatively simple test for the deconjugating capacity of these aspirates. An aliquot is passed through a Millipore filter, and the filter, which retains the bacteria in the aspirate, is incubated for 2 h with conjugated bile salts under both aerobic and anaerobic conditions. The medium is then analysed for deconjugated bile salts by thin layer chromatography. Meanwhile the bacterial population of the aspirate has been determined by counting the bacteria on another Millipore filter. Egger and Kessler obtained a positive deconjugation test in all their 38 patents, all of whom also had 10^6 bacteria per millilitre of aspirate or more. This is a remarkable achievement, and was probably the result of exceptional care in aspirating from an area close to the blind loop. A possible snag with this test is that it is too sensitive. Positive results were obtained in two out of three patients with coeliac disease, a condition in which bacterial overgrowth is seldom clinically important, and in four patients with watery diarrhoea after gastric surgery (all of whom responded to tetracycline). Further reports on this test will be awaited with interest. Meanwhile, most clinical gastroenterologists will keep the faecal response to antibiotics as the keystone of their clinical investigation, since thin layer chromatography of bile acids is not performed in routine chemical pathology laboratories.

WHEN AND HOW DO BILE ACIDS CAUSE DIARRHOEA?

The concept of bile acid-induced or cholegenic diarrhoea is not new. The laxative effect of bile acids was well known to older physicians and exploited by them in many nostrums, but it only came to prominence with the recognition that the watery diarrhoea of *ileal disorders* is associated with severe bile acid malabsorption (Hofmann, 1967). This diarrhoea is generally precipitated by meals and worst after breakfast. It often causes anal soreness or itching. Daily excretion of bile acids is increased two to ten-fold over the normal 300 to 500 mg/d, depending on the amount of ileum resected or diseased (Hofmann, 1972; Findlay, Eastwood and Mitchell, 1973). The concentration of bile acids in stool water is often over 4 and has been recorded as high as 18 mmol/litre, that is in the range of concentrations found in the duodenum (Hofmann and Poley, 1972; Findlay et al, 1973). Paradoxically, the higher concentrations are found in patients with shorter resections (40–100 cm) and little or no steatorrhoea. In these patients, the high bile acid concentrations seem to inhibit the dehydroxylating enzymes of colonic bacteria, and so the faeces contain only cholic and chenodeoxycholic acids (Hofmann and Poley, 1972; Mitchell and Eastwood, 1972). These acids remain largely in solution. With large resections dehydroxylation is for some reason unimpaired, and the faeces contain mainly the usual deoxycholic and lithocholic acids. These are more prone to precipitate than their parent acids, so the bile acid concentration in stool water is within normal limits at 1 to 3 mmol/litre (Hofmann and Poley, 1972). In these patients, who have gross steatorrhoea, diarrhoea seems to be caused mainly by unabsorbed fatty acids.

These findings have important therapeutic implications. With massive resections and gross steatorrhoea, the most effective antidiarrhoeal treatment is restriction of dietary fat, or at least replacement of the normal long-chain triglycerides with medium-chain fats. With shorter resections and bile acid diarrhoea, the most effective treatment is oral administration of a bile acid-binding resin, which greatly reduces the concentration of bile acids in faecal water (Hofmann and Poley, 1972). In practice, ordinary antidiarrhoeal agents seem often to be effective. The use of cholestyramine increases faecal fat, but not enough to have nutritional significance. On the other hand, the absorption of fat soluble vitamins is seriously compromised, and cases of osteomalacia responding to vitamin D and of hypoprothrombinaemia responding to vitamin K have been reported (Heaton, Lever and Barnard, 1972; Gross and Brotman, 1970). Patients on long-term cholestyramine therapy should be given supplements of fat-soluble vitamins.

The diarrhoea of ileal resection is considerably worse if the ileocaecal valve and ascending colon are removed as well (Cummings, James and Wiggins, 1973). The reason is not clear. It may simply be that normally the right colon is the main site of water absorption. In addition, the ileocaecal sphincter probably delays the passage of bowel contents into the colon and so allows more time for bile salt absorption in the remaining ileum.

Even with minor ileal resections, there is usually some steatorrhoea. The reason for this is that with interruption of the enterohepatic circulation there is a deficiency of bile salts available to be secreted into the duodenum. This is often described as a reduction in the bile salt pool. However, it is more accurate to say that there is no bile salt pool. The term pool implies miscibility and exchangeability between old and newly synthesised material. If there is no circulation there can be no mixing or exchange. The bile salts accumulated in the gallbladder during fasting are mostly or wholly newly synthesised. They will be used only once instead of the normal 20 times. They are all that is available for the digestion of the next meal. After a prolonged fast, for example overnight, the liver (which is synthesising bile salts at maximal rate since the normal feedback inhibition by recycled material has been lost) may be able to accumulate 2 g of bile salts in the gallbladder, which is near the 2.5 to 3 g size of the normal circulating pool (Abaurre et al, 1969). However, between later meals there is much less time for new synthesis and so, for these meals, less stored bile salt is available in the gallbladder. When the concentration of bile salts in the duodenum during digestion is measured, it is found to be only slightly subnormal after breakfast but very low after later meals, e.g. 1 to 2 mmol instead of the normal 4 to 12 mmol (van Deest et al, 1968). At these low concentrations there are insufficient bile salt micelles to solubilise the products of fat digestion, some of which therefore escape absorption (see also Chapter 2).

The *mechanism of cholegenic diarrhoea* has attracted much interest. It was shown many years ago that bile enemas caused prompt defaecation in dogs, and more recently that bile acids infused into the rabbit caecum at 2 to 4 mmol/litre concentrations increase colonic motor activity (Kirwan et al, 1974). This suggests that bile salts may cause diarrhoea by accelerating colonic transit. However, cholegenic diarrhoea is usually ascribed to the actions of bile salts on colonic absorption, the main features of which were established in a classic study by Forth, Rummel and Glasner (1966). Absorption of water from tied-off loops of rat colon was completely blocked by unconjugated deoxycholic acid (DC) in the low concentration of 1 mmol/litre. Unconjugated chenodeoxycholic acid (CDC) was also very potent. Indeed, the threshold concentration for inhibition of absorption by CDC was only 0.4 mmol/litre, whereas the concentration in normal colonic contents is up to 4 mmol/litre. Compared with these dihydroxy bile acids, the trihydroxy acid cholic acid was less effective, and conjugates of all three were ineffective.

The relevance of these findings to man was established by Mekhjian et al (1971) in an exhaustive series of experiments on 20 healthy volunteers. Test solutions were perfused via a long per-oral tube into the caecum, and the effluent collected from the rectum for analysis of water and electrolyte movement. When the test solution contained DC 3 mmol/litre or CDC 5 mmol/litre there was not merely inhibition of water absorption, but actually net secretion of water or rather of an isotonic sodium chloride solution. Unconjugated cholic acid had no effect even at 10 mmol/litre. Conjugation with glycine and taurine seemed to make no difference to the secretory effects of the dihydroxy bile acids. These findings differ somewhat from the rat data of Forth et al (1966) but have been confirmed in the dog (Mekhjian and Phillips, 1970). In the dog the colon was also observed to secrete excess mucus.

Thus, dihydroxy bile acids in physiological or near-physiological concentrations increase colonic motility, decrease absorption, stimulate secretion and possibly induce mucus production. The secretory effects, like those of cholera toxin on the small intestine, are probably mediated by stimulation of the enzyme adenylate cyclase, which catalyses the production of cyclic AMP in the intestinal mucosa (Binder et al, 1975; Conley et al, 1975).

In *small bowel bacterial overgrowth*, watery diarrhoea can be a problem. It has long been suspected that this, like the sometimes associated steatorrhoea, is caused by the toxic action of unconjugated bile acids on the small bowel mucosa. Impaired fluid absorption would cause diarrhoea if the volume of ileal effluent exceeded the absorptive capacity of the colon (normally about 1500 ml/d; Phillips and Giller, 1973). Experimentally, unconjugated bile acids certainly have powerful effects on the small intestine. With in vitro incubation, DC and CDC in low concentration inhibit all the metabolic processes of the small intestinal mucosa, including active transport of sugars and amino acids (Dietschy, 1967). However, these are non-specific cytotoxic actions and are largely an artefact of in vitro preparations, in which bile acids accumulate in the mucosa. In vivo, such actions can be demonstrated but only at much higher bile salt concentrations (Teem and Phillips, 1972). Nevertheless, bile salts do affect small intestinal function at physiological concentrations. In human volunteers, perfusion of the jejunum with 2.5 or 3 mmol/litre conjugated DC and CDC inhibited water and electrolyte absorption and at higher concentrations evoked secretion of an isotonic fluid (Wingate, Phillips and Hofmann, 1973; Russell et al, 1973). However, Wingate et al made the important observation that addition of lecithin to the perfusion fluid abolished these effects. Lecithin and similar polar lipids (such as monoglyceride) are always to be found in the jejunum during digestion, that is during the periods when bile salts are present in the small bowel. This implies that, even in vivo, the effects of pure bile acid solutions on the jejunum may be an artefact of the laboratory. On the other hand, the ileum is likely to be exposed to bile salts without the protective polar lipids being present, because lipids are largely or wholly absorbed in the jejunum, whereas bile salts remain unabsorbed until they reach the terminal ileum. Nature seems to have taken care of this problem, since in vivo perfusion studies suggest that the ileum is less sensitive to bile salts than the jejunum. Thus, Harries and Sladen (1972) found that in the jejunum of the rat DC inhibited water absorption at a concentration of 1 mmol/litre, whereas over 5 mmol/litre was required to have the same effect in the ileum. In man, perfusion of the ileum with 2.5 mmol/litre CDC or DC, or with 5 mmol/litre glycochenodeoxycholic acid (GCDC) or glycodeoxycholic acid (GDC), inhibited water and electrolyte absorption and even caused some net secretion (Krag and Phillips, 1974). Whether such concentrations of dihydroxy bile acids are ever naturally present in the ileum is unknown. They will in any case be constantly changing as bile acid absorption occurs rapidly in this part of the intestine. It is still not possible, therefore, to state definitely whether or not free bile acids cause diarrhoea by their action on the small intestine.

Postvagotomy diarrhoea has long been an enigma, but recent evidence points to bile acid malabsorption as an important cause, at least in the small minority who have persistent watery stools. In 1973, Allan, Gerskowitch and Russell reported that the mean faecal bile acid excretion in seven such patients was 2100 mg/d, compared with 688 mg/d in normal controls. The same group have gone on to show in a controlled trial that this diarrhoea is relieved by cholestyramine (Allan and Russell, 1975), which confirms the uncontrolled experience of Ayulo (1972) and of Condon et al (1975). Why patients who have undergone vagotomy and a drainage procedure should have difficulty in reabsorbing their bile acids is at present quite obscure. Further investigations of ileal function in these patients will be of interest. Meanwhile, the possibility of small bowel bacterial overgrowth must be considered since, even in vagotomy patients without diarrhoea, there is evidence of increased bacterial degradation of bile salts (Arnesjö and Stahl, 1974). However, if it occurs, this bacterial overgrowth must be limited to the ileum, since the jejunum is not colonised particularly often in vagotomy patients who develop diarrhoea (Browning, Buchan and Mackay, 1974).

Cystic fibrosis poses a similar problem (see also Chapter 11). Weber and his colleagues (1973) measured the faecal bile acids of 24 children with pancreatic insufficiency secondary to cystic fibrosis and found it to be 743 mg/d, which is much higher than in age-matched controls (110 mg/d) and not significantly different from infants with ileal resection. The most obvious explanation of these findings is malabsorption of bile acids, and this has been confirmed by reports that the half-life of isotopically labelled bile acids is abnormally short in cystic fibrosis (Weber et al, 1975; Watkins et al, 1975). Bile acid loss was proportional to faecal fat excretion, and improved when pancreatic replacement therapy was given (Weber et al, 1973). On the other hand, children with steatorrhoea due to coeliac disease did not have cholerrhoea. This led to the suggestion that bile acid absorption is inhibited by large quantities of unhydrolysed fat, or other undigested nutrients in the ileum.

This raises the question—*can diarrhoea itself cause bile acid malabsorption* by rushing bile salt molecules past the active transport sites in the terminal ileum? The only published studies bearing on this question are those of Meihoff and Kern (1968). They induced watery diarrhoea in four volunteers by giving them large volumes of 10 per cent mannitol to drink. The rate of excretion of radioactive cholic acid was doubled, but this was a trivial change compared with that observed in six patients with ileal resection. It hardly merited the term bile acid malabsorption.

The only direct *test for cholegenic diarrhoea* is a therapeutic trial of cholestyramine. Other bile acid sequestrants may be effective but have not been evaluated. When cholestyramine is given in a dose of 4 g (e.g. one sachet of Questran) with each meal, there should be an immediate reduction in the fluidity and weight of the stools. The ^{14}C-cholylglycine breath test is quick and convenient but it is non-specific and gives many false negatives (see page 208). Tests for bile acid malabsorption itself are much less convenient. The simplest is measurement of faecal radioactivity after taking a ^{14}C-labelled bile acid by mouth (as in the breath test). The most specific but also most complicated are chemical assay of faecal bile acids and measurement of biliary bile salt half-lives (fractional turnover rates) using the isotope dilution technique (Hofmann et al, 1970). Detection of a high G/T ratio in the bile has been advocated as a screening test for bile acid malabsorption (Bruusgaard and Hess Thaysen, 1970), but its specificity has not been established and it involves duodenal intubation and chromatography.

ARE GALLSTONES THE RESULT OF DISTURBED BILE SALT METABOLISM?

Most gallstones in economically developed countries are composed largely of cholesterol, with smaller amounts of calcium salts, fatty acids and bile pigment (Sutor and Wooley, 1971; Trotman et al, 1975). Their formation is rightly regarded as a metabolic disease. The essence of this disease is the production of gallbladder bile which is supersaturated with cholesterol (Bouchier, 1975). Such bile is rarely found in areas with a low incidence of gallstones such as Africa and Japan, but is common in the general population in high incidence areas (Redinger and Small, 1972). The fact that supersaturated bile is common in subjects who have not (yet) formed gallstones implies that other conditions must be satisfied as well. These are probably the provision of a nucleating or seeding agent and perhaps stasis. We are still very ignorant of these later stages in the process, but much has been discovered of the essential first stage, the formation of supersaturated bile.

By definition, supersaturated or lithogenic bile contains an excess of cholesterol in relation to its twin solubilisers, bile salts and the phospholipid lecithin. The gallbladder itself is not now thought to play any role in altering the relative proportions of these three lipids, although an inflamed gallbladder may absorb bile salts (Ostrow, 1971). The blame for producing this abnormal bile rests on the liver. Hepatic bile secreted during fasting is more saturated than gallbladder bile even in control subjects without gallstones, but it is more saturated still in patients with stones (Metzger et al, 1973).

The key question in gallstone pathogenesis however is not: 'why does the liver secrete supersaturated bile?' but rather: 'why does gallbladder bile become supersaturated?' The difference is subtle but important. It is important because it is out of gallbladder bile that gallstones form. It is subtle because it depends on the ever-changing physiology of bile secretion. To explain the argument (which, unfortunately, is overlooked by some workers in this field) it is necessary to set out some of the salient facts of bile physiology.

The formation of bile involves the transport into bile canaliculi of its three main organic solutes—bile salts (70–80 per cent), lecithin (15–25 per cent) and cholesterol (3–15 per cent). The prime mover is bile salts. By extrapolating experimental data, one can usually deduce that with no bile salt secretion there would be no phospholipid or cholesterol secretion. With increasing bile salt secretion rates, curves are obtained for the other two lipids which are

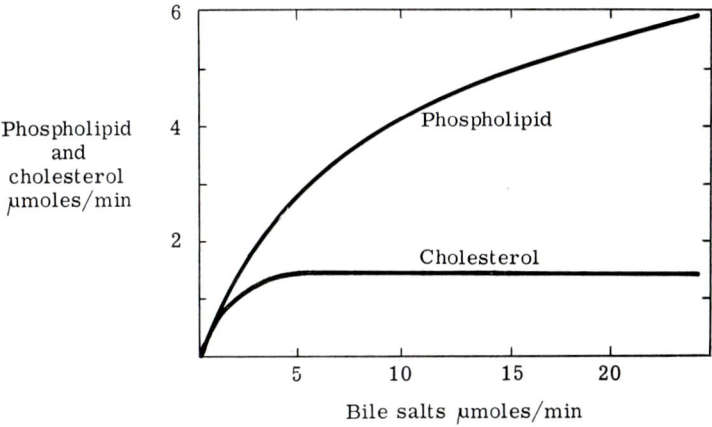

Figure 9.2 The curves which describe the relationship between bile salt secretion and the outputs of phospholipid and cholesterol in gallstone patients. Modified from Wagner et al (1973). Other workers report the phospholipid curve to be sigmoid in shape (Northfield and Hofmann, 1973)

concave downwards (Fig. 9.2). As the figure shows, cholesterol output levels off at the relatively low bile salt secretion of 5 μmol/min, whereas phospholipid output continues to rise. This implies that, once bile salt secretion rises above this level, there is a progressive increase in the ratio of the solubilisers, bile salts plus phospholipid, to cholesterol and hence a progressive fall in the saturation index of bile. Conversely, low bile salt secretion rates are dangerous because they are associated with more saturated bile. Actually, bile becomes supersaturated if bile salt output falls below about 12 μmol or 6 mg/min (Northfield and Hofmann, 1973; Wagner et al, 1973).

During the course of the day, the bile salt secretion rate varies greatly, because it depends heavily on whether the bile salt pool is circulating or not. During digestion, when the gallbladder remains contracted and the sphincter of Oddi is relaxed, bile salt secretion is high (about 50 μmol/min) because the whole bile salt pool is actively circulating. Between digestive periods, especially during the overnight fast, the majority of the pool is sequestered in the relaxed gallbladder and bile salt secretion is low. Exact figures are unavailable, but it is highly probable that secretion falls well below the critical level of 12 μmol/min. It can be predicted therefore that, during fasting, *hepatic* bile will become supersaturated even in normal subjects, precisely as found by Metzger et al (1973).

What decides whether *gallbladder* bile becomes supersaturated during the overnight fast? In the morning, the gallbladder contents may be considered as the result of the mixture of two sorts of bile. The first is the bile which has been diverted into the gallbladder as digestion of the evening meal finished. As cholecystokinin levels in the blood fall, the sphincter of Oddi closes and

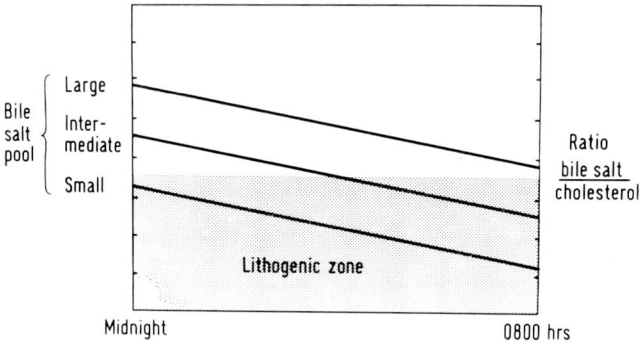

Figure 9.3 The ratio of bile salts to cholesterol in gallbladder bile during an overnight fast. A scheme to show how the addition to the gallbladder contents of supersaturated hepatic bile invariably lowers the bile salt/cholesterol ratio, but only renders the gallbladder bile supersaturated (lithogenic) if the latter starts the night with a low bile salt/cholesterol ratio. The initial ratio will depend on the 'priming dose' of bile salts, that is the size of the bile salt pool. This simplified scheme ignores the variable factor of incomplete mixing of incoming bile with resident bile

the gallbladder relaxes to accommodate the diverted bile, concentrating it up to ten-fold as it does so. This bile will contain the bile salt pool and so will have a high bile salt secretion rate. From Figure 9.2, it can be predicted that it will be undersaturated with cholesterol. Just how undersaturated it will be, will depend on the size of the bile salt pool.

Thus around midnight the bile in the gallbladder is most unsaturated. During the night it is constantly added to by hepatic bile which, as we have seen, is inevitably supersaturated. Just how supersaturated it is depends not so much on the bile salt and phospholipid secretion rates, which are bound to be low, but on the cholesterol secretion rate. Cholesterol secretion rates are relatively constant in a given individual, but vary widely between individuals.

This scheme is illustrated in Figure 9.3, which emphasises the importance of the bile salt pool in determining gallbladder bile composition. The role of cholesterol secretion rate can be defined as the factor which determines the slope of the line. A high secretion rate makes the line steeper, and so plunges the gallbladder's contents more deeply into the lithogenic zone.

If this scheme is valid, the formation of cholesterol gallstones should be accompanied by a small bile salt pool or a high cholesterol secretion rate, or preferably both. In fact both abnormalities have been identified in patients with radiolucent stones in functioning gallbladders. The bile salt pool is on average only 50 to 60 per cent of the normal size (Vlahcevic et al, 1970; Arnesjö and Ståhl, 1973; Pomare and Heaton, 1973b). It is also reduced in size in young American Indian women who have a 70 per cent expectation of developing gallstones (Vlahcevic et al, 1972a) and, in a group of subjects, there is a good correlation ($P<0.001$) between the size of the bile acid pool and the degree of saturation of gallbladder bile (Gregory, Vlahcevic and Swell, 1974). At the very least, therefore, a small bile acid pool must be regarded as a risk factor for cholelithiasis. The fact that small pools circulate more frequently, and maintain normal or near-normal bile acid secretion rates during digestion (Northfield and Hofmann, 1973, 1975; Grundy et al, 1974) is quite irrelevant to this discussion.

Increased cholesterol secretion has been demonstrated both in white and Indian American women with cholesterol stones (Grundy et al, 1974; Grundy, Metzger and Adler, 1972). During continuous infusion of a formula meal, the cholesterol secretion rates of white women with gallstones and of healthy control women averaged 56 and 29 mg/h respectively. Grundy and his coworkers have made the important discovery that cholesterol secretion is proportional to body fatness. Moreover, weight reduction leads to a fall in cholesterol secretion rates (Bennion and Grundy, 1975). This obviously helps to explain the well-known clinical association between obesity and gallstones. Increased cholesterol secretion is presumably the result of increased cholesterol synthesis by the liver. Certainly obesity is associated with high cholesterol synthesis rates (Miettinen, 1971; Nestel, Schreibman and Ahrens, 1973). In the livers of gallstone patients there is increased activity of the enzyme which controls the rate of cholesterol synthesis—HMG CoA reductase (Salen et al, 1975).

The decreased bile acid pool is less easily explained. The obvious possibility is that bile acid synthesis is suppressed. In fact, the livers of gallstone patients do show reduced activity of the enzyme which controls the rate of bile acid synthesis, 7α-hydroxylase, even though there is an excess of its substrate, cholesterol (Salen et al, 1975). Direct measurements of bile acid synthesis in gallstone patients have shown it to be normal at least in US Indians (Vlahcevic et al, 1972a; Bell et al, 1972). However, this can still indicate that the synthetic mechanism is suppressed; a fall in the circulating pool implies reduced return of bile acids to the liver, which is normally a stimulus to *increased* synthesis. The gallstone patient's liver seems not to respond to this stimulus. A similar conclusion was reached by Hepner and Quarfordt (1975) after studying the fate of ^{14}C-labelled cholesterol over a 10 week period. In four out of six gallstone patients they found not only reduced primary bile acid pools but also decreased conversion of cholesterol to bile acids. Defective cholesterol catabolism has been suggested before (Hikasa et al, 1969; Heaton, 1972) and is an attractive mechanism, because it could help to explain excess cholesterol in liver and bile as well as bile acid deficiency.

If cholesterol catabolism is suppressed, what is the cause? One suggestion is that, because the small bile acid pools of gallstone patients circulate more frequently, there is increased feedback inhibition of the liver (Northfield and Hofmann, 1973, 1975; Low-Beer and Pomare, 1973). This would make rapid circulation of the pool the primary abnormality, rather than small size of the pool. However, no adequate explanation of such rapid circulation has been put forward while, on the other hand, more frequent circulation could be the effect rather than the cause of the small pool—presumably a small amount of bile salt is reabsorbed more rapidly than a large one. This theory rests on the plausible suggestion that bile acid synthesis is controlled by the frequency with which the pool circulates. However, when all these variables were measured in 21 patients, the proposed relationships were not found (von Bergmann, Mok and Grundy, 1975). Subjects with high secretion rates were simply those who had large pools, and they showed no inhibition of bile acid synthesis.

Another explanation of suppressed cholesterol catabolism arose from the often-repeated observation that in dogs, rats, rabbits and monkeys, so-called semisynthetic diets lead to reduced bile salt synthesis and pool size. These diets are strikingly similar to those which have been used to induce gallstone formation and supersaturated bile in various species. The only feature which all these diets have in common is a high content of refined carbohydrate, especially sugar (for references, see Heaton, 1975). It was suggested, therefore, that refined carbohydrate inhibits cholesterol catabolism (Heaton, 1972, 1975). Recently Hepner (1975b) noted that human volunteers given a diet of sugary liquids failed to expand their bile salt pools as much as would be expected from the fact that they circulate these pools far less than normal. A mere 10 per cent increase was noted, whereas there is a 300 per cent increase in coleliac patients who have a naturally sluggish enterohepatic circulation (Low-Beer et al, 1971).

Much work is needed to substantiate this theory. In the meantime it has the virtue of explaining the association of gallstones with obesity, and the epidemiological pattern of the disease, namely its predilection for technological societies, in which 40 to 50 per cent of calories are obtained from refined carbohydrate (Heaton, 1973, 1975). Simply adding fibre to a refined diet does not reverse all the abnormalities. In rats, adding cellulose or psyllium hydrocolloid (Metamucil) in large amounts expands the bile salt pool (Portman and Murphy, 1958; Beher and Casazza, 1971), but in man adding quite large amounts of bran does not do so (Pomare et al, 1974). On the other hand, bran does decrease the saturation of bile in most gallstone patients, probably because it increases the endogenous synthesis of chenodeoxycholate. Studies of bile composition on refined and unrefined diets have not been reported.

The role of bile salt deficiency in causing gallstone formation is paramount in one situation, dysfunction of the terminal ileum. Here, documentation is good for each step in the following scheme: loss of ileal mucosa interrupts the reabsorption of bile salts, which reduces the amount of bile salt available to be secreted into the bile (van Deest et al, 1968; Dowling, Mack and Small, 1970), which renders the bile supersaturated with cholesterol (Dowling, Mack and Small, 1971; Dowling, Bell and White, 1972), which increases the frequency of gallstones to three to five times the expected (Heaton and Read, 1969; Cohen et al, 1971) (see also Chapter 4).

REFERENCES

Abaurre, R., Gordon, S. G., Mann, J. G. & Kern, F. (1969) Fasting bile salt pool size and composition after ileal resection. *Gastroenterology*, **57**, 679–688.

Admirand, W. H. & Bauer, K. (1971) Phenobarbital (PB): an effective form of therapy in primary biliary cirrhosis. *Journal of Clinical Investigation*, **50**, 1A (Abstract).

Allan J G., Gerskowitch, V. P. & Russell, R. I. (1973) A study of the role of bile acids in the pathogenesis of post-vagotomy diarrhoea. *Gut*, **14**, 423–424 (Abstract).

Allan, J. G. & Russell, R. I. (1975) Double-blind controlled trial of cholestyramine in the treatment of post-vagotomy diarrhoea. *Gut*, **16**, 830 (Abstract).

Allan, R. N., Carter, J. A., Yu, P. S., Thistle, J. L. & Hofmann, A. F. (1975) Effect of chenodeoxycholic acid on immunoreactive serum lithocholate in gallstone patients. *Gastroenterology*, **68**, 913 (Abstract).

Ament, M. E., Shimoda, S. S., Saunders, D. R. & Rubin, C. E. (1972) Pathogenesis of steatorrhea in three cases of small intestinal stasis syndrome. *Gastroenterology*, **63**, 728–747.

Arnsejö, B. & Ståhl, E. (1973) Taurocholate metabolism in patients with cholesterol gallstones. *Scandinavian Journal of Gastroenterology*, **8**, 369–375.

Arnsejö, B. & Ståhl, E. (1974) Taurocholate metabolism after truncal vagotomy and pyloroplasty or antral resection. *Scandinavian Journal of Gastroenterology*, **9**, 601–606.

Arnsejö, B., Ståhl, E., Sörbris, R. & Kock, N. G. (1974) Taurocholate metabolism in patients with small intestinal stagnant loops. *Scandinavian Journal of Gastroenterology*, **9**, 579–585.

Ayulo, J. A. (1972) Cholestryamine in post-vagotomy diarrhea. *American Journal of Gastroenterology*, **57**, 207–226.

Back, P. (1972) Urinary profile of bile acids in liver disease. In *Bile Acids in Human Diseases*, ed. Back, P. & Gerok, W., pp. 53–55. Stuttgart: Schattauer.

Badley, B. W. D., Murphy, G. M., Bouchier, I. A. D. & Sherlock, S. (1970) Diminished micellar phase lipid in patients with chronic non-alcoholic liver disease and steatorrhea. *Gastroenterology*, **58**, 781–789.

Beher, W. T. & Casazza, K. K. (1971) Effects of psyllium hydrocolloid on bile acid metabolism in normal and hypophysectomised rats. *Proceedings of the Society of Experimental Biology and Medicine*, **136**, 253–256.

Bell, C. C., McCormick, W. C., Gregory, D. H., Law, D. H., Vlahcevic, Z. R. & Swell, L. (1972) Relationship of bile acid pool size to the formation of lithogenous bile in male Indians of the Southwest. *Surgery, Gynecology and Obstetrics*, **134**, 473–478.

Bennion, L. J. & Grundy, S. M. (1975) Effects of obesity and caloric intake on biliary lipid metabolism in man. *Journal of Clinical Investigation*, **56**, 996–1011.

Binder, H. J., Filburn, C. & Volpe, B. T. (1975) Bile salt alteration of colonic electrolyte transport: role of cyclic adenosine monophosphate. *Gastroenterology*, **68**, 503–508.

Blum, M. & Spritz, N. (1966) The metabolism of intravenously injected isotopic cholic acid in Laennec's cirrhosis. *Journal of Clinical Investigation*, **45**, 187–193.
Bouchier, I. A. D. (1975) Gallstones. In *Modern Trends in Gastroenterology*—5, ed. Read, A. E., pp. 203–230. London: Butterworths.
Browning, G. G., Buchan, K. A. & Mackay, C. (1974) Clinical and laboratory study of postvagotomy diarrhoea. *Gut*, **15**, 644–653.
Bruusgaard, A. & Thaysen, E. H. (1970) Increased ratio of glycine/taurine conjugated bile acids in the early diagnosis of terminal ileopathy. Preliminary report. *Acta medica scandinavica*, **188**, 547–548.
Carey, J. B. (1970) Bile salts and hepatobiliary disease. In *Diseases of the Liver*, 3rd edn, ed. Schiff, L., pp. 103–146. Philadelphia: Lippincott.
Carey, J. B., Wilson, I. D., Zaki, F. G. & Hanson, R. F. (1966) The metabolism of bile acids with special reference to liver injury. *Medicine, Baltimore*, **45**, 461–470.
Cohen, S., Kaplan, M., Gottlieb, L. & Patterson, J. (1971) Liver disease and gallstones in regional enteritis. *Gastroenterology*, **60**, 237–245.
Condon, J. R., Robinson, V., Suleman, M. I., Fan, V. S. & McKeown, M. D. (1975) The cause and treatment of post-vagotomy diarrhoea. *British Journal of Surgery*, **62**, 309–312.
Conley, D. R., Coyne, M. J., Chung, A., Bonorris, G. G. & Schoenfield, L. J. (1975) Mechanism of bile acid diarrhea: the role of cyclic AMP in colonic secretion. *Gastroenterology*, **68**, 877 (Abstract).
Cowen, A. E., Korman, M. G., Hofmann, A. F. & Cass, O. W. (1975a) Metabolism of lithocholate in healthy man. I. Biotransformation and biliary excretion of intravenously administered lithocholate, lithocholylglycine, and their sulfates. *Gastroenterology*, **69**, 59–66.
Cowen, A. E., Korman, M. G., Hofmann, A. F. & Coffin, S. B. (1975b) Metabolism of lithocholate in healthy man. II. Enterohepatic circulation. *Gastroenterology*, **69**, 67–76.
Cowen, A. E., Korman, M. G., Hofmann, A. F. & Thomas, P. J. (1975c) Plasma disappearance of radioactivity after intravenous injection of labelled bile acids in man. *Gastroenterology*, **68**, 1567–1573.
Cummings, J. H., James, W. P. T. & Wiggins, H. S. (1973) Role of the colon in ileal-resection diarrhoea. *Lancet*, **1**, 344–347.
Danzinger, R. G., Hofmann, A. F., Thistle, J. L. & Schoenfield, L. J. (1973) Effect of oral chenodeoxycholic acid on bile acid kinetics and biliary lipid composition in women with cholelithiasis. *Journal of Clinical Investigation*, **52**, 2809–2821.
Dawson, A. M. & Isselbacher, K. J. (1960) Studies on lipid metabolism in the small intestine with observations on the role of bile salts. *Journal of Clinical Investigation*, **39**, 730–740.
Demers, L. M. & Hepner, G. W. (1975) Serum bile acids in patients with hepatobiliary disease. *Gastroenterology*, **68**, 881 (Abstract).
Denk, H., Greim, H. & Hutterer, F. (1971) Detergent action of bile acids on hepatocellular microsomes, and its role in cholestasis. *Gastroenterology*, **60**, 187 (Abstract).
Dietschy, J. M. (1967) Effects of bile salts on intermediate metabolism of the intestinal mucosa. *Federation Proceedings*, **26**, 1589–1598.
Donaldson, R. M. (1970) Small bowel bacterial overgrowth. *Advances in Internal Medicine*, **16**, 191–212.
Dowling, R. H., Bell, G. D. & White, J. (1972) Lithogenic bile in patients with ileal dysfunction. *Gut*, **13**, 415–420.
Dowling, R. H., Mack, E. & Small, D. M. (1970) Effects of controlled interruption of the enterohepatic circulation of bile salts by biliary diversion and by ileal resection on bile salt secretion, synthesis and pool size in the Rhesus monkey. *Journal of Clinical Investigation*, **49**, 232–242.
Dowling, R. H., Mack, E. & Small, D. M. (1971) Biliary lipid secretion and bile composition after acute and chronic interruption of the enterohepatic circulation in the Rhesus monkey. IV. Primate biliary physiology. *Journal of Clinical Investigation*, **50**, 1917–1926.
Drasar, B. S. & Shiner, M. (1969) Studies on the intestinal flora. Part II. Bacterial flora of the small intestine in patients with gastro-intestinal disorders. *Gut*, **10**, 812–819.
Egger, G. & Kessler, J. I. (1973) Clinical experience with a simple test for the detection of bacterial deconjugation of bile salts and the site and extent of bacterial overgrowth in the small intestine. *Gastroenterology*, **64**, 545–551.

Erb, W., Schreiber, J. & Walczak, M. (1972) Gas-chromatographische untersuchungen der serum-gallensäuren methodik sowie ergebnisse bei patienten mit akuter hepatitis. *Gastroenterologie*, **10**, 349–358.

Eyssen, H., Parmentier, G., Boon, J. & Eggermont, E. (1972) Trihydroxycoprostanic acid in the duodenal fluid of two children with intrahepatic bile duct abnormalities. *Biochimica et biophysica acta*, **273**, 212–221.

Findlay, J. M., Eastwood, M. A. & Mitchell, W. D. (1973) The physical state of bile acids in the diarrhoeal stool of ileal dysfunction. *Gut*, **14**, 319–323.

Fisher, M. M. & Miyai, K. (1971) Lithocholic acid induced intrahepatic cholestasis. *Gastroenterology*, **60**, 193 (Abstract).

Forth, W., Rummel, W. & Glasner, H. (1966) Zur resorptions-hemmenden Wirkung von Gallensäuren. *Archiv für experimentelle Pathologie und Pharmakologie*, **254**, 364–380.

Fromm, H. & Hofmann, A. F. (1971) Breath test for altered bile-acid metabolism. *Lancet*, **2**, 621–625.

Fromm, H., Thomas, P. J. & Hofmann, A. F. (1973) Sensitivity and specificity in tests of distal ileal function: prospective comparison of bile acid and vitamin B_{12} absorption in ileal resection patients. *Gastroenterology*, **64**, 1077–1090.

Frosch, B. & Wagener, H. (1967) Quantitative determination of conjugated bile acids in serum in acute hepatitis. *Nature, London*, **213**, 404–405.

Giannella, R. A., Rout, W. R. & Toskes, P. P. (1974) Jejunal brush border injury and impaired sugar and amino acid uptake in the blind loop syndrome. *Gastroenterology*, **67**, 965–974.

Gorbach, S. L. & Tabaqchali, S. (1969) Bacteria, bile and the small bowel. *Gut*, **10**, 963–972.

Gourgoutis, G. D. (1975) Intraduodenal concentration of bile salts and pancreatic function in patients with alcoholic liver disease and steatorrhea. *Gastroenterology*, **68**, 902 (Abstract).

Gracey, M., Houghton, M. & Thomas, J. (1975) Deoxycholate depresses small intestinal enzyme activity. *Gut*, **16**, 53–56.

Gracey, M., Papadimitriou, J. & Bower, G. (1974) Ultrastructural changes in the small intestines of rats with self-filling blind loops. *Gastroenterology*, **67**, 646–651.

Gracey, M., Papadimitriou, J., Burke, V., Thomas, J. & Bower, G. (1973) Effects on small-intestinal function and structure induced by feeding a deconjugated bile salt. *Gut*, **14**, 519–528.

Gracey, M., Thomas, J. & Houghton, M. (1975) Effect of stasis on intestinal enzyme activities. *Australian and New Zealand Journal of Medicine*, **5**, 141–144.

Gregory, D. H., Vlahcevic, Z. R. & Swell, L. (1974) Determination of the cholesterol saturation of human bile and its relevance to gallstone formation. *American Journal of Digestive Diseases*, **19**, 268–270.

Greim, H., Trülzsch, D., Czygan, P., Rudick, J., Hutterer, F., Schaffner, F. & Popper, H. (1972) Mechanism of cholestasis. 6. Bile acids in human livers with or without biliary obstruction. *Gastroenterology*, **63**, 846–850.

Gross, L. & Brotman, M. (1970) Hypoprothrombinemia and hemorrhage associated with cholestyramine therapy. *Annals of Internal Medicine*, **72**, 95–96.

Grundy, S. M., Duane, W. C., Adler, R. D., Aron, J. M. & Metzger, A. L. (1974) Biliary lipid outputs in young women with cholesterol gallstones. *Metabolism*, **23**, 67–73.

Grundy, S. M., Metzger, A. L. & Adler, R. D. (1972) Mechanisms of lithogenic bile formation in American Indian women with cholesterol gallstones. *Journal of Clinical Investigation*, **57**, 3026–3043.

Gumucio, J. J., Accatino, L., Macho, A. M. & Contreras, A. (1973) Effect of phenobarbital on the ethynyl estradiol-induced cholestasis in the rat. *Gastroenterology*, **65**, 651–657.

Hamilton, J. D., Dyer, N. H., Dawson, A. M., O'Grady, F. W., Vince, A., Fenton, J. C. B. & Mollin, D. L. (1970) Assessment and significance of bacterial overgrowth in the small bowel. *Quarterly Journal of Medicine*, **39**, 265–285.

Harries, J. T. & Sladen, G. E. (1972) The effects of different bile salts on the absorption of fluid, electrolytes and monosaccharides in the small intestine of the rat in vivo. *Gut*, **13**, 596–603.

Heaton, K. W. (1972) *Bile Salts in Health and Disease*. Edinburgh: Churchill Livingstone.

Heaton, K. W. (1973) The epidemiology of gallstones and suggested aetiology. *Clinics in Gastroenterology*, **2**, 67–83.

Heaton, K. W. (1975) Gallstones and cholecystitis. In *Refined Carbohydrate Foods and Disease; Some Implications of Dietary Fibre*, ed. Burkitt, D. P. & Trowell, H. C., pp. 173–194. London: Academic Press.

Heaton, K. W., Lever, J. V. & Barnard, D. (1972) Osteomalacia associated with cholestyramine therapy for post-ileectomy diarrhea. *Gastroenterology*, **62**, 642–646.

Heaton, K. W. & Read, A. E. (1969) Gallstones in patients with disorders of the terminal ileum and disturbed bile salt metabolism. *British Medical Journal*, **3**, 494–496.

Hepner, G. W. (1975a) Increased sensitivity of the cholylglycine breath test for detecting ileal dysfunction. *Gastroenterology*, **68**, 8–16.

Hepner, G. W. (1975b) Effect of decreased gallbladder stimulation on enterohepatic cycling and kinetics of bile acids. *Gastroenterology*, **68**, 1574–1581.

Hepner, G. W., Hofmann, A. F., Malagelada, J. R., Szczepanik, P. A. & Klein, P. D. (1974) Increased bacterial degradation of bile acids in cholecystectomised subjects. *Gastroenterology*, **66**, 556–564.

Hepner, G. W., Hofmann, A. F. & Thomas, P. J. (1972) Metabolism of steroid and amino acid moieties of conjugated bile acids in man. I. Cholylglycine. *Journal of Clinical Investigation*, **51**, 1889–1897.

Hepner, G. W. & Quarfordt, S. H. (1975) Kinetics of cholesterol and bile acids in patients with cholesterol cholelithiasis. *Gastroenterology*, **69**, 318–325.

Hikasa, Y., Matsuda, S., Nagase, M. et al (1969) Initiating factors of gallstones, especially cholesterol stones (III). *Archiv. Japanische Chirurgie*, **38**, 107–124.

Hirschowitz, B. I., Bondi, J., Beschi, R., Siegel, R. & Mihas, A. (1975) Modification of the $^{14}CO_2$ breath test for bile salt deconjugation. *Gastroenterology*, **68**, 911 (Abstract).

Hofmann, A. F. (1967) The syndrome of ileal disease and the broken enterohepatic circulation: cholerheic enteropathy. *Gastroenterology*, **52**, 752–757.

Hofmann, A. F. (1972) Bile acid malabsorption caused by ileal resection. *Archives of Internal Medicine*, **130**, 597–605.

Hofmann, A. F., Korman, M. G. & Krugman, S. (1974) Sensitivity of serum bile acid assay for detection of liver damage in viral hepatitis type B. *American Journal of Digestive Diseases*, **19**, 908–910.

Hofmann, A. F. & Poley, J. R. (1972) Role of bile acid malabsorption in pathogenesis of diarrhea and steatorrhea in patients with ileal resection. I. Response to cholestyramine or replacement of dietary long chain triglyceride by medium chain triglyceride. *Gastroenterology*, **62**, 918–934.

Hofmann, A. F., Schoenfield, L. J., Kottke, B. A. & Poley, J. R. (1970) Methods for the description of bile acid kinetics in man. In *Methods in Medical Research*, ed. Olson, R. E., Vol. 12, pp. 149–180. Chicago: Year Book Medical Publishers.

Hofmann, A. F. & Thomas, P. J. (1973) Bile acid breath test: extremely simple, moderately useful. *Annals of Internal Medicine*, **79**, 743–744.

Iser, J. H., Dowling, R. H., Mok, H. Y. I. & Bell, G. D. (1975) Chenodeoxycholic acid treatment of gallstones. A follow-up report and analysis of factors influencing response to therapy. *New England Journal of Medicine*, **293**, 378–383.

James, O. F. W., Agnew, J. E. & Bouchier, I. A. D. (1973) Assessment of the ^{14}C-glycocholic acid breath test. *British Medical Journal*, **3**, 191–195.

Javitt, N. B. & Emerman, S. (1968) Effect of sodium taurolithocholate on bile flow and bile acid excretion. *Journal of Clinical Investigation*, **47**, 1002–1014.

Josephson, B. (1941) The circulation of the bile acids in connection with their production, conjugation and excretion. *Physiological Reviews*, **21**, 463–486.

Kaplowitz, N., Kok, E. & Javitt, N. B. (1973) Postprandial serum bile acid for the detection of hepatobiliary disease. *Journal of the American Medical Association*, **225**, 292–293.

Kim, Y. S., Spritz, N., Blum, M., Terz, J. & Sherlock, P. (1966) The role of altered bile acid metabolism in the steatorrhea of experimental blind loop. *Journal of Clinical Investigation*, **45**, 956–962.

Kirby, J., Heaton, K. W. & Burton, J. L. (1974) Pruritic effect of bile salts. *British Medical Journal*, **4**, 693–695.

Kirwan, W. O., Smith, A. N., Mitchell, W. D. & Eastwood, M. A. (1974). Effect of bile acids on the motility of the colon. *Gut*, **15**, 828 (Abstract).

Korman, M. G., LaRusso, N. F., Hoffman, N. E. & Hofmann, A. F. (1975) Development of an intravenous bile acid tolerance test. Plasma disappearance of cholylglycine in health. *New England Journal of Medicine*, **292**, 1205–1209.

Korman, M. G., Summerskill, W. H. J., Go, V. L. W. & Hofmann, A. F. (1973) Sensitivity and predictive value of serum bile acid concentrations in patients with chronic active liver disease. *Gastroenterology*, **65**, 554 (Abstract).

Krag, E. & Phillips, S. F. (1974) Active and passive bile acid absorption in man. Perfusion studies of the ileum and jejunum. *Journal of Clinical Investigation*, **53**, 1686–1694.

Lack, L. & Weiner, I. M. (1961) In vitro absorption of bile salts by small intestine of rats and guinea-pigs. *American Journal of Physiology*, **200**, 313–317.

LaRusso, N. F., Hoffman, N. E., Hofmann, A. F. & Korman, M. G. (1975) Validity and sensitivity of an intravenous bile acid tolerance test in patients with liver disease. *New England Journal of Medicine*, **292**, 1209–1214.

LaRusso, N. F., Korman, M. G., Hoffman, N. E. & Hofmann, A. F. (1974) Dynamics of the enterohepatic circulation of bile acids: postprandial serum concentrations of conjugates of cholic acid in health, cholecystectomised patients, and patients with bile acid malabsorption. *New England Journal of Medicine*, **291**, 689–692.

Lenthall, J., Reynolds, T. B. & Donovan, J. (1970) Excessive output of bile in chronic hepatic disease. *Surgery, St Louis*, **130**, 243–253.

Lenz, K. (1975) An evaluation of the 'breath test' in Crohn's disease. *Scandinavian Journal of Gastroenterology*, **10**, 655–671.

Lewis, B., Panveliwalla, D., Tabaqchali, S. & Wootton, I. D. P. (1969) Serum-bile-acids in the stagnant-loop syndrome. *Lancet*, **1**, 219–220.

Low-Beer, T. S., Heaton, K. W., Heaton, S. T. & Read, A. E. (1971) Gallbladder inertia and sluggish enterohepatic circulation of bile-salts in coeliac disease. *Lancet*, **1**, 991–994.

Low-Beer, T. S. & Pomare, E. W. (1973) Regulation of bile salt pool size in man. *British Medical Journal*, **2**, 338–340.

Low-Beer, T. S., Schneider, R. E. & Dobbins, W. O. (1970) Morphological changes of the small-intestinal mucosa of guinea-pig and hamster following incubation in vitro and perfusion in vivo with unconjugated bile salts. *Gut*, **11**, 486–492.

Low-Beer, T. S., Tyor, M. P. & Lack, L. (1969) Effect of sulfation of taurolithocholic and glycolithocholic acids on their intestinal transport. *Gastroenterology*, **56**, 721–726.

Low-Beer, T. S., Wilkins, R. M., Lack, L. & Tyor, M. P. (1974) Effect of one meal on enterohepatic circulation of bile salts. *Gastroenterology*, **67**, 490–497.

McCormick, W. C., Bell, C. C., Swell, L. & Vlahcevic, Z. R. (1973) Cholic acid synthesis as an index of the severity of liver disease in man. *Gut*, **14**, 895–902.

Makino, I., Hashimoto, H., Shinozaki, K., Yoshino, K. & Nakayawa, S. (1975) Sulfated and nonsulfated bile acids in urine, serum, and bile of patients with hepatobiliary diseases. *Gastroenterology*, **68**, 545–553.

Makino, I., Nakagawa, S. & Mashimo, K. (1969) Conjugated and unconjugated serum bile acid levels in patients with hepatobiliary diseases. *Gastroenterology*, **56**, 1033–1039.

Mehta, S. J., Struthers, J. E., Kaye, M. D. & Naylor, J. L. (1974) Biliary deoxycholate in patients with alcoholic cirrhosis. *Gastroenterology*, **67**, 674–679.

Meihoff, W. E. & Kern, F. (1968) Bile salt malabsorption in regional ileitis, ileal resection and mannitol-induced diarrhea. *Journal of Clinical Investigation*, **47**, 261–267.

Mekhjian, H. S. & Phillips, S. F. (1970) Perfusion of the canine colon with unconjugated bile acids. Effect on water and electrolyte transport, morphology and bile acid absorption. *Gastroenterology*, **59**, 120–129.

Mekhjian, H. S., Phillips, S. F. & Hofmann, A. F. (1971) Colonic secretion of water and electrolytes induced by bile acids: perfusion studies in man. *Journal of Clinical Investigation*, **50**, 1569–1577.

Metreau, J.-M., Bismuth, H., Franco, D. & Dhumeaux, D. (1975) Effect of phenobarbital in a case of extrahepatic cholestasis. *Gastroenterology*, **68**, 567–571.

Metzger, A. L., Adler, R., Heymsfield, S. & Grundy, S. M. (1973) Diurnal variation in biliary lipid composition. Possible role in cholesterol gallstone formation. *New England Journal of Medicine*, **288**, 333–336.

Miettinen, T. A. (1971) Cholesterol production in obesity. *Circulation*, **44**, 842–850.

Mitchell, W. D. & Eastwood, M. A. (1972) Faecal bile acids and neutral steroids in patients with ileal dysfunction. *Scandinavian Journal of Gastroenterology*, **7**, 29–32.

Murphy, G. M., Billing, B. H. & Baron, D. N. (1970) A fluorimetric and enzymatic method for the estimation of serum total bile acids. *Journal of Clinical Pathology*, **23**, 594–598.

Nair, P. P. & Kritchevsky, D. (1971) *The Bile Acids*. New York: Plenum Press.

Neale, G., Lewis, B., Weaver, V. & Panveliwalla, D. (1971) Serum bile acids in liver disease. *Gut*, **12**, 145–152.

Nestel, P. J., Schreibman, P. H. & Ahrens, E. H. (1973) Cholesterol metabolism in human obesity. *Journal of Clinical Investigation*, **52**, 2398–2397.

Newman, A., Katsaris, J., Blendis, L. M., Charlesworth, M. & Walter, L. H. (1973) Small-intestinal injury in women who have had pelvic radiotherapy. *Lancet*, **2**, 1471–1473.

Norman, A. & Strandvik, B. (1973) Excretion of bile acids in extrahepatic biliary atresia and intrahepatic cholestasis of infancy. *Acta pediatrica scandinavica*, **62**, 253–263.

Northfield, T. C. (1973) Intraluminal precipitation of bile acids in stagnant loop syndrome. *British Medical Journal*, **2**, 743–745.

Northfield, T. C., Drasar, B. S. & Wright, J. T. (1973) Value of small intestinal bile acid analysis in the diagnosis of the stagnant loop syndrome. *Gut*, **14**, 341–347.

Northfield, T. C. & Hofmann, A. F. (1973) Biliary lipid secretion in gallstone patients. *Lancet*, **1**, 747.

Northfield, T. C. & Hofmann, A. F. (1975) Biliary lipid output during three meals and an overnight fast. I. Relationship to bile acid pool size and cholesterol saturation of bile in gallstone and control subjects. *Gut*, **16**, 1–11.

Ostrow, J. D. (1971) Absorption of organic compounds by the injured gallbladder. *Journal of Laboratory and Clinical Medicine*, **78**, 255–264.

Palmer, R. H. (1967) The formation of bile acid sulfates: a new pathway of bile acid metabolism in humans. *Proceedings of the National Academy of Sciences, Washington*, **58**, 1047–1050.

Palmer, R. H., Glickman, P. B. & Kappas, A. (1962) Pyrogenic and inflammatory properties of certain bile acids in man. *Journal of Clinical Investigation*, **41**, 1573–1577.

Panveliwalla, D., Lewis, B., Wootton, I. D. P. & Tabaqchali, S. (1970) Determination of individual bile acids in biological fluids by thin-layer chromatography and fluorimetry. *Journal of Clinical Pathology*, **23**, 309–314.

Parkin, D. M., O'Moore, R. R., Cussons, D. J., Warwick, R. R. G., Rooney, P., Percy-Robb, I. W. & Shearman, D. J. C. (1972) Evaluation of the 'breath test' in the detection of bacterial colonisation of the upper gastrointestinal tract. *Lancet*, **2**, 777–780.

Paulley, J. W. (1969) The jejunal mucosa in malabsorptive states with high bacterial counts. In *Malabsorption*, ed. Girdwood, R. H. & Smith, A. N. (Pfizer Monograph), pp. 171–176. University of Edinburgh Press.

Pedersen, L., Arnfred, T., Hess Thaysen, E. (1973) Rapid screening of increased bile acid deconjugation and bile acid malabsorption by means of the glycine-1-(^{14}C) cholylglycine assay. *Scandinavian Journal of Gastroenterology*, **8**, 665–672.

Phillips, S. F. & Giller, J. (1973) The contribution of the colon to electrolyte and water conservation in man. *Journal of Laboratory and Clinical Medicine*, **81**, 733–746.

Pomare, E. W. & Heaton, K. W. (1973a) The effect of cholecystectomy on bile salt metabolism. *Gut*, **14**, 753–762.

Pomare, E. W. & Heaton, K. W. (1973b) Bile salt metabolism in patients with gallstones in functioning gallbladders. *Gut*, **14**, 885–890.

Pomare, E. W. & Heaton, K. W. (1973c) Alteration of bile salt metabolism by dietary fibre (bran) *British Medical Journal*, **4**, 262–264.

Pomare, E. W., Heaton, K. W., Low-Beer, T. S. & White, C. (1974) Effect of wheat bran on bile salt metabolism and bile composition. *Gut*, **15**, 824–825 (Abstract).

Pomare, E. W. & Low-Beer, T. S. (1975) The selective inhibition of chenodeoxycholate synthesis by cholate metabolites in man. *Clinical Science and Molecular Medicine*, **48**, 315–321.

Portman, O. W. & Murphy, P. (1958) Excretion of bile acids and β-hydroxysterols by rats. *Archives of Biochemistry and Biophysics*, **76**, 367–376.

Redinger, R. N. & Small, D. M. (1972) Bile composition, bile salt metabolism and gallstones. *Archives of Internal Medicine*, **130**, 618–630.

Russell, R. I., Allan, J. G., Gerskowitch, V. P. & Cochran, K. M. (1973) The effect of conjugated and unconjugated bile acids on water and electrolyte absorption in the human jejunum. *Clinical Science and Molecular Medicine*, **45**, 301–311.

Salen, G., Nicolau, G., Shefer, S. & Mosbach, E. H. (1975) Hepatic cholesterol metabolism in patients with gallstones. *Gastroenterology*, **69**, 675–684.

Schaffner, F. & Popper, H. (1969) Cholestasis is the result of hypoactive hypertrophic smooth endoplasmic reticulum in the hepatocyte. *Lancet*, **2**, 355–359.

Schoenfield, L. J. (1969) The relationship of bile acids to pruritus in hepatobiliary disease. In *Bile Salt Metabolism*, ed. Schiff, L., Carey, J. B. & Dietschy, J. M., pp. 257–265. Springfield: Thomas.

Sherr, H. P., Nair, P. P., White, J. J., Banwell, J. G. & Lockwood, D. H. (1974) Bile acid metabolism and hepatic disease following small bowel bypass for obesity. *American Journal of Clinical Nutrition*, **27**, 1369–1379.

Shimoda, S. S., O'Brien, T. K. & Saunders, D. R. (1974) Fat absorption after infusing bile salts into the human small intestine. *Gastroenterology*, **67**, 7–18.

Siegel, J. H., Barnes, S., Morris, J. S. & Brooke, B. N. (1975) Bile acid metabolism in chronic bowel disease: determinations in gallbladder bile, portal blood, and peripheral blood. *Gut*, **16**, 393–394 (Abstract).

Simmonds, W. J., Korman, M. G., Go, V. L. W. & Hofmann, A. F. (1973) Radioimmunoassay of conjugated cholyl bile acids in serum. *Gastroenterology*, **65**, 705–711.

Stiehl, A. (1974) Bile salt sulphates in cholestasis. *European Journal of Clinical Investigation*, **4**, 59–63.

Stiehl, A., Earnest, D. L. & Admirand, W. H. (1975) Sulfation and renal excretion of bile salts in patients with cirrhosis of the liver. *Gastroenterology*, **68**, 534–544.

Stiehl, A., Thaler, M. M. & Admirand, W. H. (1972) The effects of phenobarbital on bile salts and bilirubin in patients with intrahepatic and extrahepatic cholestasis. *New England Journal of Medicine*, **286**, 858–861.

Sutor, D. J. & Wooley, S. E. (1971) A statistical survey of the composition of gallstones in eight countries. *Gut*, **12**, 55–64.

Tabaqchali, S. (1970) The pathophysiological role of small intestinal bacterial flora. *Scandinavian Journal of Gastroenterology*, Suppl. **6**, 139–163.

Tabaqchali, S., Hatzioannou, J. & Booth, C. C. (1968) Bile-salt deconjugation and steatorrhoea in patients with the stagnant loop syndrome. *Lancet*, **2**, 12–16.

Teem, M. V. & Phillips, S. F. (1972) Perfusion of the hamster jejunum with conjugated and unconjugated bile acids: inhibition of water absorption and effects on morphology. *Gastroenterology*, **62**, 261–267.

Toskes, P. P., Giannella, R. A., Jervis, H. R., Rout, W. R. & Takeuchi, A. (1975) Small intestinal mucosal injury in the experimental blind loop syndrome. Light- and electron-microscopic and histochemical studies. *Gastroenterology*, **68**, 1193–1203.

Trotman, B. W., Petrella, E. T., Soloway, R. D., Sanchez, H. M., Morris, T. A. & Miller, W. T. (1975) Evaluation of radiographic lucency or opaqueness of gallstones as a means of identifying cholesterol or pigment stones. *Gastroenterology*, **68**, 1563–1566.

Turnberg, L. A. & Grahame, G. (1970) Bile salt secretion in cirrhosis of the liver. *Gut*, **11**, 126–133.

van Berge Henegouwen, G. P., Brandt, K.-H., Eyssen, H. & Parmentier, G. (1975) Variations in serum and urinary bile acid patterns in patients with cholestasis. *Gastroenterology*, **68**, 1005 (Abstract).

van Deest, B. W., Fordtran, J. S., Morawski, S. G. & Wilson, J. D. (1968) Bile salt and micellar fat concentration in proximal small bowel contents of ileectomy patients. *Journal of Clinical Investigation*, **47**, 1314–1324.

Vlahcevic, Z. R., Bell, C. C., Buhac, I., Farrar, J. T. & Swell, L. (1970) Diminished bile acid pool size in patients with gallstones. *Gastroenterology*, **59**, 165–173.

Vlahcevic, Z. R., Bell, C. C., Gregory, D. H., Buker, G., Juttijudata, P. & Swell, L. (1972a) Relationship of bile acid pool size to the formation of lithogenic bile in female Indians of the Southwest. *Gastroenterology*, **62**, 73–83.

Vlahcevic, Z. R., Buhac, I., Farrar, J. T., Bell, C. C. & Swell, L. (1971) Bile acid metabolism in patients with cirrhosis. I. Kinetic aspects of cholic acid metabolism. *Gastroenterology*, **60**, 491–498.

Vlahcevic, Z. R., Juttijudata, P., Bell, C. C. & Swell, L. (1972b) Bile acid metabolism in patients with cirrhosis. II. Cholic and chenodeoxycholic acid metabolism. *Gastroenterology*, **62**, 1174–1181.

von Bergmann, K., Mok, H. Y. I. & Grundy, S. M. (1975) Regulation of bile acid pool size in man. *Gastroenterology*, **69**, 877 (Abstract).
Wagner, C. I., Soloway, R. D., Trotman, B. W. & Schoenfield, L. J. (1973) Effects of bile flow and lipid output on composition and cholesterol saturation of bile. *Gastroenterology*, **65**, 575 (Abstract).
Watkins, J. B., Tercyak, A. M., Szczepanik, P. & Klein, P. D. (1975) Bile salt kinetics in cystic fibrosis: influence of pancreatic enzyme replacement. *Gastroenterology*, **68**, 1087 (Abstract).
Weber, A. M., Roy, C. C., Lepage, G., Chartrand, L. & Lasalle, R. (1975) Interruption of the enterohepatic circulation of bile acids in cystic fibrosis. *Gastroenterology*, **68**, 1066 (Abstract).
Weber, A. M., Roy, C. C., Morin, C. L. & Lasalle, R. (1973) Malabsorption of bile acids in children with cystic fibrosis. *New England Journal of Medicine*, **289**, 1001–1005.
Williams, C. N. & Senior, J. R. (1971) ^{3}H-cholic acid and ^{14}C-chenodeoxycholic acid kinetic studies in Laennec's cirrhosis: correlation with steatorrhea and pancreatic function. *Gastroenterology*, **60**, 737 (Abstract).
Wingate, D. L., Phillips, S. F. & Hofmann, A. F. (1973) Effect of glycine-conjugated bile acids with and without lecithin on water and glucose absorption in perfused human jejunum. *Journal of Clinical Investigation*, **52**, 1230–1236.
Yoshida, T., McCormick, W. C., Swell, L. & Vlahcevic, Z. R. (1975) Bile acid metabolism in cirrhosis. IV. Characterisation of the abnormality in deoxycholate metabolism. *Gastroenterology*, **68**, 335–341.

10
SHUNTS FOR HEPATIC DISEASE
Ronald A. Malt

Logic in defining the role of portasystemic venous shunts for treatment of hepatic disease remains almost as elusive as it was a decade ago, when only four well-controlled reports were identified among 38 studied (Grace, Muench and Chalmers, 1966). Proper investigations are difficult; even those meant to be well controlled are confounded by clinical exigencies.

As a consequence of the best studies of portasystemic shunts, and of the areas of agreement among others, I conclude:

1. Successful portasystemic venous shunts reduce the likelihood of bleeding from oesophageal varices.
2. Protection from bleeding varices is virtually guaranteed after a portacaval shunt; it is less sure after other shunts.
3. Portasystemic shunts are valuable treatment for some patients who have bled from oesophageal varices—which ones remain to be defined.
4. Prophylactic portacaval shunts should not be done for patients whose varices have not bled. Under these circumstances a shunt exchanges encephalopathy for haemorrhage, without prolonging life.
5. Hypersplenism in portal hypertension is most reliably relieved by a splenectomy and shunt.
6. Shunts as treatment for bleeding varices in children should be deferred as long as possible.
7. Side-to-side portacaval shunts usually relieve intractable ascites, and end-to-side shunts are almost as effective.
8. Certain glycogen-storage diseases and homozygous familial hypercholesterolaemia are ameliorated by portacaval shunts.
9. The risk of death from hepatic coma, the depth of coma, and the frequency of coma are increased after shunts for portal hypertension caused by alcoholic cirrhosis.
10. After shunting operations for the treatment of variceal bleeding resulting from parenchymal disease of the liver, the competence of the hepatocytes is the chief determinant of encephalopathy and survival.
11. In patients with normal hepatocytes and with varices from a *preparen-*chymal block, encephalopathy will almost certainly develop after a portacaval shunt, but is less likely after a splenorenal shunt.

12. Few measurements of the rate and direction of portal blood flow are valid. Those that may be correct have no proved value in predicting the optimal shunt or the chance of encephalopathy.

PHYSIOLOGY AND NATURAL HISTORY

Before an attempt is made to justify these views, some unresolved anatomical, physiological, and epidemiological aspects of the surgical treatment of portal hypertension will be considered. Unresolved problems in deciding whether or not oesophageal varices are the source of gastrointestinal bleeding will not be discussed except in passing.

Compartmentation

Since the portal system consists of myriad elastic vessels, laws describing hydrodynamic events in rigid tubes cannot be applied to blood flow in this complex vascular network. Draining one portal vessel should not necessarily drain others, and functionally separate sectors could exist.

Clinical observations suggest that the splanchnic circulation in human beings is compartmented. Thrombosis of the splenic vein from pancreatitis may cause portal hypertension limited to the left upper quadrant of the abdomen and curable by splenectomy (Longstreth, Newcomer and Green, 1971; Yale and Crummy, 1971; Léger et al, 1974). Varices may be localised to a single segment of small bowel or colon (Rosen, Silen and Simon, 1967; Gray and Grollman, 1974; Hamlyn et al, 1974). A loop of bowel adherent to an anterior abdominal scar in a patient with mild portal hypertension may develop sharply localised bleeding varices eliminated by a resection of that loop (Moncure et al, 1976). Huge spontaneous collateral veins are sometimes present between the splenic vein and the renal vein in patients who bleed from varices. Moreover, decompression of oesophageal varices with a coronary-caval shunt can be accomplished with no effect on portal vein pressure (Inokuchi et al, 1975).

Although splanchnic compartmentation has been best documented in dogs, reservations must be held about the generality of this phenomenon since the canine intrahepatic venous sphincters have no counterparts in man and since vascular reactivity in the canine gut may be species specific. The proximal canine portal circulation has compartments that do not overflow into one another until a pressure of $70\,cmH_2O$ is reached (Waddell et al, 1972). Selective caval diversion of the coronary (left gastric) vein (Waddell et al, 1973) or of the splenic vein after ligation of the gastric vein (Teixeira et al, 1968) seems to be the most rational method of draining the oesophageal veins in this animal.

Haemodynamic Measurements

Assertions to the contrary notwithstanding, measurements of portal venous flow, portal venous pressure, and total hepatic flow do not correlate with morbidity or mortality from any shunt (LeBrec, Sicot and Benhamou, 1973; Bismuth, Franco and Hepp, 1974; Burchell et al, 1974; Charters et al, 1974; Reynolds, 1974a, b; Smith, 1974). Selection of a shunting procedure cannot be based on these haemodynamic determinations, nor upon the pressure obtained on each side of an occluding clamp placed on a portal vein during an operation. Directions and rates of flow estimated by roentgenologic techniques are no better aides in selection since these variables change depending on the rate and manner of injection, on the phase of respiration, and on the extent to which the patient deviates from haemodynamic equilibrium (Gitlin et al, 1970). Blood flow in the portal vein is often sluggish, and the flow through a completed shunt bears no relation to the cross-sectional area of the shunt (Bradley, 1963; Moreno et al, 1967).

Fortunately, the wedged hepatic vein pressure correlates well with direct transhepatic measurements of portal pressure and can be used to evaluate the degree of portal hypertension in patients with cirrhosis, whether awake or anaesthetised (Horisawa et al, 1975; Viallet et al, 1975). Cirrhotic patients with pressures in the portal system less than 10 to 12 mmHg above pressures in the inferior vena cava are unlikely to manifest gastrointestinal bleeding from varices (Reynolds, 1974a; Viallet et al, 1975).

Encephalopathy

The frequency of encephalopathy cannot be assessed accurately from retrospective reviews, from cooperative studies, or from surveys in which the investigators know how each patient was treated. The reported incidences of encephalopathy from 5 to 67 per cent after various operations strain credulity. Aside from unconscious bias, obvious sources of error are failure to apply statistical comparisons, to compare patients of equivalent physical condition, and to use defined criteria for recognising and recording encephalopathy. The depth of coma is the touchstone for some studies and the frequency of coma for others; sometimes encephalopathy as a component of terminal hepatic failure is talleyed, but sometimes not.

An exacting, prospective and randomised, but 'unblinded', study showed that an 18 per cent incidence of encephalopathy in patients with alcoholic cirrhosis increased to 38 per cent in a little over four years even without a shunt (Mutchnick, Lerner and Conn, 1974). For patients with portacaval shunts the incidence during the same period increased from 20 to 53 per cent. But despite the apparent difference between 38 and 53 per cent, the rates were statistically the same. The presence of encephalopathy before shunting was followed by encephalopathy afterward in only half the patients. However, after shunting the frequency of acute encephalopathy was more than twice as common as in patients not shunted (0.5 episodes per year vs. 0.2 per year, $P<0.001$), and severe encephalopathy was much more common (20 per cent vs. 3 per cent, $P<0.01$). When encephalopathy occurred, it was precipitated by haemorrhage in the unshunted patients and by large quantities of oral protein in those who were shunted.

Table 10.1 Diseases that may require porta-systemic shunting

I. Preparenchymal
   A. Thrombosis
      1. Congenital
      2. Acquired
         (a) Pyogenic
         (b) Haematologic disease
         (c) Extrinsic malignant disease
         (d) Pancreatitis and pseudocyst
   B. Neoplasia

II. Parenchymal
   A. Congenital fibrosis of liver
   B. Congenital atresia of bile ducts
   C. Cystic disease of liver
   D. Granulomatous disease
      1. Sarcoid
      2. Reticuloendothelioses
      3. Miscellaneous
   E. Schistosomiasis
   F. Cirrhosis
      1. Alcoholic
      2. Post-necrotic
      3. Biliary
   G. Secondary thrombosis
   H. Metabolic disorder
      1. Glycogen storage
      2. Familial hypercholesterolaemia

III. Postparenchymal
   A. Hepatic vein obstruction
      1. Thrombosis
      2. Vascular diaphragms
   B. Veno-occlusive disease

Controlled Studies

The complexities of portal hypertension confound the best-intentioned clinical trials. For studies on the therapeutic value of shunts, uniform and unequivocal diagnoses of bleeding varices are required, but have never been achieved. Prospective stratification of patients to be operated upon and control patients in a single hospital has not been feasible because the number of patients available is too small. Cooperative multicentre trials are beset by problems ranging from the differing selectivity of investigators to the criteria applied for interpreting findings. Violations of protocol because of the practicalities of clinical care bias results in ways hard to compensate.

DISEASES AND SHUNTS

Table 10.1 is a classification of the forms of hepatoportal disease that may be relieved by shunting; it is a modification for surgical purposes of schema popularised by Sherlock (1975) and others. It recognises that some preparenchymal and postparenchymal diseases may have portal hypertension associated with them relieved by natural or surgical shunts, but that the parenchymal diseases always add metabolic complexity. The variety of shunts in Table 10.2 exemplify efforts to design an operation that will be metabolically more tolerable than the others. The discussion to follow centres on the diseases (Table 10.1) for which these shunts are used.

Preparenchymal Blocks

These are mechanical obstructions of the portal vein, comprising most of the entities often called extrahepatic blocks in other classifications.

'Congenital' thrombosis

Children afflicted with thrombosed portal system may bleed from oesophageal varices massively and repeatedly, but they require operations to control bleeding less frequently than they are performed. Abundant cardiovascular reserve generally allows children and adolescents to tolerate variceal haemorrhage, and the frequency of bleeding decreases with age, stopping altogether in 20 per cent of patients. Though they tend to support these statements, data showing that only 2 of 69 patients in one hospital and 7 of 129 in another died from bleeding should be accepted with the understanding that the statistics may be weighted by inclusion of patients who had shunts to control variceal bleeding (Fonkalsrud, Myers and Robinson, 1974; Voorhees and Price, 1974).

Since the prognosis is on the whole good, operations should be delayed to late adolescence whenever possible. Shunts done by most surgeons have a greater chance of success when the blood vessels are larger, and, otherwise, extensive obliterative thrombophlebitis may require makeshift operations or splenectomy alone, with poor results. Delay also avoids the high risk of encephalopathy for the growing child, although it poses the threat of hepatitis B infection from repeated blood transfusions.

When shunting must be undertaken, a splenorenal anastomosis is the first choice (Fig. 10.1), provided the splenic vein is present and is 1 cm in diameter (~ 1.2 cm on angiograms taken with ordinary magnification). Although veins 5 mm in diameter can be used successfully (Gross, 1953; Linton, 1973) they are not for the neophyte. To obtain a length of splenic vein with maximal

Table 10.2 Types of shunts

I. Portal vein
   A. Portacaval
      1. End-to-side
      2. Side-to-side
      3. Double barrel
      4. Transposition
      5. H-graft
      6. Arterialised
   B. Portarenal

II. Mesenteric veins
   A. Mesocaval
      1. End-to-side
      2. Side-to-side
      3. H-graft
   B. Mesorenal

III. Splenic vein
   A. Splenorenal
      1. With splenectomy
         (a) Distal
         (b) Central
      2. Spleen preserved
         (a) End-to-side
         (b) Side-to-side
   B. Splenocaval

IV. Coronary (left gastric) vein
   A. Coronary–caval
   B. Coronary–renal

V. Thoracic vessels
   A. Omentopexy
      1. Intrathoracic
      2. Prethoracic
   B. Hepatophrenic poudrage
   C. Splenopexy
   D. Splanchnic vein
      1. Pulmonary vein
      2. Right atrium

VI. External via umbilical vein
   A. Jugular
   B. Saphenous
   C. Caval
   D. Cannula

diameter, after splenectomy the distal part of the vein should be followed centrally, close to its confluence with the inferior mesenteric vein (Clatworthy and DeLorimer, 1964). As an alternative, the inferior or superior mesenteric vein can be joined direct to the vena cava (Shumacker, Nahrwold and Zook, 1970).

A side-to-end (Marion–Clatworthy) mesocaval shunt (Fig. 10.2) is the first choice of some surgeons and is the option for almost everyone if the spleen has been removed, if the splenic vein is too small, or if the splenomesenteric trunk is obliterated. Unlike adults (Jochimson and Castaneda, 1968; Gliedman, 1971), children can tolerate complete interruption of the vena cava at its origin without massive oedema of the lower extremities (Zuidema and Ebert, 1967; Auvert, Farge and Weisgerber, 1973; Inberg, Harjola and Scheinin, 1974; Lambert, Tank and Turcotte, 1974).

Makeshift impromptu shunts from the splanchnic system to a peripheral vein permanently control only 30 per cent of children who bleed uncontrollably, but who lack a patent major splanchnic vein (Voorhees and Price, 1974).

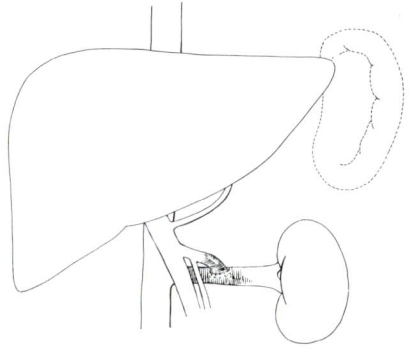

Figure 10.1 Splenorenal shunt, with splenectomy

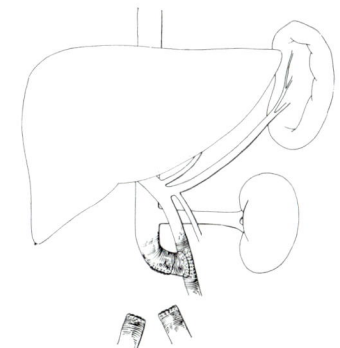

Figure 10.2 Mesocaval shunt in children

It is debatable whether these children are treated best by shunting, by complete severance of all veins between the portal vein and the oesophagus (portal-azygos disconnection) (Sugiura and Futagawa, 1973), or by gastrectomy (Rothwell-Jackson and Hunt, 1970).

Acquired thrombosis and neoplasia

The most readily cured type of portal hypertension is that produced by isolated thrombophlebitis of the splenic vein after pancreatitis. Unchecked, peripancreatic inflammation can obliterate all the major splanchnic vessels, but if thrombosis is limited to the splenic vein (which courses along the upper border of the pancreas), portal hypertension will be confined to the spleen, the short gastric veins, and the submucosal oesophageal venous plexus. Splenectomy solves the problem (Longstreth et al, 1971; Yale and Crummy, 1971; Léger et al, 1974).

Few patients with obstruction of the portal vein from neoplastic invasion compression should be considered for a shunting operation. Rarely will they live long enough to justify the attempt, and their risk of encephalopathy is great. The outlook is better when portal hypertension is a consequence of pyelophlebitis or hypercoagulation (Hamilton and Hunt, 1970; Turcotte and Child, 1972).

Parenchymal Blocks

Some congenital diseases, the granulomatous diseases, and schistosomiasis appear to obstruct inflow of the portal vein or to divert hepatic arterial blood into the portal vein by reason of their location at the entrance to the sinusoids. As they produce haemodynamic obstruction without hepatocellular dysfunction, these diseases are haemodynamically indistinguishable from those causing preparenchymal blocks. Although hepatocellular function is normal, total diversion of portal blood produces an unacceptable incidence of encephalopathy for reasons not satisfactorily explained. More commonly, cirrhosis produces the parenchymal block, with associated hepatocellular dysfunction. Spontaneous encephalopathy is not rare, but its incidence rises after shunting operations.

Congenital fibrosis, congenital atresia and cysts

Congenital hepatic fibrosis, perhaps itself a form of cystic disease, constricts the portal structures in scar tissue while sparing the hepatocytes; the mechanism by which polycystic disease occasionally produces portal hypertension is probably similar. To the contrary, biliary cirrhosis from longstanding biliary atresia damages hepatocytes, leading first to cirrhosis and then to portal hypertension.

Because of their physiological similarity to the preparenchymal block of congenital portal thrombosis, blocks from congenital fibrosis and cysts should probably be treated in the same way: by waiting as long as possible before shunting. The danger is that both children and adults with fibrosis and cysts can die from bleeding varices (Bradford et al, 1968; DelGuerico et al, 1973), and the line between operating too soon and operating too late is ill defined. No sure guides to making a decision exist.

Before portal-enterostomy became feasible for some infants with congenital biliary atresia (Kasai, 1974), any form of portal decompression could have been called meddlesome interference with an inexorable disease. If portal-enterostomy is proved to prolong life, a more aggressive attitude may be justified.

Granulomatous disease and schistosomiasis

Schistosomal liver disease is overwhelmingly the most common granulomatous disease producing portal hypertension. Despite vast numbers of patients, the reports of surgical treatment tend to be anecdotal, making assessment of benefits insecure. Definitive studies in this disease are especially difficult because of the risk of reinfection and the additional handicap imposed on patients by cardiorespiratory schistosomiasis. Since the reported risk of encephalopathy after shunting varies widely around the world, it is possible also that the ravages of the disease are different in different populations.

Mild degrees of hypersplenism and portal hypertension are reversible with effective antihelminthic therapy. Although prophylactic portasystemic shunts have been recommended for persistent portal hypertension if hepatic function is good (Kamel and Shaker, 1969), their efficacy in prolonging life has not been demonstrated. If shunts are to be done for patients who have bled from their varices the portacaval shunt should usually not be considered in the absence of alternatives, since at least two-thirds of patients with all grades of hepatic function having portacaval shunts will develop encephalopathy (Goffi et al, 1968). Provided that the good results in one study were not from inadvertent preselection of patients, the splenorenal shunt would seem preferable, since encephalopathy is rarely recognised after it was performed (Nel, Honiball and van Wyk, 1974). If a splenorenal shunt is not technically feasible, it may be possible to use a Dacron vascular prosthesis to connect the splenic vein to the vena cava as a selective drainage channel for variceal blood after the other perigastric veins are ligated (Raia and Teixeira da Silva, 1975).

Judged from published data, portal-azygos disconnection seems to offer as good palliation as the shunting operations. From 605 patients with portal-azygos disconnection, a group of uncertain size had disappearance of varices in 48 per cent, decrease in size of varices in another 44 per cent and a 41 per cent mean fall in wedged hepatic vein pressure (Hassab, 1970). For the uncommon patient with schistosomal ascites refractory to pharmacological therapy, fostering portasystemic communication by transposing the omentum into the subcutaneous tissue of the abdomen and thorax may be useful (El-Zawahry et al, 1971).

Cirrhosis

Imperfect as they are, the few prospective studies of the efficacy of shunts in controlling oesophageal varices are the measures of objectivity in a confused field. Imperfect as future studies may be, only those that attempt to follow standard statistical principles merit attention when a new form of therapy is championed.

PROPHYLACTIC END-TO-SIDE PORTACAVAL SHUNT

Four prospective studies testify there is no place for an end-to-side portacaval shunt in the management of the patient with alcoholic cirrhosis whose varices have not bled. Although shunts make varices disappear and nearly eliminate the risk of bleeding, life is not prolonged. Death from hepatic coma merely replaces death from bleeding.

The similarity in results among 12 Veterans Administration hospitals (Jackson et al, 1968), a group of Boston hospitals (Resnick et al, 1969), and the Yale–New Haven Medical Center (Conn and Lindenmuth, 1965; Conn et al, 1972) is remarkable considering the complexities of postalcoholic and postnecrotic cirrhosis. Matching patients for alternative treatments was impossible, random selection for operation itself a criterion introduced bias, since some patients selected for operation refused it, and the prevalence of fatal encephalopathy increased markedly after randomisation to either treatment group. In addition, the diagnosis of varices was not uniform; radiographical criteria alone were used in the Boston study, but endoscopical examination and radiographical criteria were used at New Haven.

THERAPEUTIC END-TO-SIDE PORTACAVAL SHUNT

Some patients with varices that have bled undoubtedly lead longer, happier, and more productive lives after portal decompression. Which ones? For a brief period, preliminary results from two controlled studies indicated greater survival rate after end-to-side portacaval shunting, leaving only the limits of statistical significance to be argued.

The final report from 13 Veterans Administration hospitals (Jackson et al, 1971) showed a 64 per cent death rate in the untreated patients vs. 34 per cent in those treated with a shunt ($P < 0.01$). But later, when the impressive survival rate among patients selected for a shunt but refusing it was considered, the significance of the difference in death rates vanished.

The final report from the Boston Interhospital Liver Group (Resnick et al, 1974) concluded that the ~60 per cent survival rate of shunted patients (life-table method) was not significantly different from the ~38 per cent survival rate of control patients because the P value was just over 0.05, although the trend was towards greater survival. Since this study was confounded by the same kinds of epidemiological problems that afflicted the prophylactic shunt studies and was concluded earlier than desired, accepting only P values below 0.05 as 'significant' may be overly severe; the practical clinical lesson seems clear. On the other hand, the conclusion from this study that the quality of life is worsened by a shunt is a clinical inference with which many will agree.

The first data from a controlled trial of end-to-side portacaval shunts for patients in Child's class A seemed another argument in favour of shunting, for they showed 60 per cent five-year survival rate, calculated by the life-table method, compared with a 10 per cent survival rate for control patients, giving a 90 to 95 per cent chance that the two groups were different (Mikkelsen, 1974). Now it seems best to suspend conclusions until the end results are known—especially since a controlled trial from France (Benhamou, unpublished) is said to have shown no difference (Conn, 1974).

Assessment of complications

As much as anything else, controlled studies have illuminated the difficulty of comparing complications of an operation with those of untreated disease (see page 234).

The prospective study of encephalopathy after portacaval shunting (Mutchnick et al, 1974) is the standard for comparison. Other surveys of the frequency of encephalopathy are more heavily influenced by preselection of the populations, causing some surgeons to report a lower prevalence of encephalopathy after a splenorenal shunt than after a portacaval anastomosis (Linton, 1974) and others to report the reverse (Riddell et al, 1972). When patients have equivalent hepatic disease, the prevalence may be the same (Malt, Szczerban and Malt, 1976). One study reported 35 per cent frequency of chronic encephalopathy in patients who were not operated upon for bleeding varices, compared with only 16 per cent in those who had an end-to-side portacaval shunt, but the difference was not significantly different (Resnick et al, 1974). If children are followed long enough after any shunt for preparenchymal portal hypertension, the prevalence of encephalopathy is 100 per cent in some hospitals (Fonkalsrud et al, 1974); in others it seems not to be a major problem (Folkman et al, 1972).

Although the clinical commonplace is that the frequency of encephalopathy increases with the age of patients who have a shunt (McDermott et al, 1968; Panke, Rousselot and Burchell, 1968; Kardel et al, 1970; Sherlock, Hourigan and George, 1970), presentation of data by the life-table method shows no difference (Maillard, Clot and Coste, 1974c).

Predictors of death after any operation on a cirrhotic patient are likely to depend more upon the patient than upon the operation performed. Many authorities would argue for the functional integrity of hepatocytes as the key factor (Hermann, Rodriguez and McCormack, 1966; Turcotte, Wallin and Child, 1969; Foster et al, 1971; Nackache et al, 1971; Léger, Delaitre and Nicodème, 1973; Campbell, Parker and Anagnostopoulos, 1973; Kanel et al, 1974; Lecompte et al, 1974; Ottinger and Moncure, 1974; Wirthlin et al, 1974; Windle and Peacock, 1975). However, in other retrospective studes the long-term death rate has been correlated with the presence of a small or large liver, muscle wasting, and alcoholism, not with most of the indices of hepatic function or with the age of the patients (Maillard et al, 1974c; Orloff et al, 1975). The histological appearance of the liver and the tests of hepatic function correlated with survival only in the first year (Maillard et al, 1974c). After that, compared with normal population of the same age, there was no difference in survival of any age group.

At the Massachusetts General Hospital a six-point scale based on bilirubin concentrations, presence of ascites, and the urgency of shunting defined a sharp boundary between 37 per cent risk of death at three points and 61 per cent risk at seven points (Malt et al, 1976). At Good Samaritan Hospital, Los Angeles, recognition of appreciable alcoholic hyaline necrosis in a frozen liver biopsy specimen portended a greater likelihood of death than of survival after a portacaval shunt (Mikkelsen, 1974); detection of hyaline necrosis only in the paraffin-embedded specimens was immaterial.

Causes of repeated bleeding leading to death after any shunt must be unequivocally proved before results can validly be compared. Oesophageal laceration, coagulopathies, peptic ulcer, gastritis, and, rarely, carcinoma of the oesophagus must be considered aside from variceal rupture (Testart and Tenière, 1974). Portacaval shunts do not increase the frequency of peptic ulcer (Phillips, Ramsby and Conn, 1975).

EMERGENCY END-TO-SIDE PORTACAVAL SHUNT

For dependable relief of portal hypertension, emergency shunts for bleeding varices must decompress the splanchnic system immediately draining into the portal vein; in practice, the options for gaining this goal are overwhelmingly the portacaval and H-graft mesocaval shunts (page 243). Peripheral splanchnic shunts are considerably less effective.

Although the quality of life after an emergency shunt compared with life after an elective shunt has not been scrutinised, it seems reasonable to recommend an urgent end-to-side portacaval shunt (within 16 h of the bleeding episode) for Child's class A patients who would otherwise be offered an elective portacaval shunt (Dustman et al, 1968; Hoffman, Jepson and Harris, 1969; Balasegaram and Damodaran, 1970; Baird, Tutassaura and Miyagishima, 1971b; Keighley, Ionescu and Wooler, 1973; Mikkelsen, 1974; Sandblom, 1974; Ungeheuer, 1974), although increased mortality has followed this course in some excellent hospitals (Herman et al, 1966). Whether a shunt should be offered as a desperate gesture to patients in Child's class C is a matter of private philosophy; their chance of death is high no matter what therapy is chosen.

The most extensive base for construction of a randomised study is the 12-year experience with emergency portacaval shunts at Harbor General Hospital and the University of California at San Diego (Orloff et al, 1975). From a group of 138 consecutive patients operated upon, a diagnosis of bleeding varices was confirmed in 75 of 76 of them studied by fibreoptic endoscopy. The mean time between admission and operation was 8.5 h. Compared with previous studies of balloon tamponade and of variceal ligation by the same group, the actual survival rate of 57 per cent following an emergency shunt and the predicted seven-year survival rate of 36 per cent were judged appreciable advances.

SIDE-TO-SIDE PORTACAVAL SHUNT

Except in the treatment of intractable ascites and the Budd–Chiari syndrome the direct side-to-side portacaval shunt is of limited use. In 21 patients in the Boston Interhospital Liver Group randomised protocol it failed to prolong survival (Resnick et al, 1974). Survival curves were practically superimposable with those of 23 surgically untreated patients.

Retrospective studies correlate survival rate with integrity of hepatic function after direct side-to-side shunting (Turcotte and Lambert, 1973). The survival rate of poor-risk patients after side-to-side shunts is less than that of those treated with end-to-side portacaval shunts (Turcotte et al, 1969), and the risk of encephalopathy is higher (Iwatsuki et al, 1973). Decreased survival rate might follow a higher rate of closure or of thrombosis, presumably caused by greater tension on the anastomosis. Perhaps many of the bad results follow loss of hepatic arterial blood via sinusoidal arteriovenous shunts retrograde through the side-to-side anastomosis.

Although an end-to-side anastomosis is an effective remedy for ascites (Barker and Reemtsma, 1960; Jackson et al, 1971; Resnick et al, 1974), truly intractable ascites is probably better managed with a side-to-side shunt or,

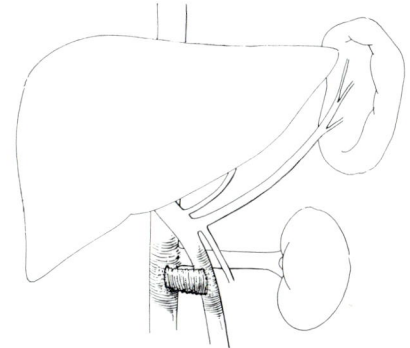

Figure 10.3 Mesocaval interposition shunt (H-graft)

possibly, a splenorenal shunt. The double-barrel portacaval shunt is a special example of the side-to-side type (McDermott, 1974). Patients too ill for venovenous shunting may be considered for a prosthetic shunt to drain ascites from the peritoneal cavity to the right atrium or the superior vena cava (LeVeen et al, 1974; Pollack, 1975).

Placing a vascular graft between the side of the portal vein and the side of the vena cava may rescue an intended end-to-side portacaval shunt otherwise impossible because of inability to approximate the vessels (Graziano and Sullivan, 1973).

MESOCAVAL SHUNT (H-GRAFT)

Enthusiastically used for certain hypothetical advantages, the only sure role for the interposition mesocaval shunt (H-graft) (Fig. 10.3) is to create decompression approximately equivalent to that of a side-to-side portacaval shunt in adults for whom a portacaval anastomosis is not feasible. H-grafts with a wide-bore arterial prosthesis, autogenous jugular vein, or arterial allograft permit mesocaval union in adults without producing incapacitating oedema of the lower extremities (Gliedman, 1971; Lord et al, 1971; Stipa et al, 1973; Rosenberg, Konigsberg and Noronha, 1974; Thompson, Read and Casali, 1975). Haemodynamic and functional advantages from the mesocaval shunt have not been incontestably proved.

Anatomical considerations arguing for a mesocaval shunt include obliteration of the portal vein with preservation of the superior mesenteric vein, extensive periportal fibrosis, a large caudate lobe overriding but not compressing the vena cava, the Budd–Chiari syndrome, extreme obesity, and pulmonary disease that might be worsened by an operation in the subhepatic region. Although some surgeons find access to the superior mesenteric vein routinely easier than to the portal vein, others do not (Malt, 1974); anatomical abnormalities probably prevent a satisfactory mesocaval shunt as least as often as a portacaval shunt (Holyoke, Davis and Harry, 1975).

Among 80 patients with mesocaval shunts with Dacron prostheses at Charity Hospital, New Orleans, there was 95 per cent rate of patency of the graft and complete prevention of variceal haemorrhage when it was open (Drapanas, LoCicero and Dowling, 1975). In patients in Child's classes B and C, the operative mortality was 9 per cent and the prevalence of encephalopathy was 11 per cent—surprisingly less encephalopathy than ordinarily described in patients with varices who do not have a shunt, for reasons that are not clear. By life-table analyses, survival rates were 100 per cent for class A patients, 85 per cent for class B, and 65 per cent for class C. Other surgeons have echoed some of these enthusiastic reports (Giles, Brennan and Losowsky, 1973; Smith et al, 1974; Huguet, Benhamida and Lévy, 1975). Although the mesocaval shunt has been said to lower mortality from emergency shunts, no difference has been seen to date at the Massachusetts General Hospital in a small prospective study of 20 emergency mesocaval and portacaval shunts in poor-risk patients (unpublished data).

PORTARENAL SHUNTS

The anatomical and haemodynamic results of these anastomoses (Fig. 10.4) are similar to those of an end-to-side or side-to-side portacaval anastomosis. If performed through the peritoneal cavity, their utility is similar to that of a mesocaval shunt. If large numbers were performed, the results would probably be the same.

What makes these anstomoses possible is the ability to divide the left renal vein in any patient between the vena cava and the gonadal vein or the adrenal vein (which then provide drainage for the kidney) or to capitalise on the rich collateral branches of the kidney in portal hypertension by ligation of the left renal vein near the hilum of the kidney (Erlik, Barzilai and Shramek, 1964; Jaffe, 1967; Simeone and Hopkins, 1967). The stump of the renal vein can be rotated forward and to the right for anastomosis to the side of an intact portal vein, to the pancreatic end of a divided portal vein, or to the side of the superior mesenteric or splenic vein (Baird, Tutassaura and Miyagishima, 1971a; Regensberg et al, 1973; Saubier et al, 1974). End-to-side anastomoses have the potential for allowing the vessels to be reconstituted.

SPLENORENAL SHUNT WITH SPLENECTOMY

Few differences appear to exist between results of portacaval and splenorenal shunts in patients of equivalent risk. The conventional splenorenal shunt was unfortunately not the object of a proper trial at its inception, and today it is difficult to concentrate a large number of patients in the hands of a few surgeons in large hospitals. Concentration is essential for valid assessment, for the splenorenal shunt is the most difficult operation thus far discussed and it cannot be safely applied except by experts (Linton, 1974). Irrespective of its merits compared with those of a portacaval shunt when each could be done with facility, the splenorenal shunt is to be preferred if dense adhesions fill the

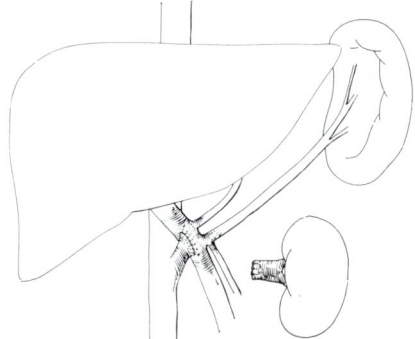

Figure 10.4 Side-to-end portarenal shunt

right upper quadrant of the abdomen. Besides the mesocaval H-graft, it is one of the obvious alternatives for relieving portal hypertension associated with obliteration of the portal vein and for relieving hypersplenism.

An extreme view holds that the splenorenal shunt and the side-to-side portacaval shunt are both of questionable value since they are either so large as to be total shunts or so small as not to provide decompression (Rueff and Maillard, 1974). Unless all patients undergo routine postoperative angiographic examination this view cannot easily be countered; in addition to the questionable ethics that would be involved, streaming and collateral flow of the contrast medium might make angiography unreliable (Castell and Conn, 1972) unless performed with special care (Nabseth et al, 1975). A closed shunt is relative protection against encephalopathy (Voorhees, Price and Britton, 1970), but it is also a predisposing cause for the greater frequency of gastrointestinal bleeding after splenorenal anastomosis than after portacaval anastomosis (Barnes et al, 1971). Attempts to improve patency by ligating the renal end of the renal vein and by forming end-to-end splenorenal anastomoses

(Simon, Brown and Ross, 1972) probably result in a situation indistinguishable from that following a portarenal shunt.

A prospective study from Hôpital Paul-Brousse, Paris, found almost no difference among the results of end-to-side portacaval shunts, small-stoma side-to-side shunts, and central splenorenal shunts (near the mesenteric axis) in 120 patients (Bismuth et al, 1974). Although non-lethal postoperative haemorrhage occurred in five patients after splenorenal shunting, there was no operative mortality and no death from recurrent bleeding in any group. Encephalopathy was present in 16 per cent of each group. Early mortality after a shunt, long-term mortality, and persistence of varices were equivalent, and haemodynamic measurements were unhelpful in predicting the chance of complications. The survival rate was actually higher in patients more than 60 years old (78 vs. 63 per cent, $P<0.05$). If a group of control patients non-operated had been included and if it were known why the numbers of patients in the three treatment groups were so different and why the mortality rates were so low, this study would settle many fruitless arguments (Benhamou, 1974).

Like the prospective survey from Paris, a retrospective survey of results from the Massachusetts General Hospital from 1959 to 1965 showed greater frequency of gastrointestinal haemorrhage after a splenorenal shunt than after a portacaval shunt (Barnes et al, 1971). There were 2.9 episodes of haemorrhage per year of follow-up after splenorenal shunting compared with 1.8 episodes per year after portacaval shunting; however, only 17 per cent of haemorrhages after a splenorenal shunt were fatal, contrasted with 38 per cent fatal after a portacaval shunt. There is probably no significant difference between the 25 per cent frequency of encephalopathy after splenorenal shunting and the 33 per cent frequency after portacaval shunting in that study. Little else can be said about the comparative merits of the two kinds of shunts because the patients with splenorenal shunts were better risks, as assessed from their serum levels of protein and albumin, their bromsulphthalein clearance, and the preoperative assessment of the anaesthetist.

But preselection can work the opposite way as well. If poor-risk patients are chosen because splenorenal shunts confer putative benefits that portacaval anastomoses do not, results will be worse. Where this policy was followed, the morality rate after splenorenal shunting was 11 per cent (compared with 1 to 2 per cent after portacaval shunting in the same hospital), and the prevalence of encephalopathy was 38 per cent (Riddell et al, 1972).

Computerised comparisons permitted inferences to be drawn in the retrospective survey of 120 patients at the Massachusetts General Hospital from 1966 to 1973. If results from emergency portacaval shunts were discounted because the physical condition of patients selected was conspicuously poor, there was no difference after splenorenal shunting and portacaval shunting in rates of operative death rates or of encephalopathy (Malt et al, 1976). To the contrary a retrospective study of patients with minimal abnormalities in hepatic function tests and patent shunts revealed a 5 per cent rate of encephalopathy after splenorenal shunts and 50 per cent after portacaval shunts (Pliam, Adson and Foulk, 1975). Less encephalopathy after any shunt than the 18 to 38 per cent rate of unshunted patients would seem remarkable.

The splenorenal shunt with splenectomy has an undeniable advantage over the portacaval shunt in definitely relieving hypersplenism. The portacaval shunt is not uniformly so effective, even though it decompresses the spleen (Mutchnick, Lerner and Conn, 1975). About 60 per cent of patients with hypersplenism and a portal pressure of less than 10 mmHg (as measured during an operation) have their hypersplenism relieved by a portacaval shunt (Felix et al, 1974).

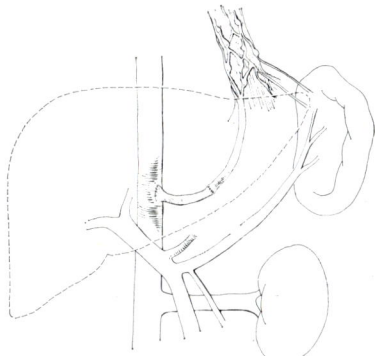

Figure 10.5 Coronary–caval shunt

CORONARY–CAVAL SHUNT

In a list of operations that should drain oesophageal varices yet interfere minimally with the portal circulation to the liver, the coronary–caval shunt (Fig. 10.5) would doubtless rank first. The coronary vein (left gastric vein) connects the oesophageal plexus with the medial wall of the portal vein, but contributes little to portal inflow. That this shunt has not been more widely exploited is testimony to the fragility of the coronary vein and to the corpulence of many patients.

With the help of a stapling device and a length of autogenous vein to bridge the gap to the vena cava, Japanese surgeons (Inokuchi et al, 1975) constructed coronary–caval anastomoses in 117 of 293 patients with portal hypertension, chiefly from postnecrotic cirrhosis. To assure preponderant drainage through the shunt, a splenectomy and ligation of all perigastric veins was performed. By these means, the coronary vein pressure was lowered from 310 to 200 cm H_2O without appreciable changes in portal vein pressure or in liver function tests. The patency rate was 90 per cent and there was scarcely any encephalopathy.

SELECTIVE SPLENORENAL SHUNT (DISTAL SPLENORENAL)

If the portal circulation is compartmented and if the coronary–caval shunt is technically not suitable for widespread use, the selective splenorenal shunt (Fig. 10.6) may represent the best compromise available in the search for an ideal operation to decompress oesophageal varices. Its intent is to drain the oesophageal plexus by the route opposite the coronary vein. The coronary vein, the gastroepiploic arcade, the umbilical vein, and any perisplenic collateral veins are ligated, with the hope of increasing venous flow through the short gastric veins. Blood is meant to flow through the short gastric veins into the intact spleen and then into the splenic vein which is decompressed by a central splenorenal shunt (Warren, Salam and Smith, 1974a; Warren et al, 1974b). In one variant of this operation designed to make it less of a technical feat, decompression is accomplished between the end of

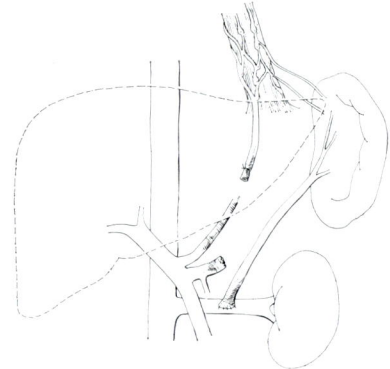

Figure 10.6 Distal (selective) splenorenal shunt

the caval side of a transected renal vein and the side of the splenic vein (Warren et al, 1972; Stoney, Mehigan and Olcott, 1975). In another, the splenorenal shunt is constructed side-to-side rather than end-to-side; the portal end of the splenic vein may be ligated (Britton, Voorhees and Price, 1970).

Apparent drawbacks to wholesale endorsement of the distal splenorenal shunt are: (1) it has not been subject to controlled trials, although one is in progress; (2) it may be suitable for only 50 per cent of the patients; (3) it cannot be used for urgent control of bleeding varices; (4) it should not be done in the presence of uncontrolled ascites; and (5) it is more difficult than the conventional splenorenal shunt, which itself is more difficult than a portacaval or mesocaval shunt.

The selective shunt has been performed in fewer than 100 patients whose results have been documented (Reichle, 1972; Silver et al, 1974; Warren et al, 1974a, b; Thomford, Sirinek and Martin, 1975). At Emory University Hospital, varices decreased in about 75 per cent of 55 patients with patent shunts, and bleeding was totally prevented at the cost of only two patients re-admitted to the hospital with encephalopathy (Warren et al, 1974b). Selective splenorenal shunts caused little change in the estimated maximal rate of urea synthesis, in contrast to decreases after non-selective or total shunts, and the maximal rate of urea synthesis may be an inverse correlate of the degree of encephalopathy (Warren et al, 1974c). At the University of Lund, however, 6 of 11 surviving patients with distal splenorenal shunts had encephalopathy (Bengmark, 1975). Ligation of the splenic artery alone to accomplish some of the goals of a distal splenorenal shunt seems an uncertain procedure (Witte et al, 1976).

In comparing distal splenorenal shunts with mesocaval shunts, a preliminary account of a randomised trial disclosed three differences in favour of the distal shunt: late mortality (5 vs. 23 per cent), encephalopathy (5 vs 32 per cent), and depression of maximal rate of urea synthesis (13 vs. 45 per cent) (Galambos et al, 1975). The absence of early postoperative mortality in either group of patients and the low prevalence of encephalopathy suggests bias in favour of good-risk patients.

ARTERIALISED PORTACAVAL SHUNT

Efforts to maintain total hepatic blood flow and sinusoidal pressure after a portacaval shunt by channelling new arterial blood into the liver have not generated widespread enthusiasm. The main arterialisation procedures studied have been an anastomosis between the gastroepiploic or splenic artery and the reopened umbilical vein (which connects with the left branch of the portal vein), a union between the splenic artery or the aorta and the hepatic side of the portal vein stump, and connection of the ileocolic artery or right common iliac artery with the portal vein stump via an autogenous saphenous vein graft (Burliu, Ratiu and Monesco, 1968; Maillard, Benhamou and Rueff, 1970; Adamsons et al, 1972; Maillard and Prandi, 1974; Maillard et al, 1974a).

Since these procedures in the hands of others than their originators would probably contribute to increased operating time and morbidity, unequivocal advantages proved in well-conducted trials are required before they warrant general application. At present, many reports are anecdotal. The methods of estimating hepatic blood flow are arguable, statistical analyses are difficult to evaluate, and too much dependence is placed on mitotic counts or DNA synthesis as indices of hepatic growth (Bucher and Malt, 1971) when they could as well be attempts to repair damage from unaccustomed perfusion pressures.

SPLANCHNO-THORACIC SHUNT

Occasionally, intra-abdominal portasystemic shunts are not feasible, and at other times they are not helpful. They are not feasible when extensive thromboses or fixation of the veins prevents even an impromptu shunt. They are not helpful when the pressure in the intra-abdominal systemic veins is so high that there is little gradient between the splanchnic and systemic circulations. Common reasons for a low gradient are compression of the inferior vena cava by cirrhotic lobulation in the caudate lobe (Welling and McDermott, 1973) and by ascites (Mullane and Gliedman, 1970), but even enlargement of the caudate lobe from Gaucher's disease can be a problem (Fellows et al, 1975). To establish a high gradient, shunts of arterial prostheses or autogenous vein must then be run between a patent branch of the portal system and a pulmonary artery or vein, the right atrium, or a major hepatic vein (Fonkalsrud, Linde and Longmire, 1966; Leger, Patel and Boury, 1966; Lataste and Albou, 1971; Vix and Payne, 1972; Luttwak et al, 1973; Maillard et al, 1974b). An alternative might be thoracic transposition of the spleen (see below).

UMBILICAL VEIN SHUNT

In general, decompression of the portal vein through its erstwhile tributary, the umbilical vein, (Piccone, Bonanno and LeVeen, 1968; White, Slapak and MacLean, 1968; McQuarrie, Nicoloff and Lunseth, 1970; Sobel et al, 1970) has more intellectual appeal than utility. These shunts decompress too little, and they are subject to occlusion as they meander through the peritoneal cavity to the vena cava or through the subcutaneous tissue to systemic veins in the neck or lower part of the abdominal wall.

SPLENOPEXY AND OMENTOPEXY

Although the neovascular channels between a displaced abdominal organ and the peripheral venous circulation can be huge, these decompressions can be useful only for elective situations since they develop slowly. During the several months necessary for appreciable shunting to develop, bleeding varices must be controlled by spontaneous cessation of bleeding or by some form of variceal occlusion.

The principle of splenopexy and omentopexy is reasonable, and it has been espoused by discriminating surgeons. It might be more widely used if a systematic long-term study proved beneficial. Until the time one does, splenopexy and omentopexy will have low priority. The omentum can be transposed to the mediastinum or fanned out between the rib cage and the skin (El-Zawahry et al, 1971; Couniard, 1973). The intact or partly resected spleen can be passed into the left pleural cavity or under the skin (Hästbacka, 1971; Benmark, Börjesson and Olin, 1973; Bengmark, 1975). Because splenopneumopexy in dogs relieves portal hypertension and hepatic damage produced by constriction of the vena cava, in human beings it may be useful in the treatment of chronic hepatic vein obstruction.

Secondary thrombosis

Thrombosis of the portal vein or its major branches in a patient with cirrhotic portal hypertension needs to be recognised chiefly because the occluded vein cannot be used for a shunt. Unlike the situation in children with primary thrombosis of the portal vein (page 238), secondary thrombosis poses little additional handicap, for the rate of blood flow in the portal vein is normally sluggish or stagnant in cirrhotic portal hypertension (Moreno et al, 1967).

Metabolic disorders

A portacaval shunt ameliorates hepatic glycogen-storage disease and the signs of homozygous type II hyperlipidaemia (familial hypercholesterolaemia) (Starzl and Putnam, 1975). Since a portacaval shunt diverts splanchnic blood of high glucose content to peripheral tissues without passing through the liver, in glycogen-storage disease the systemic effects of hypoglycaemia are reversed; by depriving the liver of splanchnic blood, glycogenolysis seems to be promoted. Of somewhat more than a dozen children treated with a portacaval shunt or portacaval transposition (caudal vena cava to cephalic portal vein, caudal portal vein to cephalic vena cava), all have benefited in some way (Starzl et al, 1965; Riddell, Davies and Clark, 1966; Hermann and Mercer, 1969; Boley, Cohen and Gliedman, 1970; Starzl et al, 1973b). Supplementary intravenous nutrition improves results and may, indeed, predict the benefit to be obtained (Folkman et al, 1972).

A portacaval shunt unquestionably reduces the synthesis of cholesterol and low-density lipoproteins, mobilising lipoprotein deposits even after conventional means of treatment have failed (Bilheimer et al, 1975; Starzl and Putnam, 1975). Its value in prolonging life is not yet established (Starzl et al, 1973a; Ahrens, 1974; Stein et al, 1975).

Postparenchymal Block

Although rapidly propagating occlusion of the hepatic veins is usually fatal, an urgent side-to-side portacaval shunt may occasionally be life-saving if the vena cava is patent. In general, operations to abort a fulminating course are unsuccessful and should probably be deferred in favour of fibrinolytic and anticoagulant therapy. Gradual occlusion from thrombosis, veno-occlusive disease, or congenital diaphragms in the vena cava or heart is compatible with a long course terminated by spontaneous improvement or death. Obstructing diaphragms are subject to direct attack (Kilman et al, 1971; Datta et al, 1972; Kimura et al, 1972; Eguchi, Takeuchi and Asano, 1974).

Chronic hepatic vein obstruction

If time, anticoagulants, and diuretic therapy fail, an operation should be considered while the liver is still capable of recovery. Provided that the vena cava is patent and that a swollen liver has not compressed the cava so much that proximal flow is impeded, a portasystemic shunt is the procedure of choice. First preference is for a side-to-side portacaval shunt because its utility in decompressing the liver; mesocaval and splenorenal shunts are alternatives

(Hoyumpa, Schiff and Helfman, 1971; Lévy and Caroli, 1974; Langer et al, 1975; Prandi, Rueff and Benhamou, 1975). If the interior vena cava cannot be used for decompression, thoracic transposition of the spleen (Schreiber and Gonzales, 1967; Strauch, 1970) or a transdiaphragmatic shunt must be considered (page 250). Anastomosis of an iliac vein stump on the vena cava to a variceal plexus at the hilum of the liver has successfully been used in one patient lacking identifiable splanchnic veins (Auvert, Vysas and Weisgerber, 1974).

CONCLUSIONS

Congenital preparenchymal (extrahepatic) portal hypertension is best treated by non-surgical means. If a shunt becomes mandatory, the choice lies between a Marion–Clatworthy mesocaval anastomosis and a splenorenal shunt. Cirrhotic patients with varices that have not bled should likewise be treated non-surgically. Although bleeding varices can be treated with an emergency portacaval or mesocaval interposition shunt, these operations should be restricted to good-risk patients, and it should be recognised that the quality of life after shunting is unknown. For elective decompression of varices that have previously bled, a coronary–caval anastomosis may be the best method. Since the universality of this operation has not been tested, selective distal splenorenal shunting may be the practical alternative, though proof is lacking. Otherwise, portacaval and conventional splenorenal shunts are satisfactory; the splenorenal shunt has no proved advantage except in unequivocally relieving hypersplenism. Splenopexies and omentopexies might be used more widely for poor-risk patients if their value were established. Portacaval shunts are effective treatment for glycogen-storage disease and may be helpful for homozygous familial hypercholesterolaemia. Shunts or splenopexies are occasionally useful for the Budd–Chiari syndrome. Patients with portal hypertension are subject to spontaneous portasystemic encephalopathy, and all shunts carry a risk of producing encephalopathy. The risk of encephalopathy for any patient undergoing any shunting operation is unknown.

ACKNOWLEDGEMENT

This manuscript benefited from the criticism of Professor Telfer B. Reynolds of Los Angeles, California.

REFERENCES

Adamsons, R. J., Kinkhabwala, M., Moskowitz, H., Himmelfarb, E., Minkowitz, S. & Lerner, B. (1972) Portacaval shunt with arterialisation of the hepatic portion of the portal vein. *Surgery, Gynecology and Obstetrics*, **135**, 529–535.

Ahrens, E. H., Jr (1974) Homozygous hypercholesteraemia and the portacaval shunt. *Lancet*, **2**, 449–451.

Auvert, J., Farge, C. & Weisgeber, G. (1973) Traitment de l'hypertension portale de l'enfant par implantation de l'axe cavo-iliaque retourné dans la veine mésentérique supérieure. Analyse de 45 dossiers. *Annales de chirurgie thoracique et cardio-vasculaire*, **12**, 165–173.

Auvert, J., Vysas, V. & Weisgerber, G. (1974) Hypertension portale par syndrome de Budd–Chiari compliqué de thrombophlébite diffusé du système porte. Guérison par implantation de l'axe cavo-iliique dans un segment de veine porte accesoire. *Nouvelle presse médicale*, **3**, 2238–2242.

Baird, R. J., Tutassaura, H. & Miyagishima, R. T. (1971a) Use of the left renal vein for portal decompression. *Annals of Surgery*, **173**, 551–553.

Baird, R. J., Tutassaura, H. & Miyagishima, R. (1971b) Emergency portal decompression. A review of 31 patients operated upon via a midline approach. *Archives of Surgery*, **103**, 73–75.

Balasegaram, M. & Damodaran, A. (1970) Emergency shunt surgery for bleeding oesophagogastric varices. *Australian and New Zealand Journal of Surgery*, **40**, 152–157.

Barker, H. G. & Reemtsma, K. (1960) The portacaval shunt operation in patients with cirrhosis and ascites. *Surgery*, **48**, 142–154.

Barnes, B. A., Ackroyd, F. W., Battit, G. E., Kantrowitz, P. A., Schapiro, R. H., Strole, W. E., Jr, Todd, D. P. & McDermott, W. V. (1971) Elective portasystemic shunts: morbidity and survival data. *Annals of Surgery*, **174**, 76–84.

Bengmark, S. (1975) Surgical management of portal hypertension. *Clinics in Gastroenterology*, **4**, 395–423.

Bengmark, S., Börjesson, B. & Olin, T. (1973) Development of portasystemic shunts after subcutaneous transposition of the spleen in the rat. *American Journal of Surgery*, **125**, 757–762.

Benhamou, J.-P. (1974) Splenorenal or portacaval shunt? *Gastroenterology*, **67**, 762–763.

Bilheimer, D. W., Goldstein, J. L., Grundy, S. M. & Brown, M. S. (1975) Reduction in cholesterol and low density lipoprotein synthesis after portacaval shunt surgery in a patient with homozygous familial hypercholesterolemia. *Journal of Clinical Investigation*, **56**, 1420–1430.

Bismuth, H., Franco, D. & Hepp, J. (1974) Portal-systemic shunt in hepatic cirrhosis: does the type of shunt decisively influence the clinical result? *Annals of Surgery*, **179**, 209–218.

Boley, S. J., Cohen, M. I. & Gliedman, M. L. (1970) Surgical therapy of glycogen storage disease. *Pediatrics*, **46**, 929–933.

Bradford, W. D., Bradford, J. W., Porter, F. S. & Sidbury, J. B. (1968) Cystic disease of liver and kidney with portal hypertension. A cause of sudden unexpected hematemesis. *Clinical Pediatrics*, **7**, 299–306.

Bradley, S. E. (1963) The hepatic circulation. In *Handbook of Physiology*, Section 2. Baltimore: Williams and Wilkins.

Britton, R. C., Voorhees, A. B., Jr & Price, J. B., Jr (1970) Selective portal decompression. *Surgery*, **67**, 104–113.

Bucher, N. L. R. & Malt, R. A. (1971) *Regeneration of Liver and Kidney*. Boston: Little, Brown.

Burchell, A. R., Moreno, A. H., Panke, W. F. & Nealon, T. F. (1974) Hemodynamic variables and prognosis following portacaval shunts. *Surgery, Gynecology and Obstetrics*, **138**, 359–369.

Burliu, D., Ratiu, O. & Monesco, G. (1968) Artérialisation portale par la veine ombilicale reperméabilisée. *Presse médicale*, **76**, 581–582.

Campbell, D. P., Parker, D. E. & Anagnostopoulos, C. E. (1973) Survival prediction in portacaval shunts: a computerised statistical analysis. *American Journal of Surgery*, **126**, 748–751.

Castell, D. O. & Conn, H. O. (1972) The determination of portacaval shunt patency: a critical review of methodology. *Medicine*, **51**, 315–336.

Charters, A. C., Chandler, J. G., Condon, J. K., Grambort, D. E., Levin, S. E., Modafferi, T. R. & Orloff, M. J. (1974) Spontaneous reversal of portal flow in patients with bleeding varices treated by emergency portacaval shunt. *American Journal of Surgery*, **127**, 25–29.

Clatworthy, H. W. & DeLorimer, A. A. (1964) Portal decompression procedures in children. *American Journal of Surgery*, **107**, 447–451.

Conn, H. O. (1974) Therapeutic portacaval anastomosis: to shunt or not to shunt. *Gastroenterology*, **67**, 1065–1073.

Conn, H. O. & Lindenmuth, W. W. (1965) Prophylactic portacaval anastomosis in cirrhotic patients with esophageal varices. *New England Journal of Medicine*, **272**, 1255–1263.

Conn, H. O., Lindenmuth, W. W., May, C. J. & Ramsby, G. R. (1972) Prophylactic portacaval anastomosis. A tale of two studies. *Medicine*, **51**, 27–40.

Couinaud, C. (1973) L'omentopexie dans les hypertensions portales. *Annales de chirurgie*, **27**, 855–858.

Datta, D. V., Saha, S., Singh, S. A. K., Gupta, B. B., Aikat, B. K., Chugh, K. S. & Chhuttani, P. N. (1972) Chronic Budd–Chiari syndrome due to obstruction of the intrahepatic portion of the inferior vena cava. *Gut*, **13**, 372–378.

DelGuerico, E., Greco, J., Kim, K. E., Chinitz, J. & Swartz, C. (1973) Esophageal varices in adult patients with polycystic kidney and liver disease. *New England Journal of Medicine*, **289**, 678–679.

Drapanas, T., LoCicero, J. & Dowling, J. B. (1975) Hemodynamics of the interposition mesocaval shunt. *Annals of Surgery*, **181**, 523–533.

Dustmann, H. O., Eckart, J., Gutzeit, H. J. & Wollmann, K. J. (1968) Infarktarige nekrosen der cirrhoseleber nach operativem portokavalem shunt. *Langenbecks archiv für chirurgie*, **323**, 124–141.

Eguchi, S., Takeuchi, Y. & Asano, K. (1974) Successful balloon membranotomy for obstruction of the hepatic portion of the inferior vena cava. *Surgery*, **76**, 837–840.

El-Zawahry, M. D., Ibrahim, M. S., Amer, Z., El-Maddawy, M. & El-Razek, A. A. (1971) Omental transposition for the relief of ascites in portal hypertension of bilharzial origin. *Bulletin de la Société Internationale de Chirurgie*, **5/6**, 499–505.

Erlik, D., Barzilai, A. & Shramek, A. (1964) Porto-renal shunt: a new technic for portosystemic anastomosis in portal hypertension. *Annals of Surgery*, **159**, 72–78.

Felix, W. R., Jr, Myerson, B. M., Sigel, B., Perrin, E. B. & Jackson, F. C. (1974) The effect of portacaval shunt on hypersplenism. *Surgery, Gynecology and Obstetrics*, **139**, 899–904.

Fellows, K. E., Grand, R. J., Colodny, A. H., Orsini, E. N. & Crocker, A. C. (1975) Combined portal and vena caval hypertension in Gaucher disease: the value of preoperative venography. *Journal of Pediatrics*, **87**, 739–743.

Folkman, J., Philippart, A., Tze, W.-J. & Crigler, J. (1972) Portacaval shunt for glycogen storage disease: value of prolonged intravenous hyperalimentation before surgery. *Surgery*, **72**, 306–314.

Fonkalsrud, E. W., Linde, L. M. & Longmire, W. P., Jr (1966) Portal hypertension from idiopathic superior vena caval obstruction. *Journal of the American Medical Association*, **196**, 115–118.

Fonkalsrud, E. W., Myers, N. A. & Robinson, M. J. (1974) Management of extrahepatic portal hypertension in children. *Annals of Surgery*, **180**, 487–493.

Foster, J. H., Ellison, L. H., Donovan, T. J. & Anderson, A. (1971) Quantity and quality of survival after portosystemic shunts. *American Journal of Surgery*, **121**, 490–501.

Galambos, J. T., Warren, W. D., Rudman, D., Millikan, W., Salam, A. & Smith, R. B. (1975) Is nonselective shunt (NSS) a justifiable operation for varices in cirrhotics when selective distal spleno-renal shunt (DSR) is possible? *Gastroenterology*, **68**, 896.

Giles, G. R., Brennan, T. G. & Losowsky, M. S. (1973) Interposition teflon mesenteric caval shunt for bleeding oesophageal varices. *British Journal of Surgery*, **60**, 649–652.

Gitlin, N., Grahame, G. R., Kreel, L., Williams, H. S. & Sherlock, S. (1970) Splenic blood flow and resistance in patients with cirrhosis before and after portacaval anastomoses. *Gastroenterology*, **59**, 208–213.

Gliedman, M. L. (1971) The mesocaval shunt for portal hypertension. *American Journal of Gastroenterology*, **56**, 323–333.

Goffi, F. S., Silva, L. C., Ferrarini, E., Juliao, A. F. & Bastos, E. S. (1968) Immediate and late effects of porto-caval and spleno-renal shunts on the hepatic function and the neurophysical behavior of patients with hepato-splenic schistosomiasis. *Revue internationale d'hepatologie*, **18**, 933–945.

Grace, N. D., Muench, H. & Chalmers, T. C. (1966) The present status of shunts for portal hypertension in cirrhosis. *Gastroenterology*, **50**, 684–691.

Gray, R. K. & Grollman, J. H., Jr (1974) Acute lower gastrointestinal bleeding secondary to varices of the superior mesenteric venous system. *Radiology*, **111**, 559–561.

Graziano, J. L. & Sullivan, H. J. (1973) Portal decompression: clinical experience with the 'H' graft. *Annals of Surgery*, **178**, 209–214.

Gross, R. E. (1953) *The Surgery of Infancy and Childhood*. Philadelphia: W. B. Saunders.

Hamilton, D. W. & Hunt, A. H. (1970) Extrahepatic portal obstruction. *Medical Journal of Australia*, **1**, 493–499.

Hamlyn, A. N., Morris, J. S., Lunzer, M. R., Puritz, H. & Dick, R. (1974) Portal hypertension with varices in unusual sites. *Lancet*, **2**, 1531–1534.

Hassab, M. A. (1970) Non-shunt operations in portal hypertension without cirrhosis. *Surgery, Gynecology and Obstetrics*, **131**, 648–654.

Hästbacka, J. (1971) Thoracic transposition of the spleen for portal hypertension. *Annales chirurgiae et gynaecologiae fenniae*, **60**, Suppl. 176, 5–51.

Hermann, R. E. & Mercer, R. D. (1969) Portacaval shunt in the treatment of glycogen storage disease: report of a case. *Surgery*, **65**, 499–503.

Hermann, R. E., Rodriguez, A. E. & McCormack, L. J. (1966) Selection of patients for portal-systemic shunts. *Journal of the American Medical Association*, **196**, 1039–1044.

Hoffman, D. C., Jepson, R. P. & Harris, J. D. (1969) Experiences with emergency porta-caval shunt. *Australian Annals of Medicine*, **18**, 238–242.

Holyoke, E. A., Davis, W. C. & Harry, R. D. (1975) Surgical anatomy of the mesocaval shunt. *Surgery*, **78**, 526–530.

Horisawa, M., Boyer, T. D., Redeker, A. G. & Reynolds, T. B. (1975) Direct measurement of portal and hepatic vein pressures using a thin transhepatic needle. *Gastroenterology*, **69**, 830.

Hoyumpa, A. M., Schiff, L. & Helfman, E. L. (1971) Budd–Chiari syndrome in women taking oral contraceptives. *American Journal of Medicine*, **50**, 137–140.

Huguet, C., Benhamida, F. & Lévy, V. G. (1975) Les anastomoses mésentéricocaves par prothèse de dacron interposée. *Nouvelle presse médicale*, **4**, 1481–1484.

Inberg, M. V., Harjola, P.-T. & Scheinin, T. M. (1974) Role of the mesentericocaval shunt in the management of portal hypertension. *American Journal of Surgery*, **127**, 529–534.

Inokuchi, K., Kobayashi, M., Ogawa, Y., Saku, M., Nagasue, N. & Iwaki, A. (1975) Results of left gastric vena caval shunt for esophageal varices: analysis of one hundred clinical cases. *Surgery*, **78**, 628–636.

Iwatsuki, A., Mikkelsen, W. P., Redeker, A. G., Reynolds, T. B. & Turrill, F. L. (1973) Clinical comparison of the end-to-side and side-to-side portacaval shunt: ten year follow-up. *Annals of Surgery*, **178**, 65–69.

Jackson, F. C., Perrin, E. B., Smith, A. G., Degradi, A. E. & Nadal, H. M. (1968) A clinical investigation of the portacaval shunt. II. Survival analysis of the prophylactic operation. *American Journal of Surgery*, **115**, 22–42.

Jackson, F. C., Perrin, E. B., Felix, W. R. & Smith, A. G. (1971) A clinical investigation of the portacaval shunt. V. Survival analysis of the therapeutic operation. *Annals of Surgery*, **174**, 672–701.

Jaffe, M. S. (1967) Fate of the left kidney after portorenal shunt. *American Journal of Surgery*, **113**, 671–675.

Jochimson, P. R. & Castaneda, A. R. (1968) Emergency mesocaval shunt performed during pregnancy, followed by arrest of variceal hemorrhage and uneventful delivery. *Surgery*, **63**, 601–603.

Kamel, R. & Shaker, A. (1969) Management of portal hypertension in hepatic schistosomiasis. *Journal of the Egyptian Medical Association*, **52**, 895–902.

Kanel, G. C., Zawacki, J. K., Callow, A. D. & Kaplan, M. M. (1974) Survival in patients with post-necrotic cirrhosis and Laennec's cirrhosis undergoing portacaval shunt. *Gastroenterology*, **76**, 801.

Kardel, T., Lund, Y., Olsen, P. Z., Möllgaard, V. & Gammeltoft, A. (1970) Encephalopathy and portacaval anastomosis. *Scandinavian Journal of Gastroenterology*, **5**, 681–685.

Kasai, M. (1974) Treatment of biliary atresia with specific reference to hepatic porto-enterostomy and its modifications. *Progress in Pediatric Surgery*, **6**, 5–52.

Keighley, M. R. B., Ionescu, M. I. & Wooler, G. H. (1973) Late results of elective and emergency portacaval anastomosis with particular reference to the type of stoma used. *American Journal of Surgery*, **126**, 601–605.

Kilman, J. W., Williams, T. E., Kakos, G. S., Molnar, W. & Ryan, J. M. (1971) Budd–Chiari syndrome due to congenital obstruction of the eustachian valve of the inferior vena cava. *Journal of Thoracic and Cardiovascular Surgery*, **62**, 226–230.

Kimura, C., Matsuda, S., Koie, H. & Hirooka, M. (1972) Membranous obstruction of the hepatic portion of the inferior vena cava: clinical study of nine cases. *Surgery*, **72**, 551–559.

Lambert, M. J., Tank, E. S. & Turcotte, J. G. (1974) Late sequelae of mesocaval shunts in children. *American Journal of Surgery*, **127**, 19–24.

Langer, B., Stone, R. M., Colapinto, R. F., Meindok, H., Phillips, M. J. & Fisher, M. M. (1975) Clinical spectrum of the Budd–Chiari syndrome and its surgical management. *American Journal of Surgery*, **129**, 137–145.

Lataste, J. & Albou, J. C. (1971) Syndrome de Budd–Chiari et thrombose cave inférieure traités par pontage spléno-mésaraic-auriculaire. *Presse médicale*, **33**, 1491–1493.

LeBrec, D., Sicot, C. & Benhamou, J.-P. (1973) Débit sanguin hépatique, hypertension portale et insuffisance hépatocellulaire chez les malades atteints de cirrhose alcoolique. *Archives francaises des maladies de l'appareil digestif*, **62**, 465–471.

Lecompte, Y., Metreau, J. M., Sancho, H. S. & Bismuth, H. (1974) Prediction of mortality in cirrhosis of the liver. *Surgery, Gynecology and Obstetrics*, **139**, 529–530.

Léger, L., Patel, J. C. & Boury, G. (1966) Dérivation veine splénique vaisseux pulmonaires pour syndrome de Budd–Chiari. *Presse médicale*, **74**, 2017–2018.

Léger, L., Delaitre, B. & Nicodème, J.-P. (1973) Hémorragies digestives chez le cirrhotique. Notre attitude thérapeutique à propos de 134 observations. *Journal de chirurgie*, **106**, 45–56.

Léger, L., Lenriot, J.-P., Chiche, B. & Lemaigre, G. (1974) Hypertension portale sectorielle. *Annales de gastroentérologie et d'hépatologie*, **10**, 497–519.

LeVeen, H. H., Christoudias, G., Ip, M., Luft, R., Falk, G. & Grosberg, S. (1974) Peritoneovenous shunting for ascites. *Annals of Surgery*, **180**, 580–591.

Lévy, V. G. & Caroli, J. (1974) Syndrome de Budd–Chiari. *Médicine & chirurgie digestives*, **3**, 389–399.

Linton, R. R. (1973) *Atlas of Vascular Surgery*. Philadelphia: W. B. Saunders.

Linton, R. R. (1974) Portal hypertension as I see it in 1973: the treatment of bleeding esophageal varices secondary to portal cirrhosis of the liver. In *Portal Hypertension*, ed. Child, C. G. III, Vol. 14, Major Problems in Clinical Surgery Series. Philadelphia: W. B. Saunders.

Longstreth, G. F., Newcomer, A. D. & Green, P. A. (1971) Extrahepatic portal hypertension caused by chronic pancreatitis. *Annals of Internal Medicine*, **75**, 903–908.

Lord, J. W., Rossi, G., Daliana, M. & Rosati, L. M. (1971) Portasystemic shunts in the management of massive hemorrhage from esophageal varices due to cirrhosis of the liver. *American Journal of Surgery*, **121**, 241–248.

Luttwak, E. M., Charuzi, I., Licht, A., Freund, H. & Borman, J. B. (1973) Emergency splenic vein–right atrial shunt for massive esophageal hemorrhage with cirrhosis of liver and inferior vena cava occlusion: report of an operation and follow-up. *Annals of Surgery*, **177**, 411–412.

Maillard, J.-N. & Prandi, D. (1974) Indications et résultats des anastomoses porto-caves chez le cirrhotique. *Annales de gastroentérologie et d'hépatique*, **10**, 521–532.

Maillard, J.-N., Benhamou, J.-P. & Rueff, B. (1970) Arterialization of the liver with portacaval shunt in the treatment of portal hypertension due to intrahepatic block. *Surgery*, **67**, 883–890.

Maillard, J.-N., Rueff, B., Prandi, D. & Sicot, C. (1974a) Hepatic arterialization and portacaval shunt in hepatic cirrhosis; an assessment. *Archives of Surgery*, **108**, 315–320.

Maillard, J.-N., Hay, J.-M., Elman, A. & Sicard, J.-L. (1974b) Coexistent inferior vena caval and portal hypertension. Splenic to left hepatic vein anastomosis in a cirrhotic patient. *Archives of Surgery*, **109**, 819–821.

Maillard, J.-N., Clot, P. & Coste, T. (1974c) Preoperative parameters influencing survival in patients with elective portacaval shunts. *Digestion*, **10**, 129–137.

Malt, R. A. (1974) Emergency and elective operations for bleeding esophageal varices. *Surgical Clinics of North America*, **54**, 561–571.

Malt, R. A., Szczerban, J. & Malt, R. B. (1976) Risks in therapeutic portacaval and splenorenal shunts. *Annals of Surgery* (in press).

McDermott, W. V., Jr (1974) *Surgery of the Liver and Portal Circulation*. Philadelphia: Lea & Febiger.

McDermott, W. V., Jr, Barnes, B. A., Nardi, G. L. & Ackroyd, F. W. (1968) Postshunt encephalopathy. *Surgery, Gynecology and Obstetrics*, **126**, 585–590.

McQuarrie, D. G., Nicoloff, D. M. & Lunseth, J. B. (1970) Sapheno-umbilical shunt. *Surgery, Gynecology and Obstetrics*, **130**, 1092–1094.

Mikkelsen, W. P. (1974) Therapeutic portacaval shunt. Preliminary data on controlled trial and morbid effects of acute hyaline necrosis. *Archives of Surgery*, **108**, 302–305.

Moncure, A. C., Waltman, A. C., Vander Salm, T. J., Linton, R. R., Levine, F. H. & Abbott, W. M. (1976) Gastrointestinal hemorrhage from adhesion-related mesenteric varices. *Annals of Surgery*, **183**, 24–29.

Moreno, A. H., Burchell, A. R., Rousselot, L. M., Panke, W. F., Slafsky, S. F. & Burke, J. H. (1967) Portal blood flow in cirrhosis of the liver. *Journal of Clinical Investigation*, **46**, 436–445.

Mullane, J. F. & Gliedman, M. L. (1970) Abdominal vena caval pressure and portal hypertension. *Archives of Surgery*, **101**, 363–365.

Mutchnick, M. G., Lerner, E. & Conn, H. O. (1974) Portal-systemic encephalopathy and portacaval anastomosis: a prospective, controlled investigation. *Gastroenterology*, **66**, 1005–1019.

Mutchnick, M. G., Lerner, E. & Conn, H. O. (1975) Effect of portacaval anastomosis on hypersplenism in cirrhosis: a prospective controlled evaluation. *Gastroenterology*, **68**, 1070.

Nabseth, D. C., Widrich, W. C., O'Hara, E. T. & Johnson, W. C. (1975) Flow and pressure characteristics of the portal system before and after splenorenal shunts. *Surgery*, **78**, 739–748.

Nackache, J. P., Hecht, Y., Georgakopoulos, H., Salmon, D., Garcon, Cl. & Giard, M. H. Le pronostic des anastomoses porto-systémiques pour cirrhose. *Acta gastro-enterologica belgica*, **34**, 248–262.

Nel, C. J. C., Honiball, P. J. & van Wyk, F. A. K. (1974) Portal hypertension in schistosomiasis. *South African Journal of Surgery*, **12**, 233–239.

Orloff, M. J., Charters, A. C. III, Chandler, J. G., Condon, J. K., Grambort, D. E., Modafferi, T. R., Levin, S. E., Brown, N. B., Sviokla, S. C. & Knox, D. G. (1975) Portacaval shunt as emergency procedure in unselected patients with alcoholic cirrhosis. *Surgery, Gynecology and Obstetrics*, **141**, 59–68.

Ottinger, L. W. & Moncure, A. C. (1974) Transthoracic ligation of bleeding esophageal varices in patients with intrahepatic portal obstruction. *Annals of Surgery*, **179**, 35–38.

Panke, W. F., Rousselot, L. M. & Burchell, A. R. (1968) A sixteen-year experience with end-to-side portacaval shunt for variceal hemorrhage: analysis of data and comparison with other types of portasystemic anastomoses. *Annals of Surgery*, **168**, 957–965.

Phillips, M. M., Ramsby, G. R. & Conn, H. O. (1975) Portacaval anastomosis and peptic ulcer: a nonassociation. *Gastroenterology*, **68**, 121–131.

Piccone, V. A., Bonanno, P. & LeVeen, H. H. (1968) Clinical and research uses of reopened adult umbilical vein. *Surgery*, **63**, 29–37.

Pliam, M. B., Adson, M. A. & Foulk, W. T. (1975) Conventional splenorenal shunts. A reconsideration. *Archives of Surgery*, **110**, 588–593.

Pollock, A. V. (1975) The treatment of resistant malignant ascites by insertion of a peritoneoatrial Holter valve. *British Journal of Surgery*, **62**, 104–107.

Prandi, D., Rueff, B. & Benhamou, J.-P. (1975) Side-to-side portacaval shunt in the treatment of Budd–Chiari syndrome. *Gastroenterology*, **68**, 137–141.

Raia, S. & Teixeira da Silva, A. (1975) Descompressao portal seletiva por anastomose esplenocava com interposicao de protese de dacron. *Revista do hospital das clinicas; Faculdade de Medicina, Universidade de Sao Paulo*, **30**, 69–76.

Regensberg, Cl., Gillot, Cl., Guez, D., Maury, D., Testas, P. & Frilleux, Cl. (1973) La dérivation porto-rénale. Intérêt d'une exploration cavorénale pré-opératoire. *Annales de chirurgie*, **27**, 139–149.

Reichle, F. A. (1972) Portal hemodynamics after distal splenorenal (Warren) shunt. *Annals of Surgery*, **176**, 195–198.

Resnick, R. H., Chalmers, T. C., Ishihara, A. M., Garceau, A. J., Callow, A. D., Schimmel, E. M., O'Hara, E. T. & Boston Inter-hospital Liver Group (1969) A controlled study of the prophylactic portacaval shunt. A final report. *Annals of Internal Medicine*, **70**, 675–688.

Resnick, R. H., Iber, F. L., Ishihara, A. M., Chalmers, T. C., Zimmerman, H. & Boston Inter-hospital Liver Group (1974) A controlled study of the therapeutic portacaval shunt. *Gastroenterology*, **67**, 843–857.

Reynolds, T. B. (1974a) The role of hemodynamic measurements in portosystemic shunt surgery. *Archives of Surgery*, **108**, 276–281.

Reynolds, T. B. (1974b) Promises! Promises! Hemodynamics of portal-systemic shunt. *New England Journal of Medicine*, **290**, 1484–1485.

Riddell, A. G., Davies, R. P. & Clark, A. D. (1966) Portacaval transposition in the treatment of glycogen-storage disease. *Lancet*, **2**, 1146–1148.

Riddell, A. G., Bloor, K., Hobbs, K. E. F. & Jacquet, N. (1972) Elective splenorenal anastomosis. *British Medical Journal*, **1**, 731–732.

Rosen, H., Silen, W. & Simon, M. (1967) Selective portal hypertension with isolated duodenojejunal varices. *New England Journal of Medicine*, **277**, 1188–1190.

Rosenberg, N., Konigsberg, S. F. & Noronha, J. (1974) Mesocaval and portacaval shunts using panelled bovine arterial H grafts. *Archives of Surgery*, **109**, 754–761.

Rothwell-Jackson, R. L. & Hunt, A. H. (1970) Proximal gastric resection in the treatment of bleeding gastro-oesophageal varices in patients with portal hypertension due to extrahepatic obstruction. *British Journal of Surgery*, **57**, 487–494.

Rueff, B. & Maillard, J. N. (1974) Portal-systemic shunts in patients with cirrhosis. The need of controlled clinical trials. *Digestion*, **11**, 414–427.

Sandblom, P. (1974) Portal hypertension as I see it. In *Portal Hypertension as Seen by 17 Authorities*, ed. Child, C. G. III, Vol. XIV, in Major Problems in Clinical Surgery Series, pp. 36–59. Philadelphia: W. B. Saunders.

Saubier, E. C., Brault, J. A., Russo, A. & Partensky, C. (1974) The role of reno-portal anastomosis in the surgical treatment of portal hypertension (with a report of 21 personal cases). *Chirurgica gastroenterologica*, **8**, 63–79.

Schrieber, J. T. & Gonzales, L. L. (1967) Thrombosis of hepatic veins and inferior vena cava. Relief by thoracic transposition of spleen. *American Journal of Surgery*, **113**, 807–811.

Sherlock, S. (1975) *Diseases of the Liver and Biliary System*, 5th edn. Oxford: Blackwell Publications.

Sherlock, S., Hourigan, K. & George, P. (1970) Medical complications of shunt surgery for portal hypertension. *Annals of the New York Academy of Sciences*, **170**, 392–405.

Shumacker, H. B., Nahrwold, D. L. & Zook, E. G. (1970) A new procedure for portal decompression: proximal splenic-caval anastomosis. *Annals of Surgery*, **171**, 465–470.

Silver, D., Puckett, C. L., McNeer, J. F., McLeod, M. E. & Sabiston, D. C., Jr (1974) Evaluation of selective transsplenic decompression of gastro-esophageal varices. *American Journal of Surgery*, **127**, 30–34.

Simeone, F. A. & Hopkins, R. W. (1967) Portarenal shunt for hepatic cirrhosis and portal hypertension. *Surgery*, **61**, 153–168.

Simon, J. S., Brown, A. A. & Ross, H. B. (1972) Ligation of the left renal vein in splenorenal anastomosis without impairment of renal function. *British Journal of Surgery*, **59**, 170–173.

Smith, G. W. (1974) Use of hemodynamic selection criteria in the management of cirrhotic patients with portal hypertension. *Annals of Surgery*, **179**, 782–790.

Smith, M., Tuft, R. J., Davidson, A. R., Laws, J. W., Dawson, J. L. & Williams, R. (1974) Mesentericocaval 'jump' graft in management of portal hypertension: experience with 24 cases. *British Medical Journal*, **2**, 705–708.

Sobel, S., Kaplitt, M. J., Popowitz, L., Girardet, R. E. & Adamsons, R. J. (1970) Omphalocaval shunt: a new procedure for portal decompression. *Surgery*, **68**, 456–460.

Starzl, T. E. & Putnam, C. W. (1975) Portal diversion. Treatment for glycogen storage disease and hyperlipemia. *Journal of the American Medical Association*, **233**, 955–957.

Starzl, T. E., Marchioro, T. L., Sexton, A. W., Illingworth, B., Waddell, W. R., Faris, T. D. & Herrmann, T. J. (1965) The effect of portacaval transposition on carbohydrate metabolism: experimental and clinical observations. *Surgery*, **57**, 687–697.

Starzl, T. E., Putnam, C. W., Chase, H. P. & Porter, K. A. (1973a) Portacaval shunt in hyperlipoproteinaemia. *Lancet*, **2**, 940–944.

Starzl, T. E., Putnam, C. W., Porter, K. A., Halgrimson, C. G., Corman, J., Brown, B. I., Gotlin, R. W., Rodgerson, D. O. & Greene, H. L. (1973b) Portal diversion for the treatment of glycogen storage disease in humans. *Annals of Surgery*, **178**, 525–539.

Stein, E. A., Mieny, C., Spitz, L., Saaron, I., Pettifor, J., Heimann, K. W., Bersohn, I. & Dinner, M. (1975) Portacaval shunt in four patients with homozygous hypercholesterolaemia. *Lancet*, **1**, 832–835.

Stipa, A., Thau, A., Cavallaro, A. & Rossi, P. (1973) A technique for mesentericocaval shunt. *Surgery, Gynecology and Obstetrics*, **137**, 285–287.

Stoney, R. J., Mehigan, J. T. & Olcott, C. (1975) Retroperitoneal approach for portasystemic decompression. *Archives of Surgery*, **110**, 1347–1350.

Strauch, G. O. (1970) Supradiaphragmatic splenic transposition. A successful option in the treatment of Chiari's disease. *American Journal of Surgery*, **119**, 379–384.

Sugiura, M. & Futagawa, S. (1973) A new technique for treating esophageal varices. *Journal of Thoracic and Cardiovascular Surgery*, **66**, 677–685.

Teixeira, E. D., Yu, H., Conn, J., Jr & Bergan, J. J. (1968) Selective decompression of esophagogastric varices. *Archives of Surgery*, **96**, 4–8.

Testart, J. & Tenière (1974) Les hémorragies digestives chez les malades porteurs d'une dérivation porto-cave efficace. *Journal de chirurgie*, **108**, 69–86.

Thomford, N. R., Sirinek, K. R. & Martin, E. W., Jr (1975) A series of 20 successful Warren shunts. *Archives of Surgery*, **110**, 584–587.

Thompson, B. W., Read, R. C. & Casali, R. E. (1975) Interposition grafting for portal hypertension. *American Journal of Surgery*, **130**, 733–738.

Turcotte, J. G. & Child, C. G. III (1972) Idiopathic extrahepatic portal hypertension in adults. *American Journal of Surgery*, **123**, 35–42.

Turcotte, J. G. & Lambert, M. J. III (1973) Variceal hemorrhage, hepatic cirrhosis, and portacaval shunts. *Surgery*, **73**, 810–817.

Turcotte, J. G., Wallin, V. W. & Child, C. G. III (1969) End to side versus side to side portacaval shunts in patients with hepatic cirrhosis. *American Journal of Surgery*, **117**, 108–116.

Ungeheuer, E. (1974) Oesophagusvarizenblutung. *Langenbecks archivs für chirurgie*, **337**, 519–526.

Viallet, A., Marleau, D., Huet, M., M. Martin, F., Farley, A., Villeneuve, J.-P. & Lavoie, P. (1975) Hemodynamic evaluation of patients with intrahepatic portal hypertension. Relationship between bleeding varices and the portohepatic gradient. *Gastroenterology*, **69**, 1297–1300.

Vix, V. A. & Payne, T. K. (1972) Elevated inferior vena cava pressure in ascites. Therapeutic implications in portacaval shunt. *American Journal of Surgery*, **123**, 721–723.

Voorhees, A. B., Jr & Price, J. B., Jr (1974) Extrahepatic portal hypertension. A retrospective analysis of 127 cases and associated clinical implications. *Archives of Surgery*, **108**, 338–341.

Voorhees, A. B., Jr, Price, J. B., Jr & Britton, R. C. (1970) Portasystemic shunting procedures for portal hypertension. A twenty-six year experience in adults with cirrhosis of the liver. *American Journal of Surgery*, **119**, 501–505.

Waddell, W. G., Bouchard, A. G., Wellington, J. L. & Ewing, J. B. (1972) Functional relations of the proximal components of the portal system. A preliminary report. *Journal of Surgical Research*, **12**, 281–289.

Warren, W. D., Salam, A. A., Faraldo, A., Hutson, D. & Smith, R. B. III (1972) End renal vein-to-splenic vein shunts for total or selective portal decompression. *Surgery*, **72**, 995–1006.

Warren, W. D., Salam, A. A. & Smith, R. B. III (1974a) The meso-splenorenal shunt procedures: a comprehensive approach to portasystemic decompression. *Annals of Surgery*, **179**, 791–798.

Warren, W. D., Salam, A. A., Hutson, D. & Zeppa, R. (1974b) Selective distal splenorenal shunt. Technique and results of operation. *Archives of Surgery*, **108**, 306–314.

Warren, W. D., Rudman, D., Millikan, W., Galambos, J. T., Salam, A. A. & Smith, R. B. III (1974c) The metabolic basis of portasystemic encephalopathy and the effect of selective vs. non-selective shunts. *Annals of Surgery*, **180**, 573–579.

Welling, R. E. & McDermott, W. V., Jr (1973) Combined caval and portal hypertension with cirrhosis of the liver: a problem in management. *Annals of Surgery*, **177**, 164–166.

White, J. J., Slapak, M. & MacLean, L. D. (1968) Extracorporeal portosystemic shunt for portal hypertension. *Surgery*, **63**, 17–28.

Windle, R. & Peacock, J. H. (1975) Prognosis after portocaval anastomosis: a 15-year follow-up *British Journal of Surgery*, **62**, 701–706.

Wirthlin, L. S., Van Urk, H., Malt, R. B. & Malt, R. A. (1974) Predictors of surgical mortality in patients with cirrhosis and non-variceal gastroduodenal bleeding. *Surgery, Gynecology and Obstetrics*, **139**, 65–68.

Witte, C. L., Witte, M. H., Renert, W., O'Mara, R. E. & Lilien, D. L. (1976) Splenic artery ligation in selected patients with hepatic cirrhosis and in Sprague–Dawley rats. *Surgery, Gynecology and Obstetrics*, **142**, 1–12.

Yale, C. E. & Crummy, A. B. (1971) Splenic vein thrombosis and bleeding esophageal varices. *Journal of the American Medical Association*, **217**, 317–320.

Zuidema, G. D. & Ebert, P. A. (1967) Mesenteric-caval anastomosis for portal decompression. *Johns Hopkins Medical Journal*, **120**, 201–209.

11
LIVER DISEASE IN INFANTS AND CHILDREN

Alex. P. Mowat

In many respects the clinical and pathological features of liver disease in children are similar to those in the adult. Advances in the understanding of the pathogenesis of liver disease in the adult, for example chronic active hepatitis, have important implications in paediatric practice, no less than the major impact studies performed in children associating serum hepatitis with the hepatitis B surface antigen (Giles et al, 1969), have made on adult hepatology. There are, however, important differences in the pathological response of the liver and bile duct in infancy and childhood which are presumed to be due to factors associated with growth and development but in fact are very poorly understood and require urgent study.

In this review the major emphasis will be on three areas in paediatric liver disease which still present many challenges for the clinician and investigator but in which significant advances have occurred in the last five years, namely, liver disease associated with genetic deficiency of the serum protein alpha-1 antitrypsin, extrahepatic biliary atresia, and Reye's syndrome. The problems of management in portal hypertension in childhood are given particular mention to emphasise the major iatrogenic element in the morbidity associated with this condition. We start with a brief consideration of the problems of unconjugated hyperbilirubinaemia in the newborn.

UNCONJUGATED HYPERBILIRUBINAEMIA IN THE NEWBORN INFANT

The most frequent cause of unconjugated hyperbilirubinaemia in childhood is 'physiological' jaundice, occurring in the first two weeks of life. Although not a manifestation of liver disease, consideration of its pathophysiology gives important insight into bilirubin metabolism and it does accentuate jaundice when liver disease is present. Considerable controversy still exists about the optimum method of management.

Pathophysiology

It is now considered likely that there is no single cause for bilirubin retention in the neonate (Lathe, 1974). The many contributory factors thought to be important are listed in Table 11.1 In the human infant there is good evidence for increased bilirubin formation (Maisels et al, 1971), and defective bilirubin glucuronide formation (Lathe, 1974). Poland and Odell (1971) observed that in full-term infants the serum bilirubin was inversely related to the amount of bilirubin in the stool suggesting that increased enterohepatic circulation may have been a factor in causing physiological jaundice. The data supporting the validity of the other factors mentioned in the table in causing neonatal jaundice is derived either from a few studies in human infants using dyes such as bromsulphthalein or experimental work in animals which do not suffer from physiological jaundice. This is particularly true for the enzyme

Table 11.1 Factors possibly contributing to physiological jaundice

Mechanisms	Causes
Increased bilirubin production	Increased red blood cell volume Decreased red blood cell survival Increased 'early labelled peak' Ineffective erythropoiesis
Increased enteric reabsorption of bilirubin	Reabsorption of bilirubin from meconium High β-glucuronidase levels in newborn gut Diminished production of glucurolactone (a specific β-glucuronidase inhibitor) Lack of bacterial degradation of bilirubin
Impaired hepatic uptake of bilirubin	Ineffective hepatic perfusion Diminished transport across the hepatocyte membrane Low ligandin concentration in cytoplasm Competition with other anions Diminished calorie intake in the first 72 h of life
Defective bilirubin glucuronide formation	Low concentration of glucuronide donor (UDPGA) due to diminished production and utilisation by other metabolic pathways Low UDP glucuronyltransferase activity Inhibition of UDP glucuronyltransferase activity by hormones, steroids, etc
Defective bilirubin excretion	

uridine diphosphoglucuronyl transferase (UDP transferase). In many species this enzyme is present in very low activity in the newborn period gradually rising to adult levels over the course of a few days.

The only study of this enzyme activity performed in human biopsy material however, showed a totally different time course of development, not reaching adult levels until around the seventieth day (Di Toni, Lupi and Ansanell, 1968). These authors, however, used methylumbelliferone as substrate rather than bilirubin. There is certainly impaired plasma clearance of bilirubin due to ineffective hepatic function but the exact mechanism of this is not clear. In newborn monkeys the hepatic cytoplasmic protein ligandin (Y), which may play a part in the transhepatic transport of bilirubin, is at low concentration at birth reaching adult levels by five days of age, coinciding with a fall in serum bilirubin concentration and normal hepatic uptake of bromsulphthalein (Levi, Gaitmaiten and Arias, 1970). Since this species also suffers from physiological jaundice a similar process could occur in the human infant. Evidence for the importance of the other mechanisms is well reviewed by Maisels (1972).

Hyperbilirubinaemia

In physiological jaundice the maximum serum bilirubin level occurs on the second to fourth day of life in full-term infants and rarely exceed 100 μmol/litre (6 mg/dl) in health. In infants born before term levels of 200 to 240 μmol/litre (12–14 mg/dl) are commonly reached on the fifth to seventh day

Table 11.2 Factors causing unconjugated hyperbilirubinaemia in newborn

Infection
Haemolytic disorders
Prematurity
Bruising
Late clamping of umbilical cord
Hypoglycaemia
Dehydration
Drugs conjugated with glucuronic acid
Meconium retention
High intestinal obstruction
Breast-milk jaundice
Crigler–Najjar syndrome
Transient familial neonatal hyperbilirubinaemia

of life. In full-term infants hyperbilirubinaemia is considered to exist if the serum bilirubin concentration exceeds 200 μmol/litre (12 mg/dl) while in prematurely born infants a concentration of more than 255 μmol/litre (15 mg/dl) is considered hyperbilirubinaemia. These definitions are important in that they alert the clinician firstly to the necessity to prevent kernicterus and secondly to investigate the infant in order to identify as early as possible such treatable conditions as septicaemia or galactosaemia. The many factors which may contribute to hyperbilirubinaemia are listed in Table 11.2.

Management

The presence of the above contributing factors may be suspected on the basis of the history together with careful scrutiny of the obstetrical case record and physical examination of the infant. It is necessary, however, to have a systematic scheme of investigation as outlined in Table 11.3 to avoid overlooking treatable factors.

The second role in management is to prevent kernicterus, a disorder in which death or permanent neurological damage follows the deposition of unconjugated bilirubin in the brain. Unconjugated bilirubin is transported in the plasma thoroughly bound to serum albumin with only a minute amount unbound. It is not yet possible to measure unbound serum bilirubin. Brain damage occurs when the serum concentration of unconjugated bilirubin exceeds the capacity of serum proteins to bind bilirubin. Albumin binding is very sensitive to hydrogen ion concentration, falling with falling pH. A wide range of endogenous anions such as haematin, bile acids and fatty acids compete with bilirubin for albumin binding as do such drugs as salicylate, sulphonamide, benzorates, novobiocin, oxacilin and cephalolithin. Tissue distribution of bilirubin is determined by the relative affinity for bilirubin of albumin and tissues. The actual concentration of free bilirubin may not be a valid index of the amount of bilirubin able to enter the brain. In full-term

Table 11.3 Laboratory investigations to determine causes of unconjugated hyperbilirubinaemia

1. Red blood cell morphology, reticulocyte count, normoblast count
2. Blood group of mother and child
3. Direct Coombs' test on infant's blood
4. Maternal blood group antibodies and haemolysins
5. Urinary microscopy and culture
6. Urinalysis for non-glucose reducing substances
7. Blood culture and other appropriate bacteriological investigations for causes of infection
8. Specific tests for abnormalities of red blood cell function, e.g. glucose-6-phosphate dehydrogenase activity
9. In vitro inhibition of bilirubin conjugation by breast milk

infants, a serum bilirubin concentration of 340 μmol/litre (20 mg/dl) or greater is associated with a significant risk of kernicterus.

But in some infants kernicterus does not occur even though the bilirubin rises as high as 680 μmol/litre (40 mg/dl). It has been suggested that the accurate estimation of the reserve capacity of serum protein to bind bilirubin may provide a more precise indication of the risk of kernicterus than serum bilirubin concentrations. The value of this approach has hitherto only been demonstrated using the salicylate saturation index method which is technically difficult and available only in a limited number of laboratories (Odell, Storey and Rosenberg, 1970). Because of difficulties using the salicylate saturation index, albumin binding by the dyes phenolsulphonphthalin (Waters, 1967) and 2-(4-hydroxybenzene)azobenzoic acid (HBABA) (Odievre et al, 1970) but the value of these has not yet been confirmed in clinical practice. The organic adsorbant gel Sephadex, which will absorb unconjugated serum bilirubin not firmly bound to albumin, has been used by a number of investigators to measure the bilirubin binding affinity of albumin but it has yet to be shown that this technique is of more predective value than measuring serum bilirubin concentration (Jirsova et al, 1967). It is very important that these methods be further developed and the laboratory findings be critically compared with the clinical observations, both in the perinatal period and at later follow-up. There are certainly several conditions in which kernicterus can occur at serum concentrations lower than indicated above. Of particular importance are prematurity, hypoalbuminaemia, asphyxia and acidosis as well as drugs which may compete with bilirubin for albumin binding.

Control of Unconjugated Hyperbilirubinaemia

In controlling unconjugated hyperbilirubinaemia and preventing kernicterus the factors which cause aggravation of physiological jaundice are firstly identified and minimised. It is particularly important to maintain an appropriate intake of both fluid and calories.

Exchange transfusion

This is a most effective means of removing bilirubin when the risk of kernicterus is high and must be undertaken when the level of unconjugated serum bilirubin exceeds 340 μmol/litre (20 mg/dl). It may be indicated at lower levels, for example 250 μmol/litre (15 mg/dl) in premature infants particularly if they are acidotic or serum albumin levels are low. In infants with haemolytic disease a rise in serum bilirubin concentration of more than 8.5 μmol/litre usually indicates that serum bilirubin will accumulate more rapidly than can be excreted and an exchange transfusion usually proves necessary.

Phototherapy

In the last decade it has been unequivocally documented that exposing a jaundiced infant to artificial light of moderate intensity is effective in preventing hyperbilirubinaemia and lowering elevated serum bilirubin. This mode of therapy has been the subject of numerous recent reviews (Lucey, 1972; Maisels, 1972; Ostrow, 1972; *British Medical Journal*, 1974). Phototherapy has been most widely used in preventing the hyperbilirubinaemia associated with prematurity. In haemolytic disorders it has been shown to decrease the number of exchange transfusions in rhesus isoimmunisation and in ABO incompatibility. In the management of infants with Crigler–Najjar syndrome, phototherapy may be invaluable in preventing kernicterus. Exposure to intense lights may be necessary for up to 12 or even 16 h per day and this condition has to be continued for life.

Light of wavelength near 450 nm is most effective but white light is to be preferred since observation of the patient is easier. Current evidence suggests that photodegradation of bilirubin occurs predominantly in the skin. The in vivo breakdown products remain ill characterised but a well-documented effect is the excretion in the bile of bilirubin which reacts chemically like unconjugated bilirubin. It is not yet known whether this is the consequence of an action of phototherapy on hepatocytes or from a photobiochemical transformation of the bilirubin in the skin. In vitro these photochemical derivatives of bilirubin are less toxic than bilirubin but it is not known whether these photodegradation products behave similarly in the intact organism.

A number of side effects have been recognised as complicating phototherapy. The most frequent is increased insensible water loss which may lead to dehydration and aggravate hyperbilirubinaemia. This must be corrected by providing an increased water intake. Diarrhoea has been reported but where detailed observations have been made with appropriate controls the incidence of loose stools has not in fact increased compared with the normal infants. Skin reactions, including maculopapular rashes, tanning of Negro infants, bronzing of the skin with acute haemolysis in infants with liver disease, occur rarely. Other possible biological effects of phototherapy must be considered. These include neuroendocrine functions mediated through the pineal gland and photoreceptors in the retina, possibly affecting growth, diurnal rhythms and sexual maturation. Direct photochemical reactions may occur with other body constituents, particularly the retina. Protection of the eyes during phototherapy is mandatory.

Thus far no permanent abnormalities have been detected in human infants treated with phototherapy. Nevertheless, the use of this agent should be limited to those infants who strictly need it. It should not be given for longer than is absolutely necessary. It has yet to be shown that the widespread use of phototherapy in the management of non-haemolytic jaundice in low birthweight infants is in the patient's best interests. Although it has been postulated that neonatal hyperbilirubinaemia may cause a continuum of brain damage extending from kernicterus to minor intellectual impairment (Lucey, 1972), this has never been confirmed in careful follow-up studies.

Phenobarbitone

Phenobarbitone, particularly if given to the mother for some days before delivery of the infant, has been shown in prospective control studies to be effective in both premature and full-term infants in controlling neonatal hyperbilirubinaemia even when caused by haemolysis due to ABO and rhesus isoimmunisation. This mode of treatment is considered in the review on phototherapy referred to above (Ostrow, 1972; Maisels, 1972). The mechanism of action of phenobarbitone is uncertain but from animal studies there is evidence that it can stimulate all three steps in bilirubin metabolism which are impaired in the neonate, namely hepatic uptake, conjugation and hepatic excretion. In addition it appears to stimulate the bile salt-independent component of bile flow. If started at birth in a dose of 8 mg/kg d^{-1} it will significantly decrease the frequency of repeat exchange transfusions in rhesus isoimmunisation and in glucose-6-phosphate dehydrogenase deficiency. Since its effect is not apparent until at least 48 h after the drug is commenced it is of little value in treating established hyperbilirubinaemia. The effect of phenobarbitone is not limited to bilirubin excretion. It increases hepatic haem synthesis thereby possibly aggravating jaundice and modifies the concentration and activity of many microsomal enzymes involved in the metabolism of drugs, vitamins, clotting factors and hormones, as well as influencing the intercellular ratios of reduced and oxidised forms of NAD and NADP.

Because of its non-specificity phenobarbitone cannot be recommended for the control of hyperbilirubinaemia in the newborn. It must be recognised, however, that many infants are born in conditions where optimum, highly technical perinatal care is not possible. In these circumstances the small chance of complications with relatively simple measures, namely phototherapy and phenobarbitone, may be discounted if they give an increased chance of survival with an intact neurological system.

HEPATITIS SYNDROMES IN INFANCY

Conjugated hyperbilirubinaemia in infancy is always abnormal. Active investigation is necessary to identify causes for which there is specific effective treatment and to exclude surgically correctable lesions. Recognition of a genetically determined cause even if no treatment is available is important because the family will require guidance on the prospects of recurrence in later siblings. In nearly all instances a raised conjugated bilirubin is accompanied by clay-coloured stools, dark bile-containing urine, and usually hepatomegaly. The onset in the vast majority of patients is in the first four weeks of life with a smaller number presenting at five to eight weeks of age and very few as late as four months (Mowat, Pscharopoulos and Williams, 1976). Splenomegaly, a mild haemolytic anaemic and failure to thrive are frequent features (Alagille, 1972). There is biochemical and pathological evidence of hepatocellular necrosis with hepatitis, i.e. inflammatory cell infiltrate in the portal tract and hepatic parenchyma, hence the terminology used in this review.

Even after full investigation there can be considerable difficulty in determining whether the lesion in these infants is primarily in the hepatic parenchyma, the portal tracts, the major intrahepatic bile ducts, or in the extrahepatic bile ducts. Disorders starting in one area are inevitably followed by changes in the others. Emery (1974) suggested that the hepatic abnormalities in such infants are produced by the interaction of a number of factors, noxious agents or infection, the effects of growth, metabolic maturity, and the subject's genetically determined metabolic variability. He also emphasised the very practical point that the left lobe of liver is frequently much more fibrotic than the right. The pathogenesis and significance of some of the histological features has also been critically reviewed by Landing (1974). In patients with marked hepatitis bile flow may be negligible and the extrahepatic bile ducts very narrow so that it is difficult to detect the lumen without destroying them. In these circumstances it may be impossible to demonstrate by retrograde radiography the intrahepatic bile ducts. Conversely, in biliary atresia the hepatocytes may show marked abnormalities including giant cell transformation. The term 'giant cell hepatitis' has little to recommend it since such transformation of hepatocytes occurs with a wide range of known causes of liver disease in this age group, as well as in the idiopathic varieties (Landing, 1974). In some instances at least, extrahepatic biliary atresia is a progressive disorder with destruction of previously normal extrahepatic ducts and perhaps a slower destruction of intrahepatic ducts. If we are to gain further insight into the pathophysiology of obstructive jaundice in this age group we must beware of too rigid a classification of such disorders, particularly if made on the basis of investigation made at one stage of its development. Many generic terminologies for this group of disorders have been introduced reflecting the instigator's concept of the likely pathogenesis, e.g. intrahepatic cholestasis, obstructive cholangiopathy of infancy, bile-retention syndrome of infancy. The author favours the term 'hepatitis syndrome' since this does not imply understanding of the cause of the inflammation, suggesting rather that this is a field requiring very active investigation.

Specific Factors Associated with Hepatitis in Infancy

Infections

Efforts to implicate infectious factors are unsuccessful in the vast majority of patients although a wide range of agents causing generalised infection of the neonate produce hepatitis as a major or minor component of the illness. Unfortunately, the majority are viral caused by rubella, cytomegalovirus, herpes simplex virus, coxsackie B and adenovirus and no specific therapy is available. In many instances, there is evidence of involvement of other organs (Dommergues, 1973). It is important to exclude listeriosis and infection with toxoplasmosis and *Treponema pallidum* since specific antibiotic therapy is available. The discovery of hepatitis B antigen (HBAg) has had less impact on this form of hepatitis than those seen in older children and in adults. It has been implicated in only a minority of cases of neonatal hepatitis (Wright et al, 1970; Alagille, 1972; Cossart, 1974). Asymptomatic transfer of antigen to the infant is more frequently recognised although the exact time of transfer is uncertain. Transplacental, intrapartum or postpartum all appear possible. The finding of the antigen in cord blood increases the likelihood of HBAg in the infant (Stevens et al, 1975) but it is not inevitable. If the mother has had symptomatic hepatitis in the last trimester of pregnancy, or early in the puerperium, there appears to be a 40 per cent incidence of hepatitis B antigenaemia in the infant. The hepatitis is in most instances mild with only moderate elevation of aspartate transaminase in the serum, but the infant may become a chronic carrier (Schweitzer et al, 1972). Not all infants have mild disease however, and further follow-up is mandatory (Kattamis et al, 1973).

In infants of mothers who are asymptomatic carriers there is a much lower incidence of infection in the infant, approximately 5 per cent only having antigenaemia and associated liver disease. In most instances this is mild but it may be severe (Schweitzer et al, 1973). Fulminant hepatitis due to hepatitis B surface antigen has been observed with an onset 59 to 150 days after birth in infants who had not had blood products but whose mothers were found to be asymptomatic carriers (Dupuy, Frommel and Alagille, 1975). Because of these observations, Kohler and his colleagues (1974) have reported an attempt to modify infection of the infant by giving immunoglobulin with a high concentration of antibody to hepatitis B surface antigen to a small number of infants 'at risk'. In Taiwan as many as 40 per cent of infants of asymptomatic carriers developed antigenaemia. In the adult population, between 5 and 20 per cent are carriers. It has been speculated that many of these date from infancy. Liver disease associated with the antigenaemia in the infant in Taiwan has not been well documented. Only a prospective controlled trial of immunoglobulin therapy in a population at high risk will show whether this measure is efficacious.

As well as the specific infection, it is well recognised that many bacterial infections, particularly *Escherichia coli* infections in the urine, septicaemia and diarrhoea, may be complicated by conjugated hyperbilirubinaemia with hepatocellular damage. The pathogenesis of the liver disease in these cases remains obscure but therapy with antibiotics gives a gratifying response.

Genetically determined metabolic disorders

Of the metabolic disorders causing neonatal hepatitis syndrome, galactosaemia, fructosaemia, and tyrosinosis are the most important to consider clinically, since specific treatment is likely to be effective in the former two and may be helpful in the third. In all of these conditions, hepatocellular damage occurs as part of a complex, metabolic derangement. The exact pathogenesis of the hepatocellular necrosis and increased mesenchymal activity in these patients is not fully understood. Galactosaemia and fructosaemia should be suspected clinically since both are associated with the appearance of the offending monosaccharide in the urine. This can easily be detected as a non-glucose reducing substance with a simple test such as Clinitest tablets or Benedict's solution but gives a negative test with glucose-oxidase testing. It must be emphasised that these tests will only be abnormal if the offending monosaccharide is being ingested at the time of the test. Patients with galactosaemia often die in the first days of life with a septicaemic-like illness, the diagnosis of galactosaemia may never be considered. Harris (1974) reported that galactosaemia may occur without galactosuria even in the first months of life, although galactosaemic patients may not produce galactosurea. We have recently investigated a patient with fructosaemia in whom classical enzymatic abnormalities were found in the liver biopsy but who did not have fructosuria when challenged at the age of 18 months with an adequate fructose load.

Deficiency of the serum alpha-1 antitrypsin

A major development in the last seven years has been the demonstration that a considerable proportion of serious paediatric liver disease is associated with deficiency of the serum protein alpha-1 antitrypsin. Since Freier and her colleagues (1968) found that genetically determined abnormality in the serum protein electrophoretic strip of two brothers with cirrhosis, this abnormality has been shown to be a frequent associated factor in neonatal hepatitis and cirrhosis in childhood (Aagenaes et al, 1972; Porter et al, 1972; Cottrall, Mowat and Cook, 1974).

FUNCTION

Alpha-1 antitrypsin is a glycoprotein with a molecular weight of between 50 000 and 56 000. It is synthesised in the liver. The concentration in serum is readily measured by immunochemical techniques, in health being between 200 and 400 mg/dl, with much lower concentration in other body fluids. Raised concentrations in serum are found with infection, after operations, during pregnancy, oral contraceptives, in the perinatal period and in many liver diseases. Low concentrations are found in infants with the respiratory distress syndrome and in advanced liver disease (Talamo, 1975). Individuals with genetic deficiency have concentrations of between 10 and 20 per cent of normal. The physiological role of alpha-1 antitrypsin has yet to be determined. As well as inhibiting the enzyme trypsin, it also inhibits elastase, collagenase, and leucocyte and bacterial proteases. It may thus have a role in controlling tissue responses in infection and inflammation and particularly in response to enzymes released from dying bacteria. In addition, it may influence both coagulation and fibrinolysis being an effective inhibitor of plasmin (Telamo, 1975). Hormonal factors influence its metabolism. The secretion in cervical mucus is low at the time of ovulation increasing to high levels at the eighteenth day of the menstrual cycle suggesting a possible role in implantation. (Fagerhol, 1975).

GENETICS

Early studies of patients with alpha-1 antitrypsin deficiency suggested that the inheritance was in a simple autosomal fashion. Its investigation using an acid starch gel electrophoretic technique demonstrated that there are many variants which can be identified on the basis of their electrophoretic mobility. Each produces eight bands, three of which are prominent. These variants are considered to be under the control of a single autosomal gene locus, Pi (protease inhibitor). They are designated alphabetically according to electrophoretic mobility, extending from Pi^B to Pi^Z, with in addition, Pi^-, a total of 24 being so far identified. In most studies approximately 80 per cent of the population have a Pi^M phenotype. Disease is associated with three rare phenotypes, Pi^{ZZ}, Pi^{Z-}, and Pi^-, the frequency of which appears to vary in different populations from around 1/3500 births in the United Kingdom, to

1/1500 births in Scandinavia. Approximately 10 to 20 per cent of deficient subjects will develop liver disease, 50 to 60 per cent will develop emphysema, and 10 to 20 per cent will escape both conditions (Aagenaes, et al, 1972). A minority will have both lung and liver disease (Glasgow et al, 1973). Case reports of cirrhosis in Pi^{SZ} individuals may represent a chance association (Wilkinson et al, 1974).

CLINICAL FEATURES

Liver disease usually starts with an acute hepatitis in the first four months of life. In 25 per cent of patients physiological jaundice merges into that due to hepatitis, and in over 90 per cent the hepatitis clears within the first four weeks. Its clinical severity is very variable. Some infants may appear well apart from icterus and slow weight gain while others show irritability, lethargy, poor feeding, vomiting, hypotension, purpura with low platelet counts and prolonged prothrombin time and septicaemia. Maximum recorded serum bilirubin concentrations can vary from 68 μmol/litre (4 mg/dl) to 340 μmol/litre (20 mg/dl), with aspartate aminotransferase levels varying in the acute stage from 80 to 600 iu/litre and the alkaline phosphatase from 150 to 1300 iu/litre. The jaundice gradually fades, the serum bilirubin eventually returning to normal after a period varying from ten days to more than six months. In contrast aspartate aminotransferase and alkaline phosphatase concentrations rarely return to normal. In those who survive the acute hepatitis features of cirrhosis and its complications may appear in the first year of life but the majority have a period of relative well-being before complications appear in late childhood or early adult life. Cirrhosis is not the invariable outcome, however, in rare instances it has not developed by the third decade (Sass-Kortsak, 1974). Very rarely cirrhosis may develop without an antecedent hepatitis in the newborn period.

PATHOLOGICAL FEATURES

Liver biopsy in the acute stage shows a variable degree of cholestasis, hepatocellular necrosis, glandular transformation of hepatocytes with inflammatory cell infiltrate in the parenchyma and portal tracts, and an increase in periportal fibrous tissue. Giant cell transformation of hepatocytes is not prominent. In some instances, the histological features may be very similar to those of extrahepatic biliary atresia. Commonly the clinical severity of the hepatitis is reflected in the degree of hepatocellular necrosis and mesenchymal proliferation, cirrhosis developing in the first year of life in infants with severe hepatitis and protracted hyperbilirubinaemia (Cottrall et al, 1974). In some instances hepatitis may be mild yet cirrhosis is evident on biopsy as early as three months of age and its complications apparent by twelve months. Cirrhosis may be macronodular, micronodular, or take a so-called biliary form. A distinctive pathological feature is the presence of diastase-resistant PAS-positive magenta-coloured globules 2 to 20 μm in diameter seen most prominently in periportal hepatocytes in Pi^{ZZ} infants but only after 12 weeks of age (Talbot and Mowat, 1975). These globules appear to correspond to the amorphous material which on electron microscopy is seen to distend the endoplasmic reticulum of some hepatocytes. Other organelles are normal. The material reacts with a specific fluorescein-tagged antibody to alpha-1 antitrypsin giving a bright fluorescence not seen in the hepatocytes of non-Pi^{ZZ} subjects. The accumulation of this material which is antigenically similar to normal (Pi^{MM}) serum alpha-1 antitrypsin occurs in Pi^{ZZ} subjects whether liver disease is present or not.

BIOCHEMICAL ASPECTS

The studies of Eriksson and Larsson, (1975) in which PAS-positive globules from cirrhotic livers were immunologically and chemically characterised, initially suggested that the material is an asialo form of alpha-1 antitrypsin. Further experiments on material made soluble by fairly vigorous chemical methods have shown that hepatic alpha-1 antitrypsin deficient individuals lacks not only sialic acid but many other carbohydrate residues. The polypeptide backbone of the alpha-1 antitrypsin is of similar size to that of serum alpha-1 antitrypsin (Pi^{MM}) although minor differences in amino acid composition are observed.

Comparison of serum alpha-1 antitrypsin from deficient (Pi^{ZZ}) individuals and normals (Pi^{MM}) show a difference in the polypeptide structure of the molecule close to the site of carbohydrate attachment, possibly due to amino acid substitution (Jeppsson and Laurell, 1975). These workers suggest that this abnormality of polypeptide structure could so change the physical properties to cause aggregation of alpha-1 antitrypsin and presumably prevent normal glycolysation of the polypeptide chain (Jeppsson, Larsson and Eriksson, 1975). The same group provide further evidence that a simple lack of sialic acid is not the full explanation of the difficulty in excretion in most instances because sialyltransferase activity in the serum of Pi^{ZZ} individuals is higher than in normals. In two Pi^{ZZ} patients, however, extremely low levels of serum sialyltransferase were found, presumably representing a genetic variant. The possibility must exist that these represent a different subgroup of Pi^{ZZ} individuals, but the pathophysiological significance of this latter observation is not clear (Eriksson and Larsson, 1975). It is noteworthy that the serum levels of alpha-fetoprotein, a glycoprotein whose production is partially regulated by sialyltransferase are minimally elevated in neonatal hepatitis syndrome in Pi^{ZZ} individuals but reach very high levels in Pi^{MM} subjects (Johnston, et al, 1976). If, as has been suggested, the high serum sialyltransferase activity commonly found represents an increase to compensate for stearic hindrance to sialyl in cooperation caused by the physical chemical changes in Pi^{ZZ} alpha-1 antitrypsin, local 'inactivation' of enzyme may affect other sialysations. The alternative suggested explanation for alpha-1 antitrypsin accumulation in hepatocytes, namely that it is an asialyl protein removed from the serum by the hepatocyte, seems unlikely since it is stored in the endoplasmic reticulum rather than in lysosomes.

The pathogenesis of liver disease associated with alpha-1 antitrypsin deficiency is at present uncertain. The storage of alpha-1 antitrypsin in the liver cells cannot be blamed since the same material is present in subjects without liver disease. Because liver disease has been found in certain families and is absent in others, Talamo (1975) suggests a second associated genetic defect may be necessary for liver disease to occur. The alternative explanation is that the liver is unable to control a damaging process initiated by infectious or toxic factors which would be rapidly controlled if normal inhibitors to bacterial, viral or inflammatory cell proteases were present. Early studies by our group suggested that hepatitis B surface antigen was an important additional factor (Porter et al, 1972) but this has not been confirmed in subsequent studies by ourselves or other workers.

Unfortunately, there is as yet no specific treatment for alpha-1 antitrypsin deficiency. Phenobarbitone given as a possible enzyme inducer had no effect on serum alpha-1 antitrypsin concentration, its functional activity, or liver function tests (Sharpe, 1971; Porter et al, 1972). Administration of exogenous alpha-1 antitrypsin is impractical since its half life is only six days (Makino and Reed, 1970). Corticosteroids and immunosuppressants do not appear to control the hepatitis. Liver transplantation has been attempted but the patient did not survive (Sharpe, 1971).

Rare chromosomal and familial causes of neonatal hepatitis syndrome
Cystic fibrosis may rarely be complicated by prolonged obstructive jaundice in the newborn period. In 50 per cent of cases the underlying cause may be readily suspected since the infant has had a meconium ileus or malabsorption due to deficiency of pancreatic enzymes, but in the remainder there will be no specific clinical features suggesting the diagnosis. Sweat sodium concentrations of greater than 70 μmol/litre are diagnostic (Valman, France and Wallis, 1971) (see Chapter 12).

The early manifestation of some sphingomyelin storage disorders (Neimann–Pick disease) may be prolonged obstructive jaundice in early infancy (Neville et al, 1973). This is seen particularly in patients with Nova Scotian ancestry and in the recently described variant associated with vertical supranuclear ophthalmoplegia here. Diagonsis at this early stage when abnormal storage is not a prominent feature and the central nervous system functions normally is particularly difficult unless there is a positive family history. Storage cells are frequently more prominent in the bone marrow than in the Kupffer cells.

Neonatal hepatitis syndrome may be slightly more common in Down's syndrome (trisomy 21) but is particularly frequent in trisomies 13 and 18 in which between 20 and 30 per cent of patients have hepatitis (Taylor, 1968). The diagnosis may be suspected clinically from the marked physical abnormalities and is confirmed by analysis of the chromosomal karyotype. Hepatitis also occurs in female phenotypes with Turner's syndrome the sex chromosome deletion disorder (Gardner, 1974).

In addition, three distinct syndromes with familial occurrence of obstructive liver disease in infancy have been described. Obstructive jaundice in infancy followed by recurrent episodes of jaundice throughout childhood and the development of unexplained oedema of the legs towards puberty has been reported in a group of children with common ancestory in south-west Norway (Aagenaes 1974). Familial neonatal liver disease with varying hepatic dysfunction and pulmonary stenosis has also been described (Watson and Miller, 1973). Alagille and co-workers (1975) have described 15 patients with hepatic ductular hypoplasia associated with a characteristic facies, vertebral malformations, retarded physical, mental and sexual development and a cardiac murmur with a positive family history of a neonatal cholestatic jaundice in siblings of three of the patients.

The occasional occurrence of familial cases without distinct clinical or metabolic features is well recognised. In some, particularly in the Byler syndrome, bile salt metabolism is very deranged but evidence as to whether this is primary or secondary is lacking (Linarelli, Williams and Phillips, 1972).

EXTRAHEPATIC BILIARY ATRESIA

Of all paediatric liver disorders extrahepatic biliary atresia (EHBA) causes most distress to the infant and his parents. The majority of infants survive long enough to become fully established as an individual in the family only to die before their second birthday (Lou, Schmutzer and Regan, 1972). During the first months of life these children often thrive satisfactorily although deeply jaundiced but as cirrhosis develops growth rate slows, ascites and bile salts accumulate. Abdominal distension, dyspnoea, and pruritus are particularly distressing symptoms. Hitherto, approximately 90 per cent of such infants had no prospect of surgical relief of their jaundice and could be offered only symptomatic measures (Danks and Campbell, 1966). The remainder had distal obstructions with patent bile-containing proximal bile ducts which could be anastomosed to the bowel to allow bile drainage to occur. Unfortunately, many of these develop cirrhosis and its complications by early childhood although occasional cases survive to adult life (Berenson, Garde and Moody, 1974). The best prospect for the patient with suspected EHBA has been that a choledochal cyst will be shown to be the cause of the jaundice.

The operation of hepatic portoenterostomy developed in Japan by Kasai and his co-workers (1957) nearly 20 years ago has given new hope for the patient with previously inoperable EHBA, survival to the age of 17 years having recently been reported (Kasai, Watanabe and Ohi, 1975). Short-term confirmation of the successful use of this procedure has now been reported from a number of centres (Bill, Brennon and Huseby, 1974; Danks et al, 1974; Lilly and Altman, 1975; Valayer et al, 1975) bringing a welcome enthusiasm for the investigation and treatment for what has for some time been regarded as an unrewarding field. New ideas on pathogenesis, considered below are emerging.

Definitions

Extrahepatic biliary atresia is characterised by complete inability to excrete bile and by obstruction, destruction, or absence of the bile ducts anywhere between the duodenum and the first or second order of branches of the right and left hepatic ducts. In distal atresia the proximal ducts are dilated together with the gallbladder if the lesion is below the junction of the cystic duct and the hepatic duct. These dilated segments contain bile being in continuity with the main intrahepatic ducts. Such cases are regarded as 'surgically operable'. The extent and site of the obstruction or absence of the bile ducts is extremely variable. The most common finding is complete destruction of all the extrahepatic bile ducts with complete obliteration of the lumen and their replacement by fibrous cords which may or may not have a microscopic lumen.

Intrahepatic biliary hypoplasia is characterised by an absence or reduction in the number of bile ducts in the portal tract within the liver substance. Diagnosis requires that in a number of portal tracts normal portal vein and hepatic artery branches can be identified with absent or disproportionately small bile ducts. Intrahepatic biliary hypoplasia is most commonly seen complicating extrahepatic biliary atresia in infants who survive beyond the age of 12 months. It also occurs as an isolated ill-understood syndrome with intact extrahepatic bile ducts. Wedge biopsy of the liver is usually necessary to establish the diagnosis.

Extrahepatic biliary hypoplasia is a term used to describe narrow extrahepatic bile ducts with patent lumen which can usually be demonstrated by operative cholangiography. These bile ducts are generally considered normal but are narrow because of reduced bile flow due to intrahepatic disease.

Aetiology and Pathogenesis of Extrahepatic Biliary Atresia

Although extrahepatic biliary atresia is commonly described as congenital, with the implication that there is a primary failure of development in the bile ducts, this now must be considered as very unlikely. It seems certain that the hepatic parenchymal cells develop as outgrowths from the primitive bile duct system (Koga, 1971). Since hepatocytes are present in abundance in biliary atresia, normal early development of bile ducts must have occurred. Further, the degree of duct involvement is very variable (Alagille, 1972) which is difficult to explain on the basis of a single antenatal insult or abnormality in organogenesis. Also some infants with classical EHBA have been described in whom there is postnatal evidence that the bile ducts were intact (Holden, 1964; Poley et al, 1972; Danks, 1974). Study of the pathological sections removed from the area of the bile ducts now suggest that the condition in the vast majority of cases results from a sclerosing inflammatory lesion initiated in the bile duct epithelium and involving part or all of the biliary tract, starting late in fetal life or early in postnatal life (Landing, 1974). In these the condition may be considered a *progressive obstructive cholangiopathy* with degeneration of bile duct epithelium, luminal obliteration and periductular sclerosis often associated with periportal lymph gland enlargement. The precise cause of this inflammatory reaction is unknown. It has been suggested that both neonatal hepatitis and extrahepatic biliary atresia may be due to the same basic disease process with in some instances the major damage occurring in the bile ducts (Strauss, Valderrama and Alpert, 1972; Alagille, 1972; Landing, 1974). Such a hypothesis is dependent upon the histological similarity of percutaneous liver biopsies in the two conditions and the recovery of putative, causative organisms such as rubella, cytomegalovirus, listeria and hepatitis B antigen. It must be stressed, however, that the extensive hepatocellular changes seen in association with such infections are not found in typical idiopathic extrahepatic biliary atresia. In a recently completed epidemiological study it was observed that short gestation and low birthweight are unusual in EHBA, occurring in only 1 of 32 patients, as opposed to 23 of 103 with hepatitis who were born prematurely, and 35 per cent who were of low birthweight (Mowat et al, 1975). Teratogenic agents interfering with different stages in pre- and postnatal development, or cholangitis destroying formed bile ducts are postulated as possible causes of the cholangiopathy but no agent has as yet been implicated. Twenty-five per cent of infants with biliary atresia have minor or major congenital malformations elsewhere but no single abnormality is associated with biliary atresia. Three of 29 children who were considered for liver transplantation were found to have a composite vascular abnormality, including absence of the inferior vena cava, a preduodenal portal vein, and anomalous hepatic arteries. A further five in this series had anomalous hepatic arterial vasculature (Lilly and Starzl, 1974). Familial cases are distinctly rare and no recognisable pattern of inheritance has been discerned.

A distinct difference between EHBA and other forms of bile duct obstructions such as choledochal cyst or gallstones is that the EHBA the proximal intrahepatic bile ducts do not dilate. Instead the sclerosing cholangiopathy appears to extend within the liver causing marked portal fibrosis and the development of angulated, distorted bile ducts showing apparently aimless proliferation. Within the lumen there are bile plugs. The hepatic arteries show medial hypertrophy. Within the hepatocytes there is prominent cholestasis and some giant cell transformation. As the disease progresses there is increasing fibrosis with a gradual decrease in the number of intrahepatic bile ducts giving the histological appearance of bile duct hyperplasia. Biliary cirrhosis with portal hypertension is the inevitable endpoint. There is considerable case-to-case variation in the rapidity with which this develops.

Clinical features

Jaundice followed by the development of pale stools and dark urine may start at birth but in 50 per cent of patients it is not evident until the child is two to three weeks old. The majority of infants had moderate hepatomegaly and the spleen is usually palpable within the first two months of life (Mowat et al, 1975). Serum bilirubin levels vary considerably from day to day but were usually less than 200 μmol/litre (12 mg/dl) in the first two months of life. Later considerably higher concentrations are found. The direct reacting bilirubin is almost always greater than 68 μmol/litre (4 mg/dl). The stool contains no bilirubin and urobilinogen is absent from both stools and urine. Bilirubin is of course present in urine and can easily contaminate stool specimens causing spurious investigation results. Liver function tests show raised aspartate amino transferase and alkaline phosphatase concentrations but are not helpful in distinguishing biliary atresia from hepatitis. Choledochal cysts may present similarly in the newborn period.

Diagnosis and management

Three main difficulties occur in the early management of the infant with potentially surgically correctable bile duct obstruction; preoperative distinction from the patient with an intrahepatic lesion, the timing of surgery, the choice of operative procedure.

The diagnosis must ultimately be established by laparotomy, operative cholangiography through the gallbladder, if it is present, and inspection of the porta hepatis. The observation that clinical features and standard tests of liver function do not distinguish EHBA from hepatitis has led a number of surgeons to advise laparotomy, open liver biopsy, and operative cholangiography as essential to the management of all infants with the neonatal hepatitis syndrome. Yet Thaler and Gellis, (1968) reported that cirrhosis was three times as common in patients with a primary intrahepatic cause of the jaundice if they had been submitted to such surgical investigation when compared to a group of infants with similar clinical and biochemical abnormalities who had not been subjected to such surgery. Certainly it is arguable that with modern techniques the results would not be deleterious but laparotomy and general anaesthesia still cause changes in hepatic blood flow and transient upset in liver function tests and those who advocate such an approach have yet to demonstrate its safety. It certainly does enable the early diagnosis of choledochal cyst but these account for only approximately 2 per cent of patients with chronic forms of neonatal hepatitis syndrome. The others are unlikely to benefit. Besides on humanitarian and economic grounds unnecessary surgery should be avoided.

From time to time many tests on blood and serum have been advocated as distinguishing extrahepatic biliary atresia from hepatitis with intact extrahepatic ducts but the value of these tests has not subsequently been confirmed in clinical practice. Recently the red cell peroxidase haemolysis test (Luben et al, 1971), the serum concentration of alpha-fetoprotein (Zelzer et al, 1974), lipoprotein-X (Campbell et al, 1974), serum bile salt ratios (Javitt et al, 1973) and 5'-nucleotidase (Sass-Kortsak, 1974) have been reported as being useful. We have not found the red cell haemolysis test of any discriminatory value nor have we been able to confirm that a high serum concentration of chenodeoxycholic acid indicates biliary atresia nor that cholic acid predominates in children with other forms of obstructive liver disease in the newborn period. Using a sensitive radioimmunoassay technique we have found considerable overlap in alpha-fetoprotein concentration in patients with EHBA and neonatal hepatitis at all ages, particularly in the first ten weeks of life (Johnston et al, 1976).

Three lines of investigation must be pursued where biliary obstruction is suspected

The first is systematic investigation to identify known causes of the neonatal hepatitis syndrome bearing in mind that bile duct lesions have occurred in a number of systemic infections. This seems to be distinctly rare and we did not find any in 32 infants with EHBA who were studied prospectively. Three had significant bacterial infection around the time of onset of jaundice (Mowat et al, 1975).

The second is percutaneous liver biopsy which is of considerable value in distinguishing biliary atresia from hepatitis. It should not be performed if the platelet count is less than 40 000 and the prothrombin time prolonged by more than 4 s. Unfortunately there is no single histological feature which is unique for either condition and in some patients there is considerable histological overlap (Brough and Bernstein, 1969). Operative biopsies are no more informative (Hays et al, 1967). EHBA can be considered the most likely diagnosis if there are widened portal tracts with prominent distorted elongated angulated bile ducts, increased fibrosis and inflammatory cell infiltrate, preservation of normal hepatic architecture with cholestasis both in the hepatocytes and in the bile ducts which commonly show bile plugs. A diagnosis of hepatitis is usually made on the basis of prominent hepatocellular necrosis, disorganisation of liver cords, giant cell transformation and inflammatory cell infiltrate in the parenchyma and portal tracts. Cholestasis is particularly prominent within the hepatocytes. While bile duct proliferation and some infiltration of the portal tracts is common in hepatitis, the severity of the portal lesion is much less than that of the hepatocellular one. In a recently completed analysis of histological data on the epidemiological study referred to above (Mowat et al, 1976), only six percutaneous liver biopsies from 82 infants with jaundice without an extrahepatic cause were considered to have pathological features consistent with atresia. Typical pathological features of extrahepatic biliary atresia were present in 15 of 20 percutaneous liver biopsies in patients with biliary atresia. The frequency of correct histological diagnosis was not influenced by the timing of the percutaneous liver biopsy in the first three months of life.

Thirdly, it is very helpful to perform an intravenous radioactive Rose Bengal faecal excretion test to demonstrate complete biliary obstruction. In this test an exactly measured amount of Rose Bengal labelled with ^{131}I or ^{125}I is given intravenously in a dose approximating 1 μCi per kilogram body weight. The Rose Bengal is rapidly taken up by the liver, excreted via the bile into the intestine, faecal recovery reflecting bile flow. Stools uncontaminated with urine must be collected over a three-day period. (Sass-Kortsak, 1974). An excretion of 10 per cent or less is indicative of marked biliary obstruction due to atresia or severe intrahepatic disease.

The results of both the percutaneous liver biopsy and the Rose Bengal excretion test must be considered together in deciding whether a laparotomy is necessary. If the excretion is less than 10 per cent and the biopsy shows features typical of extrahepatic biliary atresia, laparotomy should not be delayed. Where the histological features have been equivocal or suggested hepatitis, it has been our practice to repeat the Rose Bengal excretion test after three weeks during which the infant has taken cholesytramine in a dose of 1 g four times a day. If atresia is present excretion does not change but in hepatitis it is said to rise to greater than 10 per cent (Campbell et al, 1974). We have confirmed these observations in 12 patients with EHBA but have found that in two of four patients with intact extrahepatic ducts the excretion was still less than 5 per cent even after three weeks of cholesytramine. We would not therefore at present advise a three-week delay to repeat an ^{131}I Rose Bengal excretion test if this were to postpone laparotomy to beyond ten weeks of age (vide infra). By combining the results of liver biopsy and Rose Bengal excretion tests we have been able to advise against laparotomy in 95 infants with conjugated hyperbilirubinaemia in whom the jaundice subsequently cleared completely and have correctly advised laparotomy in all cases of biliary atresia and in two cases of choledochal cyst seen in the last five years.

SURGICAL MANAGEMENT

In between 3 and 15 per cent of cases it is possible to anastomose the gallbladder or the attendant bile duct to a Roux-en-Y loop from small bowel, thereby establishing biliary drainage. Unfortunately associated intrahepatic abnormalities, established cirrhosis, or ascending cholangitis will often prevent complete cure but prolonged survival has been reported (Berenson et al, 1974). For the remaining patients various surgical procedures such as prosthesis, resection of part of a lobe of liver with anastamosis to bowel have been tried without success. The operation hepatic portoenterostomy does produce effective bile drainage in up to 40 per cent of such patients and represents a feasible surgical advance in management at this time. In this procedure the portahepatis is explored, residual visible bile duct remnants removed, together with any fibrous tissue, and an anastamosis fashioned between the area of the portahepatis and the edges of the end of a Roux-en-Y loop from jejunum. No attempt is made to link bile ducts directly to bowel mucosa. Nevertheless, effective biliary drainage can be achieved but it is only likely to occur if microscopic patent bile duct remnants of greater than 200 μm are found in the resected tissue (Kasai 1974; Lilly and Altman, 1975). Kasai and co-workers (1975) reported that in 14 of 57 infants operated in this fashion obtained effective bile drainage with survival for more than two years after surgery. The survival period extended up to 18 years with nine surviving for five years or more. Three, however, had cirrhosis and one portal hypertension. Even more remarkable was the observation that in seven of eight infants operated on by ten weeks of age effective bile drainage was achieved. Lilly and Altman (1975) found that 90 per cent achieved bile drainage when operated on by 12 weeks of age if they had microscopic bile ductules in the tissue removed from the portahepatis. In other series, even short-term successes have been rare (Campbell et al, 1974; Danks et al, 1974; Mowat et al, 1975) but in these series surgery had generally been performed late; with early surgery between 30 and 40 per cent of patients should achieve bile drainage. Only more prolonged follow-up of these series will ascertain the final place in management of this procedure.

Just how this operation works is still controversial. Not all investigators concede that bile drains directly from bile ducts to bowel, although Lilly and Altman (1975) seem to show this in two of their patients. The other route of egress of bile from the liver may be via lymphatics. Fonkalsrud, Kitagawa and Longmire, (1966) showed that anastamosis of liver hilum to bowel caused a drop of serum bilirubin because of the establishment of lymphatics between the two areas. Schweitzer (1972) in an experimental model of biliary atresia in the newborn pig, showed that the serum bilirubin concentration returned to normal and hepatic lesions could be completely reversed by anastamosing the serous surface of a loop of bowel to the porta hepatis, facilitating lymphatic drainage from liver to bowel. The possible importance of lymphatic drainage is illustrated in another experimental model in the rhesus monkey in which a section of bile duct had been removed to produce biliary obstruction. Drainage of thoracic duct lymph to bowel prevented progressive liver damage, bile duct continuity was spontaneously re-established and normal bile flow ensued (Devadas, Templeton and Lennard, 1975).

An important clinical problem is 'ascending cholangitis' following hepatic portoenterostomy. This is usually associated with fever, a rise in serum bilirubin and a deterioration in liver function. Associated inflammatory changes often cause bile drainage to cease and may cause permanent liver damage. It is sometimes difficult to distinguish this from secondary failure of bile flow due to stenosis of the drainage system, usually at the porta hepatis, which would require further surgical correction. To try to overcome these difficulties a number of modifications of the original hepatic porto enterostomy has been devised. All include a Roux-en-Y anastamosis with a long loop going to the porta hepatis. Even with this retrograde infection may occur and to prevent this and to allow visual determination of bile flow the loop may be exterioised and its ends opened for a time. The Mikulicz technique used by Lilly and Altman (1975) is relatively simple and should be more free from complications than other described techniques. In spite of many formidable problems there is reason at present to be cautiously optimistic about the place of portoenterostomy in the management of extrahepatic biliary atresia.

TIMING OF SURGERY

Because of the dismal results of surgery in biliary atresia prior to the introduction of hepatic portoenterostomy, together with the difficulties of distinguishing biliary atresia from hepatitis and the wish to avoid laparotomy in the latter, Thaler and Gellis (1968) suggested that surgery should be delayed to four months of age. Because of developments in the last seven years already outlined this is now considered too late and laparotomy should not be delayed when the diagnosis is strongly suspected. Every effort must be made to complete these investigations by 10 weeks of age. Clinicians must be reminded that any hyperbilirubinaemia is abnormal and that if it persists for *more than two weeks biliary atresia* should be suspected.

LIVER TRANSPLANTATION

If effective bile drainage cannot be established, the prognosis is indeed grim. This has led to a number of groups investigating the possibility of performing liver transplantation for such children. Foremost amongst these are Starzl and his co-workers who have carried out liver transplantation in 40 patients with biliary atresia (1975). Eleven of these achieved a one year survival, seven having normal liver function, and one is alive five and a half years after transplantation. Such children have all the problems of any other recipient of a transplant, requiring immunosuppressant drugs. There is as yet an unacceptable mortality from a variety of technical difficulties causing either vascular thrombosis or haemorrhage within a few days of operation, or bile duct complications, usually within a few months. Failure to control rejection and to detect and eliminate infection has also been a problem. Because of these difficulties liver transplantation is not being attempted for this condition by the Cambridge/King's transplantation group. Liver transplantation is clearly a very formidable undertaking which should only be pioneered in units with all the necessary expertise and facilities.

MEDICAL MANAGEMENT

Close attention to details in management can do much to prevent unnecessary suffering in the patient with extrahepatic biliary atresia. Bile salt retention often causes considerable pruritus. This can often be minimised by administering cholestyramine in a dose of between 6 and 16 g/d usually in the form of Questran. Folic acid deficiency, the only recognised complication of this form of therapy, can be prevented by administering adequate amounts of vitamin. A major problem is fat malabsorption due to absent bile flow and the lack of bile salt participation in fat digestion and absorption. This leads to calorie malnutrition and deficiencies of fat-soluble vitamins. These effects may be mitigated by substituting medium-chain triglycerides for ordinary fat in the milk or diet. Fat-soluble vitamins must be given in doses considerably larger than the normal requirements and often parentally. It is necessary to repeat serum calcium, phosphate and prothrombin time regularly. When ascites complicates cirrhosis it may often be controlled for some months with thiazides and spironolactone together with potassium supplements. Febrile illnesses deserve adequate investigation and vigorous treatment. If surgery has produced bile drainage cholangitis must be considered. Repeat blood cultures may be necessary to identify the pathogen. When features of irreversible hepatocellular failure have developed, e.g. hypoalbuminaemia, and vitamin K resistant prolongation of the prothrombin time, the paediatrician's main effort should be concentrated on keeping the patient comfortable.

ENCEPHALOPATHY AND FATTY DEGENERATION OF THE LIVER (REYE'S SYNDROME)

In the last 13 years the pathological features of this syndrome have been clearly defined as an encephalopathy with cerebral oedema without cellular infiltration or demyelination and diffuse fatty infiltration of the liver and to a lesser extent, other organs (Mann et al, 1962; Reye, Morgan and Baral, 1963; Chaves-Carbalo, Gomez and Sharbrough, 1975). Most pathologists and paediatricians now accept the syndrome as a clinical entity, possibly of multiple causes to be suspected in any infant or child in whom an encephalopathy develops after a few days of mild non-specific prodromal illness. Considerable problems still remain regarding many aspects of this disorder. The aetiology is unknown; clinical diagnosis is difficult and pathological diagnosis in life may be impossible; the spectrum of severity may vary from mild to universally fatal; the frequency varies from time to time and from area to area; indices of prognosis have yet to be defined; are the brain and liver primarily affected? does encephalopathy follow disordered hepatic function? last, but not least, what treatment should be used to mitigate the high morbidity and mortality?

Clinical Features

The disorder occurs in children aged two months to fifteen years. A typical patient presents as an acute encephalopathy developing in a child who seems to be recovering from a mild illness. The usual course is fluctuating lethargy and disturbed behaviour with disturbances of consciousness proceeding rapidly to deep coma with death in 24 to 48 h. It is punctuated by sustained seizures with periods of tonic posturing of the limbs with flexed elbows, clenched fists and extended legs progressing to decerebrate rigidity. Hyperpnoea or irregular respiration may suggest the diagnosis. There are no focal neurological signs nor features of meningeal irritation. Mild to moderate hepatomegaly is the only clinical evidence of visceral disease and is often lacking especially in the early stages. The cerebrospinal fluid is normal or may show a low sugar concentration. Raised aspartate aminotransferase levels, prolonged prothrombin time and high blood ammonia and particularly in a child of less than two years, hypoglycaemia should suggest the diagnosis (Glasgow, Cotton and Dhiensiri, 1972). Hyperbilirubinaemia is distinctly rare. Hypoxia, acidosis and raised serum potassium concentrations are commonly found. Liver biopsy is required for confirmation but may be impossible because of the prolonged prothrombin time.

Pathological Features

The liver grossly is yellow-orange, pale yellow or white. Haematoxylin and eosin stained paraffin sections show uniform foaminess of the liver cell cytoplasm with centrally placed nuclei, no hepatocellular necrosis and a singular absence of inflammatory change (Bove, et al, 1975). Frozen sections stained with Sudan show triglycerides throughout the hepatic lobule mainly in small droplets. Birefringent lipid is not seen. Electron microscopic examination shows that all hepatocytes are affected by a process which causes changes in many organelles and much glycogen accumulation. The principal changes are in the mitochondria. In clinically mild cases there is pleomorphism, slight swelling and rarefaction of the matrix. In more severe cases the mitochondria have an amoeboid appearance with distorted limiting membrane. In severe or fatal cases the mitochondria are markedly distended with dense bodies. During recovery the mitochondria seem to divide, bud or branch, the matrix being normal by the fourth day (Schubert, Partin and Partin, 1972). Other striking features include proliferation of the smooth endoplasmic reticulum in all cases, areas of rough endoplasmic reticulum proliferation, a great increase in peroxisomes and decreased low-density lipoprotein particles. Schubert and co-workers (1972) consider that these ultrastructural changes may be unique to Reye's syndrome and that mitochondrial abnormalities are crucial in the pathogenesis. Fat deposition is found in other organs including the kidney, myocardium and pancreas (Brown, Madge and Schiller, 1971). The brain in fatal cases shows oedema and anoxic neural changes (Evans et al, 1970).

Aetiology

Epidemiology. The incidence of this syndrome is difficult to assess varying from isolated occurrences to suggestions that it is a leading cause of death in children aged one to six years in Thailand (Olson et al, 1970). The total number of recorded cases exceeds 500. Between December 1973 and March 1974,

286 suspected or confirmed cases were reported to the Centre for Disease Control in North America (Morbidity and Mortality—Weekly Report, US Dept of Health, 1974). Cases appear to occur in minor outbreaks in a fairly wide area, usually without any recognised link between individual cases. Rarely more than one child may be affected in a family.

No known infectious or toxic agent or metabolic abnormality has been recognised which will consistently cause the clinical, biochemical and histopathological lesions. The characteristic prodrome in some patients suggests that a viral infection may be related in some undetermined way to the development of the syndrome. Viruses have been isolated from tissue in a small number of patients. Varicella and other exanthemas have been prodromal illnesses. The incidence of the syndrome has increased concurrently with influenza epidemics (Glick et al, 1970; Reynolds et al, 1972; Morbidity and Mortality—Weekly Report, US Dept of Health, 1974). It should be stressed that there is no evidence of direct viral invasion of liver or brain.

Toxins which have been considered in the aetiology include salicylates (Norman, 1968; Reynolds et al, 1972), pteridines (Curry, Guttman and Price, 1962) and isopropyl alcohol (Silverman, Roy and Cozzetto, 1971) but the association is limited to only a few cases. There is considerable evidence linking a variety of Reye's syndrome in Thailand with aflatoxin ingestion (Bourgeois et al, 1971). Epidemiological studies show that the disease is prevalent during the rainy season in areas of the country where contamination of foodstuffs with aflatoxin is frequent. There is, however, striking lack of family or village epidemics which suggest that some additional factor may be necessary to produce the disease. There is considerable species differences in the hepatic response to aflatoxin but administration of this agent to young female Macaque monkeys produces the clinical, laboratory and pathological features of Reye's syndrome except that hepatic necrosis is marked and there is bile duct hyperplasia (Bourgeois et al, 1971). It is noteworthy that the greatest hepatic sensitivity to this agent is in the young (Wogan and Pong, 1970).

A further biological toxin which must be considered is hypoglycin, a toxin found in the unripe fruit of the Ackee tree which is considered to be responsible for vomiting sickness of Jamaica (Tanaka, Isselbacher and Shin, 1972). This disorder is characterised by vomiting, hypoglycaemia, depletion of liver glycogen, fatty infiltration of the liver and kidney, coma and death in up to 80 per cent of cases. The incidence is related to age, being highest in younger children and those with a poor nutritional state. It seems unlikely that Reye's syndrome in most parts of the world could result from hypoglycin ingestion but other chemically related substances may require consideration.

The possible importance of a synergistic action of two agents producing this syndrome has been demonstrated in a recent study from Canada (Crocker et al, 1974). An apparent concentration of 13 patients were noted to have occurred in an area which had been heavily sprayed with insecticide. This led to an interesting experiment in which encephalopathy and fatty infiltration of the liver very similar to that seen in Reye's syndrome was induced in young mice by the synergistic action of insecticide and virus. DDT and/or fenitrothion were applied to the skin of the mice for 11 days prior to exposure to sublethal concentrations of an encephalomyocarditis virus. Neither the insecticides alone or in combination or the virus alone caused similar pathological features. Such associations would be difficult to establish by epidemiological studies in man particularly since these insecticides may be stored for a long time in plants, animals and human tissue, but should give a valuable clue to further studies.

A unique pattern of hyperaminoacidanaemia has been reported in this syndrome (Hilty, Romshe and Delamater, 1974) with high alanine, glutamine lycine and alphamino-butyrate being most frequently elevated. Low levels of ornithine transcarbamylase and carbamyl-phosphate-synthetase have been reported in some patients (Thaler, Hoogenraed and Boswell, 1974). It has been suggested therefore that a spectrum of heritable defects in the conversion of ammonia to urea may underly the clinicopathological abnormalities of Reye's syndrome. This hypothesis has not been supported as yet by family studies but it is noteworthy that relapses of Reye's syndrome have been reported (Bove et al, 1975).

The cause of the encephalopathy is undetermined. A toxic factor acting directly on the brain as well as the liver has been suggested but at present it would seem more likely that the encephalopathy is secondary to metabolic effects of the hepatic lesion. Many of the biochemical abnormalities, with the exception of the lack of hyperbilirubinaemia, are similar to those found in acute hepatic failure. Correction of hypoglycaemia rarely reverses the coma. Hyperammonaemia and raised concentrations of non-esterified fatty acids have been implicated (Bourgois et al, 1971). It is noteworthy in experimental animals that these two biochemical abnormalities have an additive effect in causing coma (Zieve et al, 1972).

TREATMENT

Treatment of Reye's syndrome is supportive and empirical. The acute nature of this syndrome, its sporadic occurrence and variable severity, causes great difficulties in assessing the efficacy of other therapeutic regimens which have been advocated from time to time. A major difficulty is in determining objective criteria for severity of the illness in any particular case. The degree of hyperammonaemia has been suggested, levels of more than 200 mmol/litre (300 µg/dl) usually progressing to death, but the blood ammonia level varies a great deal during the course of the illness and may fall to normal concentrations when the patient passes into deep coma and dies. Sequential electroencephalography has been advocated by Aoki and Lombroso (1973) as a useful method of determining the deterioration or improvement of the patient's neurological status. Lovejoy et al (1974) combined the EEG findings with clinical observations, finding that when the patient developed the decorticate rigidity and marked slowing of the EEG recovery without serious neurological sequalae was very unlikely. With such difficulties in assessing prognosis it is not surprising that many forms of treatment have been introduced with early successes that have not subsequently been confirmed. Peritoneal dialysis introduced on the hypothesis that it may remove the toxins and be useful in correcting refractory metabolic abnormalities seemed an important advance (Samaha, Blaue and Berardinelli, 1974) to be denied shortly afterwards (Samaha, 1974). Exchange transfusion which has similar theoretical benefits as well as correction of abnormal clotting factors has not proved to be so efficacious (Lovejoy et al, 1974) as earlier suggested (Huttenlocher, 1972). Glucose and insulin administered together in an attempt to correct the increased levels of free fatty acids has been associated with recovery (Brown and Madge, 1974) but it, like L-citrulline therapy (Delonge, Glick and Shannon, 1974) and nicotinic acid (Powell and Rosenberg, 1972) must also be considered of unproven value.

Therapeutic efforts currently are aimed at correction of hypoglycaemia, electrolyte abnormalities, acidosis and hypoxia. A reduced fluid intake of approximately 1 to $1.2\,\text{litres}/\text{m}^2\,24\,\text{h}^{-1}$ as 10 per cent dextrose with maintenance electrolytes, is generally recommended to try to minimise the risks of cerebral oedema. This regimen will of course, have to be modified depending on the clinical condition particularly if dehydration is present or if there is inappropriate antidiuretic hormone release. Protein is removed from the diet and neomycin given by nasogastric tube together with laxatives and enemata to minimise ammonia absorption from the gut, but this is of no proven value in this condition. It is common also to use dexamethazone to minimise cerebral oedema if increased intracranial pressure is diagnosed. A cooperative multicentric study comparing results of such supportive treatment with the additional effects of peritoneal dialysis, exchange transfusion or glucose and insulin therapy has been initiated. Further studies in the pathophysiology of this condition will, however, be a necessary requisite in developing rational forms of therapy.

ASPECTS OF PORTAL HYPERTENSION IN CHILDHOOD

There are important differences in the causes and management of portal hypertension in children from those in adults; they demand special consideration. Portal hypertension in childhood is fortunately rare. The clinical features and essential pathophysiology are similar to the adult but the causes and thus the prognosis are frequently different. In considering possible surgical intervention a knowledge of the natural history of the various forms of portal hypertension seen in childhood is essential. There are formidable technical difficulties in creating effective portasystemic shunts and portal decompression in infancy and childhood. Splenectomy must be avoided under the age of 10 years since it significantly predisposes the child to the risks of overwhelming infection. Modes of treatment based on experience in the management of portal hypertension in the adult may be ill-advised in the child. Inappropriate investigation and surgery adds significantly to the morbidity and mortality associated with portal hypertension in childhood, even in centres with considerable experience with this condition. Surgery may have been advocated with excessive zeal in children because portal diversion is less commonly followed by hepatic encephalopathy than in the adult, this being particularly so in extrahepatic portal hypertension. It is now appreciated, however, that it may occur even in the non-cirrhotic patient (Voorhees and Price, 1973). Any procedure which decompresses the portal circulation and diverts blood from the liver may cause deterioration of liver function. A most important observation of recent years is that operations to produce portasystemic shunts in children with extrahepatic portal hypertension often are followed by complications requiring further surgery. For many children conservative management is attended with less morbidity and mortality. Irreversible surgical procedures must be postponed until the patient is completely evaluated. As in the adult, portal hypertension usually results from impeded blood flow in the portal venous system which may be due to obstruction of the portal vein or its tributaries, a variety of lesions within the liver or obstruction of venous outflow from the liver. Rarely it results from increased blood flow to or within the liver due to arteriovenous malformations. Portal hypertension may on occasions affect only part of the portal system. Specific therapy may be available for some of the causes of these various forms of portal hypertension. Even when portal hypertension is known to be present, alimentary bleeding may have other causes. Endoscopy is essential. Precise diagnosis is essential if correct management is to be planned and the prognosis assessed.

Investigations

Minimal initial investigations in a child with suspected portal hypertension must include laboratory studies to document the degree of anaemia or hypersplenism, the presence of biochemical evidence of liver disease and barium meal to demonstrate varices in the oesophagus, stomach or duodenum. It must be noted that varices may not be obvious if the patient is hypotensive. Barium studies may also exclude peptic ulcer which occurs more frequently in children with portal hypertension whether due to liver disease or from an extrahepatic cause. Endoscopy is essential if bleeding continues and surgery has to be considered. A liver scan may be helpful in indicating the presence of significant intrahepatic disease. Non-invasive investigations should be undertaken to exclude treatable forms of liver disease.

Definitive steps in the diagnosis are the demonstration of the portal venous anatomy and histological assessment of a liver biopsy specimen. It is usually necessary to perform biopsy and venography under general anaesthetic. Debate continues as to which form of radiological investigation is most helpful.

In a child of greater than five years portal venous anatomy should be demonstrated during the venous phase following selective angiography of the coeliac and superior messenteric arteries performed with catheters inserted via the femoral arteries. The splenic vein and superior mesenteric veins are very satisfactorily demonstrated by this technique together with the portal vein and its intrahepatic branches if they are patent. Where the portal vein is blocked and replaced by a sheet of capillaries the associated collaterals are often poorly demarcated and precise vascular arrangement may be difficult to ascertain. More satisfactory resolution can be obtained by splenic puncture and splenic venography in which a bolus of dye is injected into the spleen and followed towards the liver. This will generally show very clearly the splenic vein and the varices but blood flow from the superior mesenteric vein will dilute the dye and obscure the distal end of the portal vein and associated vessels.

Splenic vein puncture does allow measurement of portal hypertension but has a major disadvantage of occasionally causing subcapsular and intraperitoneal haemorrhage necessitating splenectomy in some infants. It, therefore, should not be undertaken unless the surgeon is prepared to proceed to splenectomy in conjunction with some shunt procedure. If the patient is less than 10 years of age this is a disservice, predisposing the patient to infection as well as resulting in a shunt which is very likely to thrombose. In addition splenectomy removes the portasystemic anastomoses which serve as a bypass to the coronary-oesophageal drainage system. For the child of less than five years small femoral arteries make arterial thrombosis a distinct risk; the prospects of successful surgery are so small that it may be correct to delay angiography either splenic or arterial, until the child is larger and procedures safer. If surgery becomes likely a useful alternative method of demonstrating the portal venous anatomy is to cannulate the umbilical vein by exposing it in its extraperitoneal course 1 to 2 cm above the umbilicus. The portal venous system may then be shown radiographically. This approach is preferential to venography performed at the time of laparotomy by cannulating an intraabdominal vessel immediately prior to carrying out a shunting procedure.

Percutaneous liver biopsy using a Trucut needle is an essential investigation to establish the histological condition of the liver, ascertaining whether or not cirrhosis is present, or whether treatable forms of liver disease, such as chronic active hepatitis or Wilson's disease underly the portal hypertension. Congenital hepatic fibrosis may not be detected on percutaneous liver biopsy, particularly if the Menghini technique is used. Laparoscopy may be helpful in establishing this diagnosis.

The measurement of wedged hepatic vein pressure, which reflects postsinusoidal pressure and is normal in extrahepatic portal hypertension, is rarely employed in paediatric practice although it is a relatively safe procedure. It must be noted that some forms of intrahepatic disease, such as congenital hepatic fibrosis and schistosomiasis, may also have a normal wedged hepatic pressure. High values in the absence of ascites indicates that other intrahepatic causes must be excluded but these can often be suspected on the basis of liver function tests.

Obstruction of Extrahepatic Portal Vein

The portal vein may be obstructed anywhere between the porta hepatis and the hilum of the spleen. It may be replaced by a fibrous remnant, contain an organised blood clot, be compressed from outside, obstructed by a web of diaphragm, or be replaced by a sheet of small channels usually described as cavernous transformation (Myers and Robinson, 1974). Omphalitis, peritonitis, umbilical vein catheterisation, have been incriminated as possible causes but these rarely account for more than 30 per cent of cases in most series (Voorhees et al, 1965). In older children abdominal trauma, duodenal ulcer, pancreatitis, parasitic infection and localised lymph gland enlargement, have on occasions been found to be responsible for portal hypertension.

CLINICAL FEATURES

The majority of patients present with haematemesis and/or melaena caused by bleeding from oesophageal varices. A smaller number have asymptomatic splenic enlargement. Less commonly, abdominal distension, ascites and hypersplenism may be the initial features. The majority present in the first 12 months of life but patients continue to present regularly throughout childhood (Myers and Robinson, 1974).

Abnormal physical findings are limited to those of anaemia and splenomegaly but even this may be absent in the hypotensive patient following bleeding. Similarly varices may not be demonstrated at barium meal at this time. Indeed in some patients the varices will only be obvious if the patient cooperates in a Valsalva manoeuvre or if intramuscular Buscapan (hyoscine-N-butyl bromide) is given. Endoscopy may be necessary to confirm the presence of varices. Standard tests of liver function are normal although bromsulphthalein clearance and hepatic storage decreases with age (Maddrey et al, 1968).

Episodes of bleeding frequently follow upper respiratory tract infections particularly if associated with aspirin administration. With bed rest, sedation and oral antacid, bleeding usually stops spontaneously but blood replacement may be required. Rarely is it necessary to control haemorrhage with a Sengstaken–Blakemore tube. Deaths from haemorrhage are very rare and occurred in only 2 of 338 episodes of haemorrhage in the cases reviewed by Fonkalsrud, Myers and Robinson (1974). Relapses occur at irregular intervals and are much less frequent as the patient reaches his late teens. Encephalopathy rarely complicates alimentary bleeding.

SURGERY

Because bleeding due to portal hypertension is the main symptom, surgical decompression of the portal venous system by creating an effective portasystemic shunt is an attractive mode of therpy particularly since acute portasystemic encaphalopathy is so rare as to be a minor risk. It may however, be a significant late complication (Voorhees and Price, 1973). The major difficulty is in creating an effective shunt which will remain patent. In most instances the portal vein becomes occluded or replaced by multiple small channels which cannot be used for anastamosis. In some instances, however, the distal end is patent, connecting with the coronary, right gastric and pancreatico-duodenal veins, and may be utilised to form a portacaval shunt (Martin, 1972). The operation is technically difficult requiring a retropancreatic approach. The absence of alimentary bleeding afterwards may be due to the ligation of the coronary and gastric veins which is a necessary step in mobilising the portal vein. In the majority of patients the portal vein is not available and one of a variety of shunt procedures has to be considered. A mesocaval shunt with or without a graft joining the superior mesenteric vein to the interior vena cava is currently the procedure of choice if surgery is really necessary (Lampert, Tank and Turcotte, 1974). Like any other shunt it is unlikely to succeed if the shunt diameter is less than 1 cm. Although this procedure in the cirrhotic has been claimed to minimise the risks of portasystemic encephalopathy, this does occur (Smith et al, 1974). The only other shunt procedure which must be considered seriously is a centrally placed splenorenal shunt; but in this too a wide shunt is necessary if early thrombosis is to be avoided. In most series up to 50 per cent of such shunts thrombose (Fonkalsrud et al, 1974). It has been suggested that many thrombose at or shortly after the anastomosis has been created and this can be prevented by local installation of heparin for 48 h after surgery. Venography should be performed at the end of the procedure to determine that the shunt is patent. Excellent short-term results have been reported using this technique (Bismuth and Franco, 1975). Unfortunately rebleeding following a shunt tends to be more severe. This is not, however, the only problem arising from shunt procedures. In a series of cases from two units, one in Los Angeles the other in Melbourne, Fonkalsrud et al (1974) found that 53 of 59 patients with extrahepatic portal hypertension required a total of 164 operations, one patient having 25 in all. Thirteen patients required further shunts. Almost all who had only splenectomy, ligation of varices, gastric diversion, splenic transposition, or make-shift shunts, bled again. No less than 78 operations were required for non-haemorrhagic complications of surgery. In this series those patients treated conservatively with portal hypertension of similar severity to those subjected to surgery, rebled no more frequently than the surgical series.

Splenectomy has no place in the management of the patient with portal vein obstruction except in fashioning a shunt, and possibly in decreasing abdominal distension. In segmental portal hypertension due to splenic vein thrombosis with a patent portal vein, splenectomy is curative. With that single exception, therefore, there is much evidence that with currently available techniques, the child with extrahepatic portal hypertension should be treated conservatively for as long as possible and that certainly shunt procedures should not be undertaken until a shunt diameter of more than 1 cm can be guaranteed. Only rarely may it be necessary to consider an oesophageal transection or injection of varices with sclerosing material. Haematemesis is rarely exsanguinating. It is a dramatic manifestation of disease which is always alarming to the patient, parent and physician. The surgeon, however, has every reason to dissuade them from reacting to this by demanding heroic surgery when the correct advice is to tell the patient to avoid aspirin.

Surgical Management of Intrahepatic Portal Hypertension in Children and Adolescents

In children, as in adults, there are no controlled studies which show portal diversion leads to increased length of survival. It is essential to identify the cause of the liver disease so that specific therapy may be made available, for example surgical drainage of a choledochal cyst. The decision to carry out a shunt procedure has to be made in the light of what is known about the natural history of the particular condition as it affects individual patients, the risk of recurrent haemorrhage and those of surgery. Any procedure causing diversion of portal blood into the systemic circulation may have detrimental effects on both the liver and the rest of the body. The rate of liver decompensation frequently increases after surgery.

A major difference from adults is that portasystemic encephalopathy is less frequently observed in the short-term children except where liver disease is due to schistosomiasis. Conversely, the patient with congenital hepatic fibrosis has a very good prognosis after surgery.

A particularly difficult problem of increasing frequency is the management of portal hypertension in the patient with *cystic fibrosis* (see Chapter 12). Cor pulmonale or pulmonary insufficiency confining the patient to bed are certainly contraindications to surgery. Where features suggesting advanced cirrhosis, such as albumin of less than 3 g/dl, a prothrombin time prolonged by more than 4 s or persistent jaundice with a serum bilirubin of more than 34 μmol/litre are present, these constitute relative hepatic contraindications giving an increased risk of hepatic encephalopathy. A further complication in these patients is that portacaval shunting may be difficult because of associated retroperitoneal oedema and fibrosis. For that reason the operation of choice is probably a mesocaval shunt, if one of sufficient diameter to give effective portal decompression can be guaranteed. If hypersplenism is present splenectomy is necessary to reverse this. It must be recognised, however, that this is a major procedure with increased risks of chest complications. Very careful pulmonary and hepatic assessment is therefore necessary for these patients. They need vigorous physiotherapy before and for a prolonged period following surgery. Nevertheless in carefully selected patients, effective surgery may be followed by a number of years of good life (Tyson, Schuster and Schwachman, 1968) and may even influence survival favourably (Schuster, 1975).

REFERENCES

Aagenaes, Ø., Matlery, A., Elgjo, K., Munthe, E. & Fagerhol, M. (1972) Neonatal cholestasis in alpha-1 antitrypsin deficient children. *Acta paediatrica scandinavica*, **61**, 632–642.
Aagenaes, Ø. (1974) Hereditary recurrent cholestasis with lymphoedema—two new families. *Acta paediatrica scandinavica*, **63**, 465–471.
Alagille, D. (1972) Clinical aspects of neonatal hepatitis. *American Journal of Diseases of Children*, **123**, 287–291.
Alagille, D., Odivere, M., Gautier, M. & Dommergues, J. P. (1975) Hepatic ductular hypoplasia associated with characteristic facies, vertebral malformations, retarded physical, mental and skeletal development, and cardiac murmur. *Journal of Pediatrics*, **86**, 63–71.
Aoki, Y. & Lombroso, C. T. (1973) Prognostic value of electroencephalography in Reye's syndrome. *Neurology (Minneapolis)*, **23**, 333–343.
Berenson, M. M., Garde, A. R. & Moody, F. G. (1974) Twenty-five year survival after surgery for complete extrahepatic biliary atresia. *Gastroenterology*, **66**, 260–263.
Bill, A. H., Brennon, W. S. & Husheby, T. L. (1974) Biliary atresia. New concepts of pathology, diagnosis and management. *Archives of Surgery*, **109**, 367–372.
Bismuth, H. & Franco, D. (1975) Portal hypertension in children under age 6. *International Meeting on Liver Disease in Childhood*. Paris (in press).
British Medical Journal (1974) Leading article. Management of neonatal jaundice. **1**, 469–370.
Bourgeois, C. H., Shank, R. C., Grossman, R. A., Johnsen, E. O., Wooding, W. L. & Chandavimol, P. (1971) Acute aflatoxin B1 toxicity in the Macaque and its similarities to Reye's syndrome. *Laboratory Investigation*, **24**, 206–216.
Bove, K. E., McAdams, A. J., Partin, J. C., Partin, J. S. & Schubert, W. C. (1975) The hepatic lesion in Reye's syndrome. *Gastroenterology*, **69**, 685–697.
Brough, A. J. & Bernstein, J. (1969) Liver biopsy in the diagnosis of infantile obstructive jaundice. *Pediatrics*, **43**, 519–526.
Brown, R. E., Madge, G. E. & Schiller, H. M. (1971) Observations on the pathogenesis of Reye's syndrome. *Southern Medical Journal*, **64**, 942–946.
Brown, R. E. & Madge, G. E. (1974) Therapeutic considerations in Reye's syndrome. *Pediatrics*, **48**, 162–166.
Campbell, D. P., Poley, J. R., Bhatia, M. & Smith, E. I. (1974) Hepatic portoenterostomy—is it indicated in the treatment of biliary atresia? *Journal of Pediatric Surgery*, **9**, 329–333.
Chaves-Carballo, E., Gomez, M. R. & Sharbrough, F. W. (1975) Encephalopathy and fatty infiltration of the viscera (Reye–Johnson syndrome). *Mayo Clinic Proceedings*, **50**, 209–215.
Cossart, Y. E. (1974) Acquisition of hepatitis B antigen in the newborn period. *Postgraduate Medical Journal*, **50**, 334–337.
Cottrall, K., Cook, P. J. L. & Mowat, A. P. (1974) Neonatal hepatitis syndrome and alpha-1 antitrypsin deficiency; an epidemiological study in South-east England. *Postgraduate Medical Journal*, **50**, 3376–3380.
Crocker, J. F. S., Rozee, K. R., Ozere, R. L., Bigout, S. G. & Hutzinger, O. (1974) Insecticide and viral interaction as a cause of fatty visceral changes and encephalopathy in the mouse. *Lancet*, **2**, 22–24.
Curry, A. S., Guttman, H. E. M. & Price, D. E. (1962) Urinary pteridine in a case of liver failure. *Lancet*, **1**, 855–886.
Danks, D. M. & Campbell, P. E. (1966) Extrahepatic biliary atresia; comments on the frequency of potentially operable cases. *Journal of Pediatrics*, **69**, 21–29.
Danks, D. M., Campbell, P. E., Clarke, A. M., Jones, P. G. & Soloman, J. R. (1974) Extrahepatic biliary atresia. The frequency of potentially operable cases. *American Journal of Diseases of Children*, **128**, 684–689.

Danks, D. M. (1974) Discussion of pathology of the bile retention syndrome. *Postgraduate Medical Journal*, **50**, 347.
Delong, G. R., Glick, T. H. & Shannon, D. C. (1974) Citrulline for Reye's syndrome. *New England Journal of Medicine*, **290**, 1488.
Devadas, M., Templeton, A. & Leonard, A. (1975) Restitution of bile duct after ligation and excision on Rhesus monkey. *Journal of Pediatric Surgery*, **10**, 511–513.
Di Toni, R., Luapi, L. & Ansanell, V. (1968) Glucuronation of the liver of premature babies. *Nature*, **212**, 265–269.
Dommergues, J. P. (1973) Hepatites infectieuses non virales du nourrisson. *La Revue du Praticien*, **23**, 4941–4954.
Dupuy, J. M., Frommel, D. & Alagille, D. (1975) Severe viral hepatitis type B in infancy. *Lancet*, **1**, 191–193.
Emery, J. L. (1974) Pathology with reference to the bile retention syndrome. *Postgraduate Medical Journal*, **50**, 344–347.
Eriksson, S. & Larsson, C. (1975) Purification and partial characterisation of PAS-positive inclusion bodies from the liver in alpha-1 antitrypsin deficiency. *New England Journal of Medicine*, **292**, 176–180.
Evans, H., Bourgeois, C. H., Corner, D. S. & Keschamras, N. (1970) Brain lesion in Reye's syndrome. *Archives of Pathology*, **90**, 543–552.
Fagerhol, M. (1975) Alpha-1 antitrypsin. *Unigate Paediatric Workshop* (in press).
Fonkalsrud, E. W., Kitagawa, S. & Longmire, W. P. (1966) Hepatic lymphatic drainage to the jejunum for congenital biliary atresia. *American Journal of Surgery*, **112**, 188–194.
Fonkalsrud, E. W., Myers, N. A. & Robertson, M. J. (1974) Management of extrahepatic portal hypertension in children. *Annals of Surgery*, **180**, 487–493.
Freier, E., Sharp, H. L. & Bridges, R. A. (1968) Alpha-1 antitrypsin deficiency associated with familial infantile liver disease. *Clinical Chemistry*, **14**, 782–783.
Geardner, L. I. (1974) Intrahepatic bile stasis in 45X Turner's syndrome. *New England Journal of Medicine*, **290**, 406–407.
Giles, J. P., McCullum, R. W., Berndston, L. W. & Krugman, S. (1969) Viral hepatitis: relationship of Australia/SH antigen to the Willobrook MS-2 strain. *New England Journal of Medicine*, **281**, 119–122.
Glasgow, A. M., Cotton, R. B. & Dhiensiri, K. (1972) Reye's syndrome. Blood ammonia and consideration of the non-histologic diagnosis. *American Journal of Diseases of Children*, **124**, 827–833.
Glasgow, J. F. T., Lynch, M. J., Hercz, M. J., Levison, H. & Sass-Kortsak, A. (1973) Alpha-1 antitrypsin deficiency in association with both cirrhosis and chronic obstructive lung disease in two siblings. *American Journal of Medicine*, **54**, 181–194.
Glick, T. H., Likosky, W. H., Levitt, L. P., Mellin, H. & Reynolds, B. W. (1970) Reye's syndrome: an epidemiological approach. *Pediatrics*, **46**, 371–375.
Hilty, M. D., Romshe, C. A. & Delamater, P. V. (1974) Reye's syndrome and hyperaminoacidaemia. *Journal of Pediatrics*, **84**, 362–365.
Harris, R. C. (1974) Negative urine surgars in galactosaemia. *Pediatrics*, **53**, 768.
Hays, D. M., Wolley, M. M., Snyder, W. H., Reed, G. B., Gwinn, J. L. & Landing, B. H. (1967) Diagnosis of biliary atresia: relative accuracy of percutaneous liver biopsy, open liver biopsy, and operative cholangiography. *Journal of Pediatrics*, **71**, 548–607.
Holden, T. M. (1964) Atresia of the extrahepatic bile ducts. *American Journal of Surgery*, **107**, 458–460.
Huttenlocher, P. R. (1972) Reye's syndrome: relation of outcome to therapy. *Journal of Pediatrics*, **80**, 845–850.
Javitt, N. B., Morrissey, K. P., Siegal, E., Goldberg, H., Gartner, L. M., Hollander, M. & Kok, E. (1973) Cholestatic syndromes in infancy: diagnostic value of serum bile acid patterns and cholestryamine administration. *Pediatric Research*, **7**, 119–125.
Jeppsson, J. O. & Laurell, C. B. (1975) Function and chemical composition of alpha-1 antitrypsin. Proteases and biological control. *2nd Coldspring Harbour Symposium in Quantitatve Biology* (in press).
Jeppsson, J. O., Larsson, C. & Eriksson, S. (1975) Characterisation of alpha-1 antitrypsin in the inclusion bodies from the liver in alpha-1 antitrypsin deficiency. *New England Journal of Medicine*, **293**, 576–579.

Jirsova, V., Jirsa, M., Heringova, A., Koldovsky, O. & Weirichova, J. (1967) The use and possible diagnostic significance of Sefadex gel filtration of serum from icteric newborn. *Biologica neonatorum*, **11**, 204–209.
Johnston, D. J., Mowat, A. P., Orr, H., & Kohn, J. (1976) Alpha-fetoprotein in the diagnosis of obstructive jaundice. *Acta Paediatrica Scandinavica* (in press).
Kasai, M. & Suzuki, S. (1957) A new operation for 'non-correctable' biliary atresia; hepatic portoenterostomy. *Shujutsu*, **13**, 733–739.
Kasai, M. (1974) Hepatic portoenterostomy and its modifications for 'non-correctable' biliary atresia. *Pediatrician*, **3**, 204–212.
Kasai, M., Watanabe, I. & Ohi, R. (1975) Follow-up studies of long-term survivors after hepatic portoenterostomy for 'non-correctable' biliary atresia. *Journal of Pediatric Surgery*, **10**, 173–182.
Kattamis, C., Demetriou, D., Karamula, K., Davri-Karamouzi, Y. & Matsaniotis, N. (1973) Neonatal hepatitis associated with Australian antigen (AU-1). *Archives of Disease in Childhood*, **48**, 133–136.
Koaga, A. (1971) Morphogenesis of intrahepatic bile ducts of the human fetus. *Zeitschrift für Anatomie und Entwicklungsgeschichte*, **153**, 156–184.
Kohler, P. F., Dubois, R. S., Merrill, D. A. & Bowes, W. A. (1974) Prevention of chronic neonatal hepatitis B virus infection with antibody to hepatitis B surface antigen. *New England Journal of Medicine*, **291**, 1378–1380.
Lampert, M. J., Tank, E. S. & Turcotte, J. G. (1974) Late sequelae of mesocaval shunt in children. *American Journal of Surgery*, **125**, 19–25.
Landing, P. H. (1974) Consideration of the pathogenesis of neonatal hepatitis, biliary atresia, and choledochal cyst—the concept of infantile obstructive cholangiopathy. *Progress in Paediatric Surgery*, **6**, 113–139. Berlin: Munchen.
Lathe, G. H. (1974) Newborn jaundice; bile pigment metabolism in the fetus and newborn. *Scientific Foundation of Paediatrics*, ed. Davis, G. A. & Dobbing, J., pp. 105–191. London: Heinemann.
Levi, A. J., Gaitmaiten, Z. & Arias, I. M. (1970) Two hepatic cytoplasmic proteins and their possible role in the hepatic uptake of bilirubin bromsulphthalein and other anions. *New England Journal of Medicine*, **283**, 1136–1138.
Lilly, J. R. & Altman, R. P. (1975) Hepatic portoenterostomy (the Kasai operation), for biliary atresia. *Surgery*, **78**, 76–86.
Lilly, J. R. & Starzl, T. E. (1974) Liver transplantation in children with biliary atresia and vascular anomalies. *Journal of Pediatric Surgery*, **9**, 707–713.
Linarelli, L. G., Williams, C. N. & Phillips, M. J. (1972) Byler's disease: fatal intrahepatic cholestasis. *Journal of Pediatrics*, **81**, 484–492.
Lou, M. A., Schmutzer, K. J. & Regan, J. F. (1972) Congenital extrahepatic biliary atresia. *Archives of Surgery*, **105**, 771–774.
Lovejoy, S. H., Smith, A. L., Brennan, M. J., Wood, J. N., Victor, B. I. & Adams, P. C. (1974) Clinical staging in Reye's syndrome. *American Journal of Diseases of Children*, **128**, 36–41.
Lubin, B. H., Baehner, R. L., Schwartz, E., Shohet, S. B. & Nathan, D. G. (1971) The red cell hemolysis test in the differential diagnosis of obstructive jaundice in the newborn period. *Pediatrics*, **48**, 562–565.
Lucey, J. F. (1972) Neonatal jaundice and phototherapy. *Pediatric Clinics of North America*, **19**, 827–839.
Maddrey, W. C., Gupta, K. P. S., Mallik, K. C. B., Iber, M. L. & Basu, A. K. (1968) Extrahepatic obstruction of the portal venous system. *Surgery, Gynecology and Obstetrics*, **127**, 989–998.
Makino, S. & Reed, C. E. (1970) Distribution and elimination of exogenous alpha-1 antitrypsin. *Journal of Laboratory and Clinical Medicine*, **75**, 742–751.
Maisels, M. J., Pathak, A., Nelson, N. H., Nathan, D. G. & Smith, C. A. (1971) Exogenous production of carbon monoxide in normal and erythroblastic newborn infants. *Journal of Clinical Investigation*, **50**, 1–11.
Maisels, M. J. (1972) Bilirubin; on understanding and influencing its metabolism in the newborn infant. *Pediatric Clinics of North America*, **19**, 447–501.
Mann, T., Nash, F. W., Elliott, R. I. K. & Sherlock, S. (1962) Liver disease in infancy. *Postgraduate Medical Journal*, **384**, 642–652.

Martin, L. W. (1972) Changing concepts of management of portal hypertension in children. *Journal of Pediatric Surgery*, **7**, 559–564.

Mowat, A. P., Pscharopolous, H. & Williams, R. (1976) Extrahepatic biliary atresia contrasted with neonatal hepatitis; pathogenesis, early diagnosis and management. *Archives of Diseases in Childhood* (in press).

Myers, A. & Robinson, M. J. (1974) Extrahepatic portal hypertension in children. *Journal of Pediatric Surgery*, **8**, 467–473.

Neville, B. G. R., Lake, B. D., Stephens, R. & Saunders, M. D. (1973) A neuro-visceral storage disorder with vertical supranuclear ophthalmoplegia and its relationship to Neimann–Pick disease. *Brain*, **96**, 97–120.

Norman, M. G. (1968) Encephalopathy and fatty degeneration of the viscera in childhood. *Canadian Medical Association Journal*, **99**, 522–534.

Odell, G. B., Storey, G. N. B. & Rosenberg, L. A. (1970) Studies in kernicterus. 3. The saturation of serum proteins with bilirubin during neonatal life and its relationships to brain damage at five years. *Journal of Pediatrics*, **76**, 12–23.

Odievre, M., Pinon, F., Schirar, M., Luzeau, R. & Sauvageot, M. (1970) The fraction of bilirubin not conjugated and the place of albumin in hyperbilirubinaemia in the newborn. *Archives Français Pediatrie*, **27**, 225–231.

Olson, L. C., Bourgeois, C. H., Keschamres, N. & Dhiensiri, K. (1970) Encephalopathy and fatty degeneration of the viscera in Thai children. *American Journal of Diseases of Children*, **120**, 1–2.

Ostrow, J. D. (1972) Photochemical and biochemical basis of the treatment of neonatal jaundice. *Progress in Liver Diseases*, ed. Popper, H. & Schaffner, F., Vol. 4. Ch. 26, pp. 447–462. New York and London: Grune & Stratton.

Poland, R. D. & Odell, G. B. (1971) Physiologic jaundice: the intrahepatic circulation of bilirubin. *New England Journal of Medicine*, **284**, 1–4.

Poley, J. R., Smith, E. I., Booth, B. J. & Campbell, D. P. (1972) Lipoprotein-X and the double ^{131}I Rose Bengal test in the diagnosis of prolonged infantile jaundice. *Journal of Pediatric Surgery*, **7**, 660–669.

Porter, C. A., Mowat, A. P., Cooke, P. J. L., Haynes, D. W. G., Shilkin, K. B. & Williams, R. (1972) Alpha-1 antitrypsin deficiency and neonatal hepatitis. *British Medical Journal*, **3**, 435–439.

Powell, H. C. & Rosenberg, R. M. (1972) Encephalopathy and fatty degeneration of the viscera. *Lancet*, **1**, 1292.

Reye, R. D. K., Morgan, G. & Baral, J. (1963) Encephalopathy and fatty degeneration of the viscera; a disease entity in childhood. *Lancet*, **2**, 749–752.

Reynolds, D. W., Reiley, H. D., Lafont, D. S., Vorse, H., Stout, C. & Carpenter, R. L. (1972) An outbreak of Reye's syndrome associated with influenza B. *Journal of Pediatrics*, **80**, 429–432.

Samaha, F. J., Blau, A. & Berardinelli, J. L. (1974) Reye's syndrome; clinical diagnosis and treatment with peritoneal dialysis. *Pediatrics*, **53**, 336–340.

Samaha, M. J. (1974) Therapeutic riddle in Reye's syndrome. *Pediatrics*, **54**, 265.

Sass-Kortsak, A. (1974) Management of young infants presenting with direct-reacting hyperbilirubinaemia. *Pediatric Clinics of North America*, **21**, 777–799.

Schubert, W. C., Partin, J. C. & Partin, J. S. (1972) Encephalopathy and fatty liver (Reye's syndrome) *Progress in Liver Disease*, ed. Popper, H. & Schaffner, F., Vol. 4, pp. 489–510. New York: Grune & Stratton.

Schuster, S. (1975) Indications and results of surgical treatment of portal hypertension in childhood. *Proceedings of the 9th European Federation Congress of the International College of Surgeons*.

Schweitzer, I. L., Wing, A., McPeak, C. & Spears, R. L. (1972) Hepatitis and hepatitis associated antigen in 56 mother and infant pairs. *Journal of the American Medical Association*, **220**, 1092–1095.

Schweitzer, I. L., Dunn, A. E. G., Peter, R. L. & Spears, R. L. (1972) A new procedure for drainage in bile duct atresia; an experimental study. Doctoral thesis.

Silverman, A., Roy, C. C. & Cozzetto, F. J. (1971) *Paediatric Clinical Gastroenterology*, **3**, 705.

Schweitzer, I. L., Dunn, A. E. G., Peter, R. L. & Spears, R. L. (1973) Viral hepatitis B in neonates and infants. *American Journal of Medicine*, **55**, 762–771.

Schweizer, P. (1972) A new procedure for drainage in bile duct atresia: an experimental study. Doctoral thesis, University of Tubingen.
Sharpe, H. L. (1971) Alpha-1 antitrypsin deficiency. *Hospital Practice*, **6**, 83–96.
Silverman, A., Roy, C. C. & Cozzetto, F. J. (1971) Reye's syndrome. *Paediatric Clinical Gastroenterology*, p. 345. St Louis: Mosby.
Smith, M., Tuft, R. J., Davidson, A. R., Laws, J. W., Dawson, J. L. & Williams, R. (1974) Mesentericocaval 'jump' graft in management of portal hypertension: experience with 24 cases. *British Medical Journal*, **3**, 705–708.
Starzl, T. (1976) Liver transplantation in management of biliary atresia. *International Meeting on Paediatric Liver Disease*, Paris, 1975 (in press).
Stevens, C. E., Beasley, T. R., Tsuy, J. & Lee, W. (1975) Vertical transmission of hepatitis B virus in Taiwan. *New England Journal of Medicine*, **292**, 771–774.
Strauss, L., Valderrama, E. & Alpert, L. I. (1972) Biliary tract anomalies: the relationship of biliary atresia to neonatal hepatitis. *Birth Defects: Original Article Series*, **1**, 135–148.
Talamo, R. C. (1975) Basic and clinical aspects of the alpha-1 antitrypsin. *Pediatrics*, **56**, 91–99.
Talbot, I. C. & Mowat, A. P. (1975) Liver disease in infancy: histological features and relationship to alpha-1 antitrypsin phenotype. *Journal of Clinical Pathology*, **28**, 559–563.
Tanaka, K., Isselbacher, K. J. & Shin, V. (1972) Isovaleric and alpha-methyl butyric acidaemia induced by hypoglycin A: mechanism of Jamaican vomiting sickness. *Science*, **175**, 69–71.
Taylor, A. (1968) Autosomal trisomy hepatitis syndromes. *Journal of Medical Genetics*, **5**, 2227–2235.
Thaler, M. M. & Gellis, S. S. (1968) Studies in neonatal hepatitis and biliary atresia. *American Journal of Diseases of Children*, **116**, 257–279.
Thaler, M. M., Hoogenraed, M. J. & Boswell, M. (1974) Reye's syndrome due to a novel protein tolerant variant of ornithine transcarbamylase deficiency. *Lancet*, **2**, 438–439.
Tyson, K. R. T., Schuster, S. R. & Shwachman (1968) Portal hypertension in cystic fibrosis. *Journal of Pediatric Surgery*, **3**, 271–277.
US Department of Health (1974) Morbidity and Mortality—Weekly Report, **23**, 115.
Valayer, H. S. (1975) Hepatic portoenterostomy for biliary atresia. Presented at an International Meeting on Paediatric Liver Disease, Paris (in press).
Valman, H. B., France, N. E. & Wallis, P. G. (1971) Prolonged neonatal jaundice in cystic fibrosis. *Archives of Disease in Childhood*, **46**, 805–809.
Voorhees, A. B. J., Harris, R. C., Britton, R. C., Price, J. B. & Santulli, T. V. (1965) Portal hypertension in children. *Surgery*, **58**, 540–552.
Voorhees, A. B. J. & Price, J. B. (1973) Portosystemic encephalopathy in non-cirrhotic patient. *Surgery*, **107**, 659–661.
Waters, W. J. (1967) The reserve albumin binding capacity as a criterion for exchange transfusion. *Journal of Pediatrics*, **70**, 185–192.
Watson, G. H. & Miller, V. (1973) Arterio-hepatic displasia. *Archives of Disease in Childhood*, **48**, 459–466.
Wilkinson, E. J., Raab, K., Browning, C. A. & Hosty, T. A. (1974) Familial hepatic cirrhosis in infants associated with alpha-1 antitrypsin SZ phenotype. *Journal of Pediatrics*, **85**, 159–164.
Wogan, G. N. & Pong, R. S. (1970) Aflatoxins. *Annals of the New York Academy of Sciences*, **174**, 623–635.
Wright, R., Perkins, J. R., Bower, B. D. & Jerrome, D. W. (1970) Cirrhosis associated with the Australia antigen in an infant who acquired hepatitis from her mother. *British Medical Journal*, **4**, 719–721.
Zeive, L., Zeive, F. J., Doizaki, W. M. & Gilsdorf, R. B. (1972) Studies on the production of coma by toxic substances abnormally present in liver failure. *Abstracts Book of the Fifth Meeting of the International Association for the Study of the Liver*, Paris, p. 71.
Zeltzer, P. M., Neerhout, R. C., Fonkalsrud, E. W. & Stiehm, E. R. (1974) Differentiation between neonatal hepatitis and biliary atresia by measuring serum alpha-fetoprotein. *Lancet*, **1**, 373–375.

12
CYSTIC FIBROSIS OF THE PANCREAS

Charlotte M. Anderson

Perhaps the excuse for the inclusion of a chapter on cystic fibrosis of the pancreas in a volume of 'Recent Advances' is to allow the natural history and management of this disorder, particularly in the years after childhood, to be brought to the closer attention of gastroenterologists and others caring for adult patients. Recognition of the disease entity (now usually known simply as *cystic fibrosis* or just CF) dates back only to the late 1930s and although knowledge of its primary metabolic basis remains scanty information regarding the natural history in childhood, and more recently in adolescence and adulthood, is more complete. Until the early 1950s expectation of life except in rare instances was very short. Since then both treatment and earlier diagnosis have led to a considerable change so that clinicians caring for considerable numbers of CF patients are able to predict that 60 to 80 per cent will now reach adult life (Shwachman and Holsclaw, 1969; Warwick and Pogue, 1969; Huang et al, 1970; Gurry, 1975).

In cystic fibrosis the major clinical features are considered to be consequent upon a generalised disturbance of exocrine secretory tissue function in that exocrine secretions manifest abnormal physicochemical properties which are particularly evident in the respiratory, gastrointestinal and reproductive tracts, but also in sweat and saliva. The condition is believed to be the commonest *inherited* disorder presenting in populations of Caucasian origin; the most frequent cause of chronic suppurative lung disease in children and young adults in 'developed countries'; responsible for over 90 per cent of malabsorptive problems associated with pancreatic exocrine insufficiency in the young; and a numerically important cause of liver cirrhosis and portal hypertension in teenage and early adulthood. Therefore the disease merits consideration by gastroenterologists because it will with increasing frequency, in the future, call upon their expertise for its continuing management. This chapter will discuss the pathogenesis of the condition emphasising gastroenterological aspects; the clinical features and methods of treatment emphasising those concerned with adolescence and adulthood and, lastly, indicate avenues of past and current research into the basic defect.

INCIDENCE
CF has been described most often in people of Caucasian origin and is

therefore widespread in Europe, the American continent, Australia, New Zealand and South Africa but it is not confined to this ethnic group although present data indicate a much lower incidence in other races. Earlier studies in the USA (Kramm et al, 1962), Australia (Danks, Allan and Anderson, 1965) and England (Hall and Simpkiss, 1968) showed a minimum incidence to be between 1:2000 and 1:2500 live births. Recent evidence from studies of meconium protein levels in newborns with subsequent confirmation of the diagnosis of CF by the 'sweat test' suggest incidence figures in those of Caucasian origin of 1:1850 (Prosser et al, 1974) and 1:1800 (Stephan et al, 1975). This newborn screening test probably detects less than 85 per cent of cases and therefore the true incidence may be nearer to 1:1500 live births. An incidence of 1:100 000 has been calculated for Mongoloid races (Wright, 1969) and 1:17 000 for Negroid races (Kulczycki and Schauf, 1974) but studies of the latter in most detail are reported from America where admixture with the white race makes it difficult to interpret incidence figures. It seems possible from recent reports (Reddy et al, 1969; Goodchild et al, 1974a) that the incidence among Pakistanis and Indians is greater than has been suspected hitherto, although of course these races have a Caucasian origin.

INHERITANCE

CF is inherited in an autosomal recessive way (Danks et al, 1965). There is no difference in sex incidence at birth and chromosomal number and structure are considered normal. Chromosome banding techniques have not shown a marker for the defective gene, nor any strong evidence for linkage between CF and other disorders or markers (Goodchild et al, in press).

The *gene carrier frequency* in a community of Caucasian origin is calculated to be 1:25, the highest frequency for an abnormal gene in such a community. As more CF children survive to adult life and marry, the genetic risk to their children comes into question but this is not great. These survivors will transmit the gene to all their children but, for the disease to be manifest, the other parent must also be a carrier. The risk to children of those affected has been estimated to be 1:40 to 1:50.

Carriers of the gene (heterozygotes) show no symptoms of cystic fibrosis. At the time of writing they cannot be distinguished reliably from non-carriers nor is there a published reliable method for detection of the disease in utero, although these problems are being actively studied (Conover et al, 1973b; Wilson, Fudenberg and Jahn, 1975).

Because until recently the condition has been lethal before the reproductive age, the continuance of a high gene carrier frequency has led geneticists to postulate an advantage in being a heterozygote. Some studies show an increased birth rate in preceding generations of known heterozygotes (Danks et al, 1965; Knudson, Wayne and Hallett, 1967) but this aspect needs further study.

PATHOGENESIS

The pathological changes in CF are notable for their widespread extent and enormous variability. Throughout the body there is an alteration in the nature of mucous, macromolecular-containing and serous secretions in that the first of these are abnormally sticky or dry and the latter two are concentrated. These characteristics hinder dispersion of the secretions and allow blockage of ducts or ductules from the consequences of which much of the organ abnormalities are derived. These abnormalities, apparent in a number of organs (Fig. 12.1) are particularly important in the lungs and pancreas, leading to the cardinal clinical features of the disease: a progressive obstructive suppurative chest disorder, together with malabsorption due predominantly to an insufficiency of pancreatic digestive enzyme secretion.

The sweat is the most obviously abnormal of the serous secretions in that the sodium and chloride content is three to four times that of normal; other serous secretions such as those of the salivary glands show a similar alteration of electrolyte content but this is less marked and not apparent clinically.

Descriptions of the morbid pathology of CF substantially unaltered by treatment are to be found in earlier publications such as those of Andersen (1938), Zuelzer and Newton (1949) and in Bodian's classic monograph (1952).

Figure 12.1 illustrates the pathogenesis based on a generalised abnormality of exocrine gland secretions, relates the final symptomatology to relevant organ pathology and suggests a means by which this was produced.

Alimentary System

Pathological change of varying degree occurs in exocrine secretory cells and organs along the alimentary tract. The degree of change depends to a large extent on whether secretions are delivered from cells with narrow necks (goblet cells), from wide-mouthed ducts (Brunner's glands) or along narrow ducts and ductules (pancreas, liver, salivary glands), the dry sticky secretions more easily blocking the latter with resultant structural change in distal tissue.

Pancreas

This organ shows the greatest structural alteration with maximal alteration in function. Secretions precipitate within the lumen of the ducts causing blockage and duct dilatation which may, on histological section, look like small cysts. Destruction of exocrine secretory tissue and replacement with fibrous and fatty tissue ensues.

Structural and functional changes are evident from birth and the former have been described in premature infants dying of meconium ileus although they were of a somewhat lesser degree than in later infancy. Figure 12.2 illustrates the progression of events in the pancreas. The islets of Langerhans

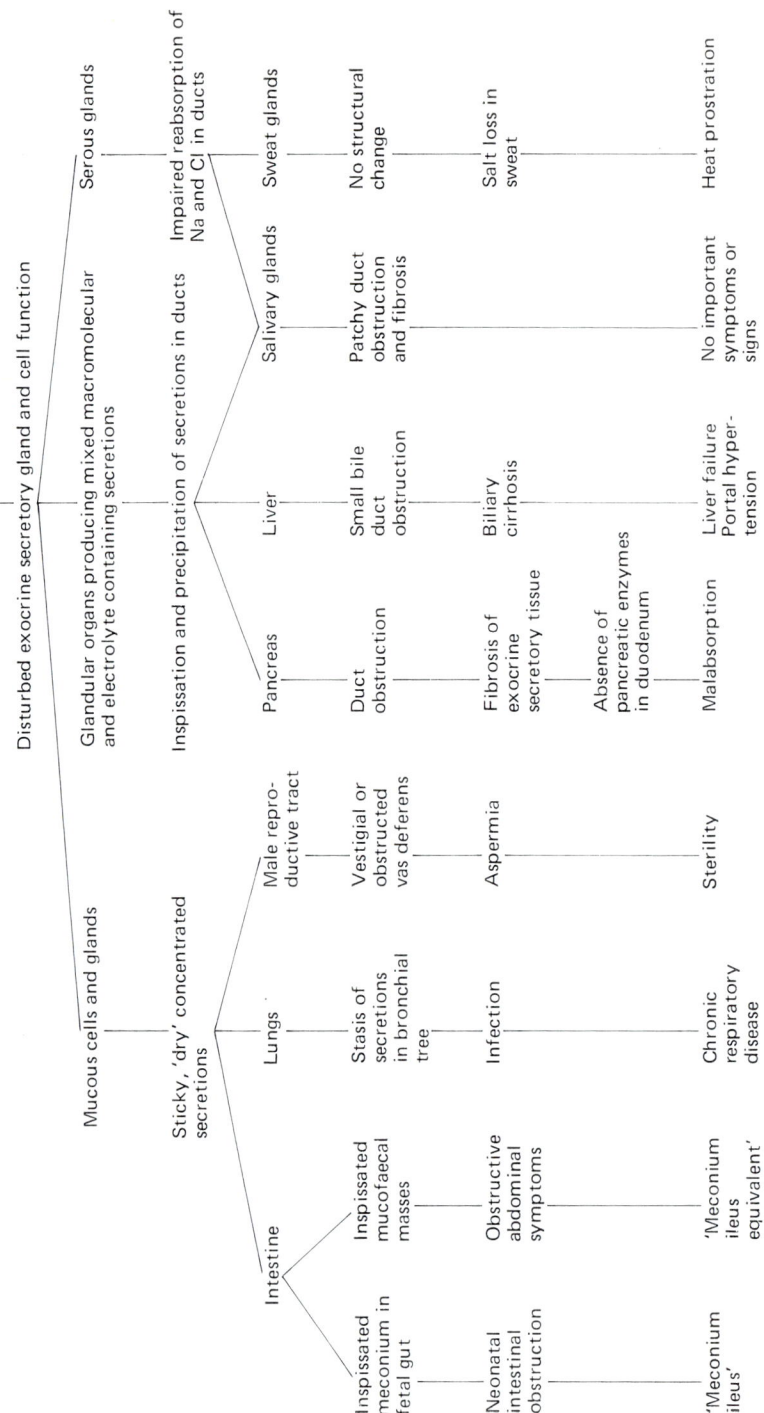

Figure 12.1 Pathogenesis of cystic fibrosis of the pancreas

are usually normal to light microscopy but the development of diabetes mellitus in some older patients has led to the suggestion that blood supply to the islets may become impaired by progressive fibrosis.

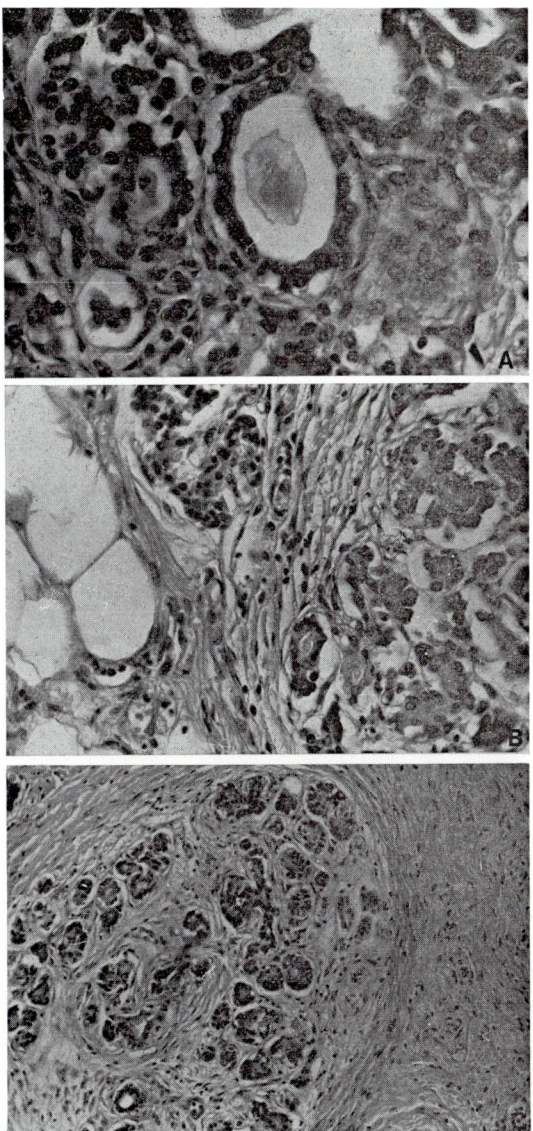

Figure 12.2 Histological appearance of pancreas in cystic fibrosis illustrating the progression of the changes. A: Inspissated material in ducts—'casts'. B: Fibrosis, lipomatous replacement tissue and inspissated secretion in ducts. C: Advanced fibrotic changes
(Reproduced, with permission, from Hadorn (1975) in *Paediatric Gastroenterology*, ed. Anderson and Burke. Oxford: Blackwell)

Steatorrhoea and creatorrhoea are usually present from birth because lipolytic and proteolytic enzymes fail to reach the duodenum via the pancreatic ducts. Duodenal content is scanty, mucosy, rarely alkaline and contains negligible amounts of lipase, trypsin, chymotrypsin and amylase. Stools are characteristically bulky, oily and offensive, the latter being contributed to by bacterial breakdown products of proteins. Fat appears in the faeces largely as fat globules while starch grains and meat fibres are obvious in older patients.

PARTIAL PANCREATIC INSUFFICIENCY

In some infants stools are normal after birth for a few weeks or months, indicating the temporary presence of some pancreatic exocrine secretion. Evidence from studies of large groups of patients indicates that 10 to 15 per cent retain some functioning pancreatic tissue throughout life because they do not show steatorrhoea or creatorrhoea. Investigation of pancreatic function in such patients (Hadorn, Johansen and Anderson, 1968) indicates that, although the duodenal juice is of low volume and 'mucosy' in nature, enzymes are present which increase after i.v. pancreozymin, often to normal concentration. However the usual volume and bicarbonate response to i.v. secretin is almost or completely, absent, indicating that although some acinar function may be retained ductular function in these patients is not normal. Such observations led Johansen, Anderson and Hadorn (1968) to postulate that inspissation and precipitation of secretions in pancreatic ducts were a consequence of the failure of production of a watery secretion which normally flushed the macromolecular acinar secretion along the ducts into the duodenum. They suggested that the marked damage of pancreatic acinar tissue compared with that in salivary glands was related to the proteolytic enzyme content of obstructed pancreatic secretions which, even prenatally, could initiate destruction of acinar cells and stimulate fibrosis.

Pancreatic calcification does not seem to occur but recently Shwachman, Lebenthal and Khaw (1975) have observed recurrent attacks of *acute pancreatitis* in patients with *partial pancreatic insufficiency*.

The liver

Pathological changes in the liver were described in the early writings of both Andersen (1938) and Bodian (1952) and have been elaborated by Craig, Haddad and Shwachman (1957), Webster and Williams (1953), and di Sant'-Agnese and Blanc (1956). Minor changes can be demonstrated in almost all young infants dying of CF and may even be present at birth (Campbell and Anderson, unpublished observations). These consist predominantly of bile ductule plugging with inspissated material (Fig. 12.3A) but small scattered foci of fibrosis and pericholangitis are also present. Later the portal tracts become prominent, bile ducts more numerous and periportal fibrosis increases (Fig. 12.3B). In most patients these changes progress slowly, the rate of progress being variable and unpredictable. In about 10 to 15 per cent of

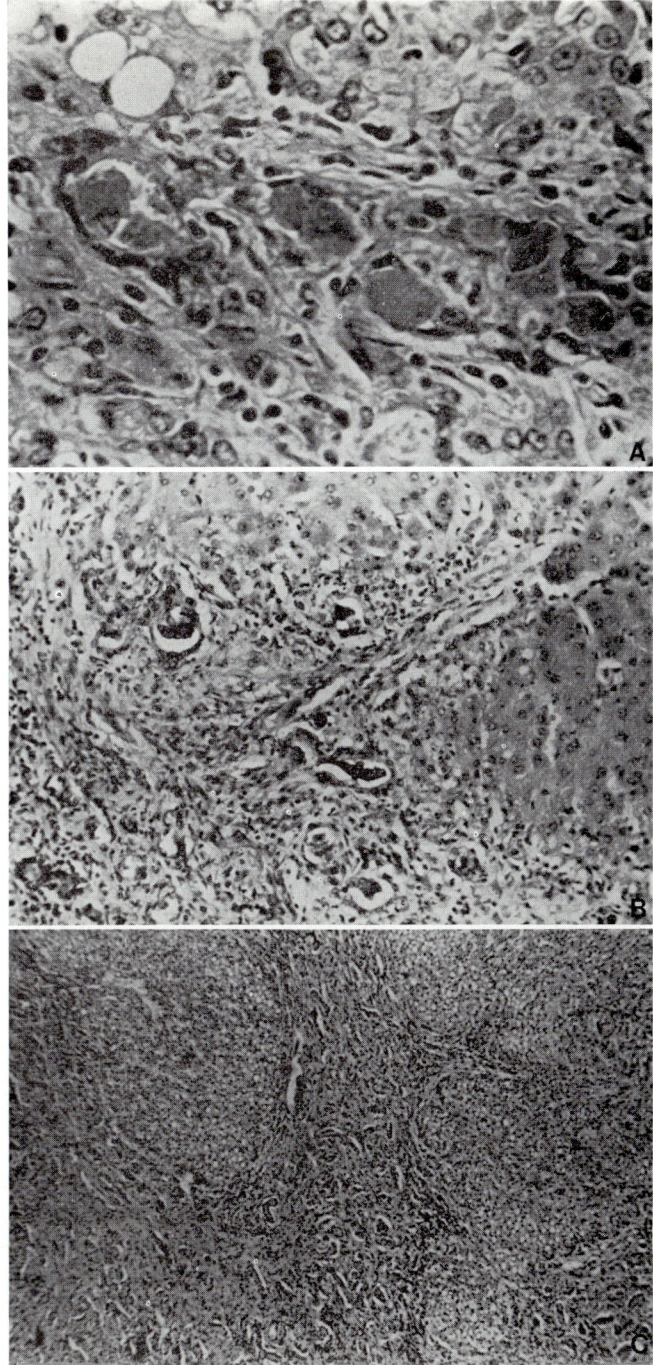

Figure 12.3 Histological appearance of liver in cystic fibrosis. A: Bile ductule plugging. B: Periportal fibrosis and multiplication of bile ducts which contain inspissated material. C: Advanced biliary cirrhosis and fatty infiltration

patients, a destructive type of multinodular biliary cirrhosis results eventually (Fig. 12.3C). The liver becomes smaller, grossly lobulated and firm. *Portal hypertension* supervenes and haemorrhage from oesophageal varices may be a presenting symptom. *Chemical evidence of liver dysfunction* is usually lacking until the cirrhotic changes are well advanced. Conventional liver function tests (Feigelson et al, 1975) and liver scans (Goodchild et al, 1975) have little predictive value. Death from hepatic failure or uncontrollable haemorrhage may be the outcome but rarely occurs before late teenage when it is claimed to occur in about 10 per cent of patients. Patients dying from advanced suppurative lung disease often show evidence of severe inanition and in these gross fatty infiltration of the liver may be apparent. However, the severity of chest disease bears little relation to the cirrhotic changes. The author has observed teenage patients who are of normal height and weight but who, despite escaping persistent chest infection, develop portal hypertension. The unpredictability of the development of cirrhosis and its inexorable progression once clinically manifest is one of the most disappointing features of cystic fibrosis in adolescence.

The aetiology of the liver pathology is not clear. Early changes may be related to bile ductule blockage but there is no ready explanation for the marked progression of cirrhosis in only certain patients. The author has not seen clinical liver disease in patients with partial pancreatic insufficiency although such patients are relatively few in number. In this regard it would be of interest to collect clinical observations of others.

Johansen et al (1968) in formulating their hypothesis that disturbed water and electrolyte movement in exocrine tissues was responsible for inspissation of secretions considered that the initial problem in the liver may also be related to this. Secretin is known to stimulate a flow of water and bicarbonate in the biliary system and from Brunner's glands. Neither CF patients with complete nor incomplete pancreatic insufficiency show any significant response to i.v. secretin in regard to volume or alkalinity of duodenal contents. If the pancreas alone is unresponsive to secretin because of gross structural damage leading to poor blood supply, following i.v. secretin there should at least be some increase in the volume of duodenal contents coming from the biliary tract and Brunner's glands. This does not seem to occur.

In a significant number of patients bile from the liver is prevented from entering the gallbladder because of blockage of the cystic duct by white mucous material. The cystic duct may become stenosed and the gallbladder small and functionless. *Cholecystitis* (Kissane and Smith, 1967) and *cholelithiasis* have both been recorded in children with CF.

Bile salt metabolism

In the past three to four years the enterohepatic bile salt circulation in CF has come under scrutiny, and the possibility that changes in this may be related to the progression of liver disease and may contribute to malabsorption of fat and vitamins is currently being investigated. Several groups, including Weber et al (1973) and Goodchild et al (1975) have demonstrated increased bile salt loss in the stools in CF. These workers suggest that this is compensated for in the early years of life by an increased rate of hepatic bile salt synthesis. However Goodchild et al (1975) found that older CF patients, particularly those with overt liver disease, had 'normal' or less than 'normal' levels of faecal bile acids with a negative correlation between faecal bile salt values and age, suggesting that the bile salt pool may be depleted in such patients. This could aggravate malabsorption. In a small number investigated, these workers have shown that duodenal fluid bile salt concentrations, at least in the morning, are within normal limits. However, no information is available in regard to levels later in the day. To date there is no evidence of the presence of unusual bile salts in the serum of CF patients although total levels rise when liver cirrhosis is severe (see also Chapter 9).

Mucous glands and goblet cells of the gastrointestinal tract

Distension of these is found to a varying degree from oesophagus to rectum and is particularly obvious in histological sections of the duodenum, small intestine and appendix. Figure 12.4 illustrates goblet cell appearances and the presence of 'stringy' mucus in the crypts of ileal mucosa from an autopsy specimen. The 'dumb-bell' shape of the extruding mucus is a characteristic feature.

Clinical presentations related to these characteristics of intestinal mucous secretions include *meconium ileus* and the '*meconium ileus equivalent*' *syndrome* (Fig. 12.1). Some 10 to 15 per cent of CF babies show symptoms of intestinal obstruction within 24 h of birth because the small intestinal content, particularly that in the ileum, is thick, sticky and dry and unable to be evacuated voluntarily per anus. The bowel is dilated proximal and collapsed distal to the blockage so that the colon appears reduced in size and is often filled with tenacious white mucus. Meconium peritonitis, volvulus and atresia are often found in association with meconium ileus. The reason why only some babies present in this way is not clear nor is there a firm explanation for the presence of inspissated meconium although the sticky, tenacious character of the mucus, together with the lack of pancreatic proteolytic enzymes to effect its digestion, have been suggested as contributory factors.

'*Meconium ileus equivalent*' is a term coined to describe a clinical presentation involving abdominal features which becomes more frequent after early childhood and in which tough, gum-like mucofaeculent masses tend to collect in the caecum and large gut or, less commonly, in the distal ileum (Hunton, Long and Tsumagari, 1966). These masses seem difficult for the gut to propel onwards; they sometimes become adherent to the wall of the caecum near the appendix, and occasionally partially calcify. They produce a variety of troublesome symptoms ranging from bouts of abdominal pain to acute or subacute intestinal obstruction, intussusception, obstructive appendicitis with abscess formation and bowel perforation. The reason for the formation of these masses is not clear but they occur in patients with complete as well as in those with partial pancreatic insufficiency and become more common in older patients.

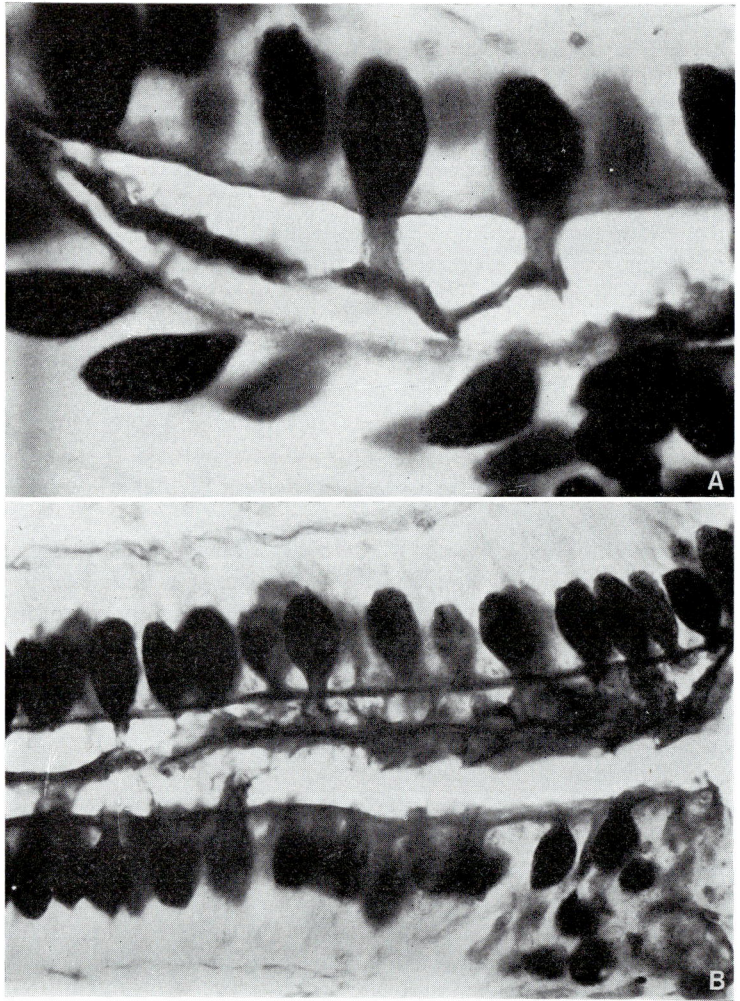

Figure 12.4 Ileal mucosa in cystic fibrosis. A: Distended goblet cells and dumbell appearance of mucus extruding from cells. B: Stringy mucus in crypts. (Acknowledgement is made to D. Barry and S. Morrissey, Queen Elizabeth College, London, for these photographs)

The author has seen this syndrome be the initial presenting symptom in several late teenage patients who had escaped severe chest infection in early life. One 19-year-old boy had a calcified rounded mass in the caecum.

Respiratory System

Both upper and lower respiratory tracts are involved, the changes being related to the presence of mucous secreting glands and cells with thick and sticky mucus which appears to allow stasis.

The lungs are structurally normal at birth but rapidly the tenacious mucus in distal bronchioles becomes infected. Infection stimulates further mucus secretion and a vicious circle develops. Infected sticky secretions, difficult to expectorate, become widespread throughout the bronchial tree and produce an obstructive suppurative chest illness. If untreated the changes become progressive and generalised leading eventually to patchy but widespread bronchiectasis, pulmonary fibrosis and finally cor pulmonale, cardiac failure and death.

Chronic respiratory disease is the major cause of morbidity and mortality and is the most difficult aspect of the condition to control consistently throughout life. It aggravates considerably the nutritional problems which may be almost non-existent until chest infection supervenes.

At autopsy the lungs are grossly overinflated and on macroscopic section bronchioles and bronchi can be seen to exude thick, tenacious, purulent material. The changes are widespread and never confined to single lobes. Peribronchial fibrosis is extensive and the walls of pulmonary arteries are thickened. The lung surfaces may show emphysematous bullae which occasionally rupture leading to pneumothorax or pyopneumothorax.

It is noteworthy that infiltration of the lung tissue by infective changes is generally confined to the area immediately surrounding the bronchial tubes and the parenchyma of the lung is largely unaffected. Classical lobar pneumonia is rarely seen and despite the constant presence of *Staphylococcus aureus* in the bronchial secretions, the pattern of illness characteristic of staphylococcal pneumonias of infancy in non-CF patients does not occur.

The organism most commonly isolated from purulent secretion is *Staph. aureus*. *Escherichia coli* and *Haemophilus influenzae* are often isolated from the younger patients and *Pseudomonas aeruginosa* from older patients, particularly the 'mucoid' form.

In the upper respiratory tract *nasal polyps* occur with increased frequency and often in association with sinus infection which is very common.

The Genital Tracts

Abnormalities of the male tract have only recently been defined in autopsy material (Kaplan et al, 1968; Oppenheimer and Esterly, 1969). There is evidence that all structures derived from the Wolffian duct are poorly differentiated, namely the seminal vesicles, vas deferens, epididymis and vasa efferentia. In the majority of patients the vas is atretic or absent precluding the passage of sperm and the abnormality is present from the first few months of life. The epididymis is often poorly defined. Whether the anatomical changes are a developmental anomaly of the mesonephric ducts or analogous to the blockage of ducts which occurs in other parts of the body associated with abnormal secretions is not clear. In support of the latter concept the bulbo-urethral glands are found to be distended with mucus and inspissated secretions occur in the prostate. The anatomical changes indicate that if blockage of ducts is the cause of the changes then secretions must have an abnormal character early in fetal life.

Although testicular histology is usually normal in the prepubertal boy small and immature testes occur in the older patient and spermatogenesis is decreased or absent.

The majority of males with CF will be sterile although isolated examples of fertile males have been recorded (Taussig et al, 1972).

In the female mucus producing glands of the cervix uteri are also distended and contain inspissated material. Puberty is usually delayed in the female. Fertility is almost certainly reduced but female patients have given birth to children, who are normal.

The Sweat Glands

No structural abnormalities have been found in the sweat gland coil or duct despite the high electrolyte content of the sweat (di Sant'Agnese et al, 1953) and the defect of sodium and chloride resorption in the sweat duct (Mangos and McSherry, 1968; Schultz, 1969).

It is clear from the foregoing that primary structural alterations in this disease are largely confined to organs where exocrine secretory tissue produces secretions containing macromolecular material such as mucopolysaccharides, mucoprotein or digestive enzymes.

CLINICAL AND DIAGNOSTIC FEATURES

In the majority the diagnosis is made in early childhood and with increasing frequency in the first months of life because of early signs of the characteristic chest disorder, with or without failure to thrive and evidence of malabsorption. Currently, evidence of high protein content of meconium is allowing detection of many during the first 24 h of life (Prosser et al, 1974) in the presymptomatic (chest) stage. However, there is no doubt that the diagnosis may be made for the first time at any age. Possibly the wide variety of clinical symptoms and the apparent differences in the severity of these, particularly in relation to the chest disorder, determine the mode and age of presentation—certain features characterise the neonatal period, early infancy and the toddler age. The more unusual clinical features and some of the secondary complications characterise presentation in later childhood and adult life. Therefore a comprehensive

Table 12.1 Features of clinical history

In the neonatal period	In infancy	Later features
Abdominal distension, bile stained vomiting and lack of passage of meconium, i.e. signs of intestinal obstruction (meconium ileus)	Abnormal stool (usually from birth) Slow weight gain (usually from birth) Large appetite	Persistent cough with purulent sputum Dyspnoea—at first with exercise only 'Fatty diarrhoea'
Occasionally, prolonged neonatal jaundice of obstructive type which usually resolves, may occur alone or may accompany meconium ileus	Harsh cough (sometimes paroxysmal) Vomiting with coughing (after paroxysms) Recurrent or persistent bronchitis Noisy, wheezy breathing (secretions in larger airways)	Recurrent abdominal pain with palpable faecal masses in abdomen, sometimes associated with attacks of subacute intestinal obstruction Haematemesis
Testing of meconium for protein content may have been used as 'screening method' to diagnose asymptomatic newborns	Rectal prolapse 'Salty taste' when kissed Family history of deaths in infancy or of living children with similar features Heat prostration or dehydration in hot weather	Progressive thirst, polyuria and weight loss due to diabetes mellitus Chronic sinusitis Delayed puberty Sterility in males Rarely, symptoms of peptic ulcer Haemoptysis

Table 12.2 Clinical examination

Early signs	Later signs
Poor growth for age and appetite	In patients with well-controlled disease or in formerly unrecognised patients there may be little to find except perhaps minor evidence of emphysema, mild finger clubbing and weight on lower centiles
Rancid smelling, greasy stools	
Abdominal distension	
Harsh choking cough	In those with progressive or untreated disease, the following may be present:
Emphysematous shape of chest	Evidence of marked malnutrition if respiratory function deteriorates
Persistent lower rib retraction (often slight)	Increasing evidence of respiratory disease and pulmonary insufficiency:
Evidence of secretions in bronchial tree on auscultation (often minimal)	Productive cough
	Sputum—yellow or green, thick and sticky, often copious
Bronchospasm	Increasing chest deformity (increase in anteroposterior diameter and fixity of upper chest)
Early finger clubbing	Lower rib retraction
Dry mottled skin	Variable degrees of cyanosis
Rapid finger wrinkling in water	Progressive finger clubbing
	Pneumothorax–pyopneumothorax
	Pulmonary osteoarthropathy
	Signs of cardiac failure (cor pulmonale)
	Liver enlargement (firm, may be irregular) ⎫ Each may be a presenting sign in older patients
	Signs of portal hypertension ⎬ and sometimes the only sign
	Palpable faecal masses in abdomen
	Signs of subacute intestinal obstruction ⎭
	Delay in appearance of secondary sexual characteristics

Table 12.3 Confirmatory investigations

	Initial		Additional
Stool microscopy	Numerous fat globules (starch grains and meat fibres after babyhood)	Chemical estimation of fat in faeces	Marked steatorrhoea (usually below 50 per cent absorption)
Chest x-ray	*Generalised* changes { Horizontal ribs / Emphysema { Flattened diaphragm / Increased A–P diameter } Thickened bronchial markings / Diffuse patchy consolidation or areas of collapse / Increasing peribronchial fibrosis	Duodenal intubation for pancreatic function studies	In the majority scanty mucosy juice pH 7 or lower—enzymes and bicarbonate in negligible quantities
Cough swab or sputum	Early { *Staph. aureus* / *Haemophilus influenzae* / *E. coli* } Later { *Pseudomonas aeruginosa*—often mucoid strain / *Staph. aureus* }		

Sweat sodium and chloride—CF levels above 60 mmol/litre

knowledge of relevant symptomatology is necessary so that the condition will receive consideration at all stages of life. Tables 12.1 to 12.3 list important clinical features, physical signs and confirmatory investigations. The following comments will refer to the particular features which characterise the disease and the mode of presentation in teenage or adult life.

The Diagnosis in Adolescence and Adulthood

It is uncommon for the diagnosis to be made for the first time in adult life (Rizk and Kissane, 1959; di Sant'Agnese and Andersen, 1959; Thomashefski, Christoforidis and Abdullah, 1970). A man of 46 years described by Marks and Anderson (1960) presented with chronic respiratory symptoms which had been thought to be due to bronchiectasis. In other patients chronic emphysematous bronchitis or asthma with infection have been diagnosed as the cause of such symptoms because the individual was considered 'too well and too old to have CF', or because growth and nutrition were little impaired, or the presence of fatty diarrhoea was not revealed by the patient or sought by the doctor. Growth may be normal in those with only partial pancreatic insufficiency and there is no clinical history relevant to malabsorption. Important features which may help to differentiate the chest illness of CF from other pulmonary disorders include: an emphysematous shaped upper chest rather than a pigeon chest; little in the way of auscultatory signs despite the presence of a productive cough: *generalised* radiological changes and areas of bronchial dilatation on bronchography which are widespread, seldom gross and do not predominate in basal areas. The sputum is tenacious, often sticking to the sides of a receptacle, and *Staph. aureus* is isolated more frequently than other organisms. The presence of *Ps. aeruginosa* should arouse suspicion of the diagnosis. Addington et al (1971) have compared pulmonary manifestations in children and young adults. Figure 12.5, the chest x-ray of one of my own patients, illustrates the relatively minor changes in the chest of a 19-year-old CF patient who leads a relatively normal life.

Some patients escape chest infection in youth and may present with later characteristics listed in Tables 12.1 and 12.2, for instance liver disease, features of the 'meconium ileus equivalent syndrome' (Jensen, 1962), diabetes or sterility. Liver and splenic enlargement of obscure origin in young adult life should lead to a search for other possible clinical manifestations of CF, as should symptoms of otherwise unexplained subacute or even acute intestinal obstruction which may be due to the 'meconium ileus equivalent syndrome'.

Confirmation of the diagnosis is more difficult in adults as the sweat test is a less reliable diagnostic aid after puberty, levels above 60 mmol/litre for Na or Cl being relatively frequent in normal subjects (Anderson and Freeman, 1960; McKendrick, 1962).

Pancreatic function studies may be necessary both in those with and without steatorrhoea. In patients with partial pancreatic insufficiency, although the enzyme response to pancreozymin may be adequate, duodenal juice will be scanty and 'mucosy' with no increase in volume or rise in bicarbonate content following i.v. secretin (Hadorn et al, 1968).

Before a final diagnosis of cystic fibrosis is accepted, all clinical features should be considered carefully together with all investigational criteria available. In the author's experience, there has always been more than one characteristic feature in each case when these were carefully sought.

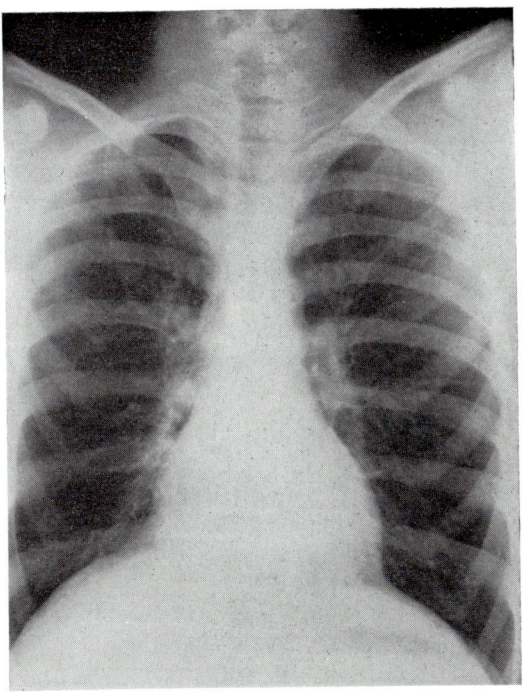

Figure 12.5 Chest x-ray of 16-year-old boy with cystic fibrosis. Some fibrosis in upper lobes and bronchial wall thickening in other areas. He has minimal cough and good exercise tolerance. His height is at the 50th centile and weight at the 10th centile. He has a full-time job and hobbies involving physical activity

Prognosis in older patients

It is clear that many patients diagnosed in childhood now survive to reach young adult life but in a state of health that varies considerably. There are several reports which describe the varied clinical characteristics of such older patients (Shwachman, Kulczycki and Khaw, 1965; Gracey and Anderson, 1969; Shwachman, Redmond and Khaw, 1970; Shwachman, Kowalski and Khaw, 1974). The latter workers report on 70 patients now over 25 years of age. Some details of this report are of interest and give an indication of the quality of life to be expected at present in adulthood. Of 3000 patients studied by Dr

Shwachman over 37 years in Boston, 800 are still living and 70 have survived beyond their twenty-fifth birthday. Of the 70 patients, 14 are over 30 and 5 over 35 years of age; the oldest is 44 years. Males predominate (47 to 23) as they do in the report of Gracey and Anderson (1969). Some of Shwachman et al's (1974) comments about the long term survivors might indicate that they had a milder form of the disease, for instance 16 did not show malabsorption, 13 were diagnosed as a result of family screening, 20 were over 10 years of age when diagnosed and 10 were over 20 years. However, the report states that the severity at diagnosis varied considerably and not all cases were mild. With regard to marriage and reproduction, 22 males are married but none has children and all those examined were aspermic; 6 women have 7 children. In regard to achievement in life, over 42 patients attended college and 40 graduated; 13 have a master's degree; 1 is a doctor of medicine, 2 are lawyers, 3 nurses, 1 a physiotherapist, 1 an engineer and 3 research workers in physics. Of 70 people, this is a high proportion with professional qualifications and illustrates the good intellect and considerable drive and ambition of these individuals, commonly noted by most clinicians who care for large numbers of such patients.

The record of *complications* among the 70 patients of Shwachman et al (1974) is of particular interest. In order of frequency these were stated to be as follows: sterility in males (100 per cent), nasal polyposis (50 per cent), faecal impaction or meconium ileus equivalent (15 per cent), diabetes mellitus (15 per cent), pneumothorax (10 per cent) and salt depletion (10 per cent). This brief report does not state that any of the patients showed clinical evidence of liver cirrhosis or portal hypertension. From the present author's own experience, death from liver disease in CF occurs most commonly in teenage and one wonders whether those who have reached adulthood have escaped this complication. The author has not seen liver complications in subjects with partial pancreatic insufficiency.

MANAGEMENT

Because the basic defect is still unknown treatment is not curative but is aimed at controlling the development of secondary and, in some cases, tertiary consequences of the exocrine secretory function abnormality. As the pathological changes in important organs are progressive and lethal unless modified, treatment should commence very early in life, preferably at birth. With regard to the respiratory system treatment must be preventative. It must be applied consistently throughout life and be of the very best quality. Inadequate treatment may do little but prolong life in a state of discomfort and misery. Some clinicians maintain that this will be so in any case, but there is no doubt that conscientious application of the currently available treatment improves the quality of life in childhood to a very great extent. Information is emerging from the follow-up of patients diagnosed at birth in Cleveland, USA, before the development of any respiratory symptoms or signs, that such children are now approaching adolescence with little lung disease and in a state of good nutrition (Gurry, 1975). Their chance of further survival to adulthood in good health seems likely. However, many patients now reaching adult life did not have the benefit of the full range of modern treatment when they were children.

Because of the chronic nature of the condition and the varied aspects of medical treatment many other facets of management must be considered: psychological, social, genetic, educational and occupational. Therefore the clinician embarking on the management of CF patients shoulders a considerable responsibility and may find that over the years he comes to play a very important role in the life of both the patient and his family. Varied members of the 'caring' professions will also have contact at some time with CF patients and their families and will be vitally concerned in aspects of overall management.

The prognosis for longevity has completely altered during the past 25 years but it is still difficult to predict the outcome in any individual patient. Intrinsic variations in the disease are considerable and together with the degree and type of organ pathology existing at the time of diagnosis, will play a major role in determining the maintenance of life and good health.

There is no doubt that longevity will depend to a large extent on the *maintenance of adequate pulmonary function and nutrition* towards which much of the treatment is directed; but there are other factors which play a part in successful management. These include: early diagnosis and treatment, preferably before any evidence of chest infection; knowledgeable and consistent medical care; a stable family setting with two parents, both of whom understand the condition and share in its management at home; immunisation against measles in early childhood; the good fortune to avoid the unpredictable and irremediable complication of liver cirrhosis; good psychological support during the difficult period of adolescence and continuation of treatment during this time.

Management of Respiratory Disease

Removal of bronchial secretions and control of infection in these secretions are the primary goals of treatment and these are achieved by the following means to a greater or lesser degree: *the administration of antibiotics orally or, at times intravenously; chest physiotherapy with coughing, breathing exercises and postural drainage; and intermittent inhalation of moisture, antibiotics, mycolytic agents.*

Uniform agreement does not exist among those caring for CF patients regarding the detailed application of all these measures. Reviews of respiratory management may be found in Mearns (1972), Shwachman and Khaw (1972),

Lloyd-Still, Khaw and Shwachman (1974), McCrae (1974) and Anderson and Goodchild (1976). Long-term antibiotic therapy is necessary for all those with persistent chest symptoms and signs with the choice being related to periodic checking of the sensitivity of the organisms. There is less agreement in regard to the use of prophylactic antibiotics but if these are given they should be in full dosage and have antistaphylococcal activity. Infants diagnosed within the first hours of birth by 'meconium screening tests' should be given prophylactic antistaphylococcal agents, otherwise there is little point in making the diagnosis at this stage. In most patients chest infection supervenes quickly if they are untreated. Continuous antibiotic treatment until after school entrance is common practice in England with intermittent use thereafter as determined by clinical need.

The efficacy of inhalation treatment is debatable. Experimental studies show little penetration of inhaled particles into the periphery of the lung (Motoyama, Gibson and Zigas, 1972; Chang et al, 1973; Alderson et al, 1974). Although sleeping in a mist of water vapour at night has been popular in the USA the difficulties of maintaining this in adolescence has caused reconsideration of its value. It has never been a popular mode of therapy in England and its use is declining elsewhere. Intermittent inhalations direct into the mouth using normal saline and a wetting agent and given before physiotherapy are more popular. In the short term they aid in attenuating an acute respiratory illness; in the long term they aid considerably in clearing sputum from the chest in children with established chest infection. Antibiotics can be added to the inhalation fluid and neomycin is popular and effective. The choice of dosage varies and high frequency deafness is undoubtedly a complication of the use of higher dosages (Anderson and Goodchild, 1976).

Management of chest disease in adolescence and adulthood will depend on the degree of damage that has become established by that stage. Perhaps the most dangerous problem at this time is complacency and lack of continuation of therapy. Because of the sticky, tenacious pulmonary secretions it is important to continue the physical measures of control and give antibiotics readily for each upper respiratory infection, intensifying physiotherapy and antibiotic course if symptoms do not clear. Suppurative chest disease in CF is more difficult to control than that of bronchiectasis. The young adult patient is often only too eager to give up treatment when he passes out of the hands of his paediatrician and his family and only too often the adult physician concurs with the frequent development of a progressively downhill course. Respiratory complications are more common in older patients, for example, pneumothorax (Levy, 1966; Mitchell-Heggs and Batten, 1970), haemoptysis (Holsclaw, Grand and Shwachman, 1970), cor pulmonale and cardiac failure. The latter may be insidious and hard to recognise because the classical physical signs may not be easy to elicit (Siassi, Moss and Dooley, 1971). Management of cardiac failure is also complicated by the sweat sodium losses and diuretics should be given with care (Whitman et al, 1975).

Management of Nutrition

Nutritional impairment may not be severe and in some patients it may not be noticeable unless chest infection is present; but as this progresses nutrition suffers and in the presence of gross pulmonary insufficiency it may be impossible to repair nutrition even by heroic measures such as artificial diets (Allan, Mason and Moss, 1973; Berry et al, 1975). The chief means of avoiding nutritional impairment is to prevent chronic chest infection but the additional use of a high calorie, high protein, moderate fat containing diet, pancreatic and vitamin supplements, particularly A, D and E, will help considerably. There is no indication for severe dietary fat restriction. Unnecessary dietary modifications are only a source of irritation to a child and certainly to an adolescent who must cope with many medicaments and other forms of treatment.

Pancreatic supplements are widely used but do not completely control steatorrhoea, even in high dosage (Lapey et al, 1974; Goodchild et al, 1974b). However, the stools become less socially offensive and this helps the patient considerably. Care should be taken in the means of administration to obtain the maximum benefit (Anderson, 1972; Anderson and Goodchild, 1976).

Medium chain triglycerides (MCT) may be a useful form of dietary fat in CF (Gracey, Burke and Anderson, 1969a, 1970) used either as a dietary additive or a partial replacement of long-chain fat. Malabsorption can be controlled best by using a diet reduced in long-chain fat and supplemented with MCT together with pancreatic supplements (unpublished observations from the author's department). MCT provide calories in small bulk, relieve abdominal distension, help rectal prolapse and alleviate the tendency to 'meconium ileus syndrome'. Milk preparations and MCT oil are available on prescription and the latter can be used in cooking, frying, etc.—for details and recipes, see Anderson and Burke (1975), Anderson and Goodchild (1976).

Nutritional supplementation. Recently some workers have recommended the complete or partial replacement of the patient's usual diet by an artificial one, if nutrition is falling off (Allan et al, 1973; Berry et al, 1974; Barclay and Shannon, 1975). These diets consist of protein hydrolysates, glucose polymers and MCT with vitamins, minerals and essential fatty acid supplements. Such a diet, if accepted by the patient, may be useful following severe bouts of illness but there has been no significant improvement in respiratory disease attributable to the improved nutrition which may be only temporary. The results of controlled trials are awaited.

Management of salt losses. Sweat sodium chloride loss is about four times normal. Daily salt supplements and copious fluids are advised for all who live in hot countries, during hot summers in cooler countries, during physical exercise or manual work involving sweating and during febrile or dehydrating illnesses even if these are mild (Anderson and Goodchild, 1976). Mucus secretions become even more sticky in the presence of dehydration and exacerbations of chest symptoms often follow hot conditions or excessive sweating. Weight gains are usually less in summer than winter.

Management of Other Gastrointestinal Problems

'Meconium ileus equivalent' syndrome. This is proving to be a common and troublesome feature of the older patient. The condition bears little relationship to whether the patient is well or ill from chest disease or whether there is

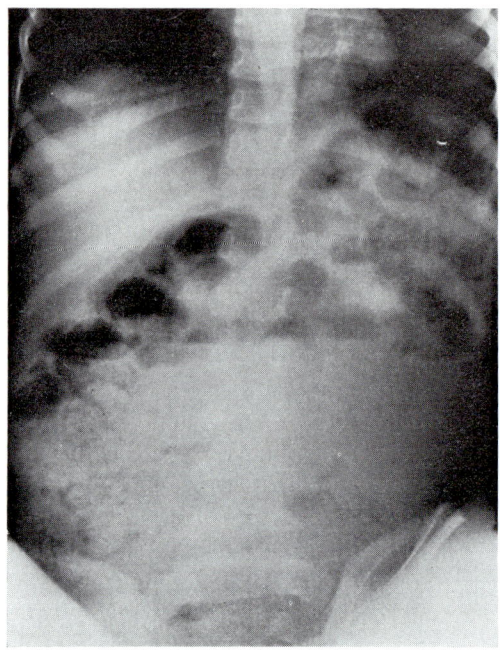

Figure 12.6 Plain abdominal x-ray (erect film) of a 6-year-old child, showing features of the 'meconium ileus equivalent' syndrome—fluid levels in small bowel and faecal mottling in colon

partial or complete pancreatic insufficiency. The syndrome is more likely to occur if pancreatic preparations are given in excessive dosage, following febrile illnesses, bouts of dehydration or during hot weather.

Bouts of colicky pain are common in patients past school age and become more frequent later. At times there may be vomiting or signs of intestinal obstruction. Plain abdominal x-ray examination may reveal fluid levels in the small intestine and faecal masses in the caecum and large gut (Fig. 12.6). Intussusception occurs in younger patients (Brown et al, 1960; Tucker et al, 1973). Calcified masses or tumours may be found in the caecum (Brown and Wilson, 1961) and these may obstruct the appendix or erode the bowel wall.

Appendicitis and appendicular abscess are sometimes difficult to differentiate from this condition or they may be a complication of it.

In management of the mild case, oral n-acetyl cysteine, a mucolytic agent usually used by inhalation, is helpful (Lillibridge, Docter and Eidelman, 1967; Gracey, Burke and Anderson, 1969b) in a dose of 5 to 10 ml t.d.s. increasing to 15 ml t.d.s. For an obstructive episode it may be given as an enema (100–200 ml of a 10 per cent solution run along the colon to the caecum). A gastrografin enema under fluoroscopic control may also be successful in stimulating evacuation but precautions against dehydration should be taken. Operation to remove masses should not be undertaken lightly as faecal fistulae can occur.

Liver disease—biliary cirrhosis and portal hypertension. Treatment is on the whole unsatisfactory but does not differ essentially from that of other types of cirrhosis.

Haematemesis from bleeding oesophageal or stomach varices is evidence of portal hypertension and indicates the severity of the cirrhosis. Treatment should be conservative by careful sedation, blood transfusion and vitamin K; if unsuccessful intravenous vasopressin is used. In most instances bleeding will cease.

Portacaval shunt operations have been carried out but results have not been encouraging. Of 10 such patients operated on in Boston, USA (Tyson, Schuster and Shwachman, 1968), 6 died within six months. However of 7 patients with hypersplenism and varices that had not bled, 6 were alive three years after operation. Personal experience has been small but not encouraging. Periods of recumbency following operation encourage stagnation of pulmonary secretions, aggravating chest infection.

Management of Social and Psychological Aspects

Recent work has emphasised the psychological difficulties associated with CF these being especially marked in the adolescent patient (Rosenlund and Lustig, 1973; Gayton and Friedman, 1973). These problems are largely related to the effects of chronic ill health and those that are of particular concern to the adolescent include small stature, easy fatigability, continuance of chest physiotherapy and numerous medications, limited peer activities, delayed appearance of secondary sexual characteristics, reduced marriage prospects, the eventual knowledge of sterility in the male adult, and the health danger to the female who wishes to have children. For the adolescent with CF and his family, the achievement of identity and autonomy—difficult enough normally—are made more so by the additional complication of a chronic and potentially fatal disease. Knowledge of the latter fact cannot help but become known to the older child if only from publicity in the media regarding the disease. This and many other worries may not be fully expressed by the patient and care should be taken to discuss each of them at an appropriate stage.

Studies have also centred around the families of these patients and the impact of the disease upon them (Turk, 1964; Meyerowitz and Kaplan, 1967; McCollum and Gibson, 1970; McCrae et al, 1973; Burton, 1973a; Allan, Townley and Phelan, 1974). Data available in the USA have been reviewed by Gayton and Friedman (1973) and Burton (1973b) has reported on studies in Northern Ireland. Although differences in the handling of the condition occur in the USA and the UK there is no doubt that the disease is a great challenge to family strength. Gayton and Friedman (1973) stress that management of CF should be orientated towards preventing the secondary social and psychological complications that are often associated with chronic illness and Burton (1975) discusses these problems in a recently published monograph. With a specific cure not yet available total family management will continue to be very important to the care of these children.

The CF child should obtain a good education and there is no place for special educational treatment simply on account of the diagnosis. This should be reserved for those with considerable impairment of health. These children are of normal intelligence but have considerable drive and enthusiasm for learning which should be encouraged strongly.

Transfer of Medical Care from Paediatrician to Physician Caring for Adults

It is fair to say that this problem could be handled better than it is at present. Only relatively recently has this change of medical care become common. It is difficult to decide to which consultant in adult medicine the condition should be referred. Continuing care of the chest is very important but gastroenterological complications become more frequent in later life. What the patient really needs is *'his doctor'* to whom he can relate about all facets of his disease. This doctor will need advice and help from a number of specialists but the patient must not run the risk of becoming lost amongst experts. By the time the patient is adult both he and his family understand the disease thoroughly. The latter have probably belonged to CF parent groups. Because of long association the tie between paediatrician and patient is often hard to break and it is my experience and that of others that the patient and family find this break rather like a bereavement and there may well be a period of depression and deteriorating health on the part of the patient. This difficulty must not be allowed to arise and there should be joint consultation of paediatrician and adult physician with the patient and parents for some time before transfer so that all aspects of management can be understood and discussed. Too often one sees the problem of a new doctor abruptly changing or stopping certain facets of treatment to which the patient has become very accustomed. This may be justified but is confusing to patient and family.

Assessing Prognosis and Comparing Treatment Regimes (Scoring Systems)

The varying manifestations and degrees of severity of CF make it difficult to assess the effects of various forms of treatments especially in the long term. Several centres have developed scoring systems in an attempt to measure these effects. The 'Shwachman score' (Shwachman and Kulczycki, 1958) was one of the earliest and is based on an assessment of four aspects: general activity, physical findings, nutritional status and chest x-ray appearances. With 25 points for each category, a high score indicates a good clinical state. The system has been modified by others (Cooperman et al, 1971; Taussig et al, 1973) particularly to take into account the increasing age of surviving patients and the increasing prevalence of complications both of the respiratory tract and of other affected organs such as the liver.

Although most clinicians experienced in caring for CF patients are able to make an assessment of prognosis on clinical grounds scoring systems such as the above are a useful discipline. They ensure a more critical approach to assessing the value of various treatments both in the short and long term and in evaluating the progress of each individual patient. It is useful to record a 'score' each year, perhaps when a radiological review is made. The European Working Group for Cystic Fibrosis is attempting to collect data relating to treatment and to the natural history of the condition. Such studies are extremely important; they attempt to rationalise aspects of management and to seek answers to the following: is very early diagnosis and prophylactic treatment the most important factor in determining prognosis?; what are the most effective methods of controlling chest disease?; is survival in good health more dependent on intrinsic lack of severity of the disease?

Neonatal Screening Procedures

In recent years methods have been developed to enable infants with CF to be detected before symptoms cause their presentation to a doctor. Opinion is not uniform that the case has been made for 'screening', at least not until answers to the questions just outlined have been found (Brimblecombe and Chamberlain, 1973). On the other hand, some maintain that the way to answer such questions is to identify newborn cases and follow them carefully. However a dilemma then arises as to whether prophylactic chest treatment including antibiotics and chest physiotherapy should be commenced in all cases. Evidence accumulating over 12 years from a Cleveland, USA, clinic (Gurry, 1975) where prophylaxis has been undertaken in a substantial group of newborn CF sibs of known CF patients indicates that the health of these individuals is good. Indeed it is considerably better than that of patients presenting for diagnosis because of symptoms arising at varying ages during that time. The outcome of such a study when the patients reach young adult life will be of great interest.

Methods of screening

Because the basic defect is still unknown all screening methods suggested so far test a secondary manifestation of the disease. Identification at or shortly after birth is necessary to justify the reasons put forward for screening. The method should give a high yield of accurate results with a minimum number of false negatives but more importantly a minimum number of false positive results so as to arouse as little parental anxiety as possible. Cost must be considered carefully in relation to benefit and the method must be acceptable to patient and parents.

The method that fulfils the greatest number of these criteria adequately is the testing of meconium for albumin (Wiser and Beier, 1964; Green and Shwachman, 1968). Meconium from normal newborns seldom contains more than 3 mg of albumin per gram meconium; that from the CF infant contains in the region of 80 mg. The presence of increased protein is related to its lack of digestion by pancreatic proteolytic enzymes so therefore those 10 to 20 per cent of patients with residual pancreatic function at birth will give false negative results. Other sources of protein such as blood or mucus in meconium will give false positives. However, the test is simple, can be done without concerning parents of normal babies at all and there is a 'captive' population. The test is currently being evaluated in a number of centres in different countries (Prosser et al, 1974; Brune et al, 1974; Stephan et al, 1975) and one commercial firm is marketing a test strip.[1] In all these studies there were 1 per cent false positives when the strip tests were carried out by nursing personnel as suggested by the makers. False negatives are revealed later and Prosser et al (1974) considered their detection rate to be only 60 per cent. Refinements of the method of testing for albumin (Ryley et al, 1974) reduce the false positive rate but add considerably to expense.

Obviously the ideal method has yet to be found and the case for whole population screening yet to be made. It is important however to continue to search as newborn testing is necessary for all new sibs in known CF families, and the availability of intrauterine testing important for such families. A chemical method of identifying the serum factor might help (Wilson et al, 175) but discovery of the basic defect should be the ultimate aim.

AETIOLOGY OF CYSTIC FIBROSIS—RESEARCH INTO THE BASIC DEFECT

New observations and comments regarding possible metabolic abnormalities in cystic fibrosis appear with unfailing regularity in the medical journals, many bringing conflicting data. As yet none has successfully indicated a specific primary metabolic error which explains the varied pathological and clinical phenomena: for instance, why structural changes relevant to the disease and

---

[1] The Boehringer Corporation (London) Ltd, Oxbridge Road, Ealing, London W5 2TZ, England.

not to secondary complications are confined to exocrine secretory tissue; why the characteristics of the secretions allow them to precipitate or aggregate rather than to disperse; why such secretions are altered from early fetal life as evidenced by gross antenatal changes in the pancreas and male reproductive tract where they appear to be associated with the early stages of development of the Mullerian duct system. The higher concentrations of electrolytes in serous secretions such as sweat and saliva must be linked in some way with the altered characteristics of macromolecular or zymogen containing secretions.

The basic defect may have a more widespread effect in other body tissues but at present there is no clinical or pathological evidence of this, at least at the primary level. The possibility that both the disease and its treatment have secondary metabolic effects on other tissues is considerable and must be taken into account when interpreting observations on the function of the tissue under investigation, such as red cells, fibroblasts, etc. (McEvoy, 1975). Clarification of the basic defect has been hampered by this problem and others including: the limited basic knowledge available regarding normal composition, production and mechanism of expulsion of exocrine gland secretions particularly mucus; the difficulty of obtaining such secretions undiluted or uncontaminated during life; the lack of an animal model condition and the considerable ethical problems involving research in children.

This chapter cannot critically analyse all the data available and only the chief avenues of past and current investigations will be mentioned with illustrative references. Search for the explanation of the secretory abnormalities has been concentrated largely around the following: studies of the structure, mechanism of synthesis and secretion of glycoproteins and of the composition, both organic and inorganic, of zymogen containing secretions; studies of membrane transport, seeking an explanation for altered electrolyte content of secretions; observations regarding autonomic nervous control of secretory activity and isolation of circulating factors which might exert an influence on secretory mechanisms.

Mucus secretions. These are difficult to obtain in the 'pure' state but no consistent abnormality of the structure of the component glycoproteins has been demonstrated. The review by di Sant'Agnese and Talamo (1967) summarises studies up to that time. Conflicting evidence exists regarding the clinical observations that mucus secretions are more viscous than normal (Denton, 1960; Feather and Russell, 1970). In the lung viscosity of secretions is now considered to have a greater relationship to the degree of accompanying infection (Sturgess, 1969) certainly when the 'mucoid' strain of *Ps. aeruginosa* is present. Duodenal fluid is observed to be viscous (Lorin, Denning and Mandel, 1972) but, on the whole, conventional means of measuring viscosity have not added to an understanding of the sticky nature of mucus secretions.

Zymogen containing secretions. Secretion from salivary glands (Chernick, Barbero and Parkins, 1961) and pancreas (Hadorn et al, 1968) have been noted to possess an increased organic content relative to their water content

(Chernick, Eichel and Barbero, 1964). Increased concentrations of inorganic ions, particularly calcium (Chernick and Barbero, 1967; Gugler et al, 1967; Mandel et al, 1969; Blomfield, Warton and Brown, 1973b; Boat, Wiesman and Pallavicini, 1974) have been observed in salivary secretions. The concept that an insoluble complex formed between glycoprotein (zymogen) and calcium may be responsible for glandular ductule blockage is attractive (Warton and Blomfield, 1971; Blomfield et al, 1973a). On the other hand insufficient dilution of the zymogen secretions by water and electrolytes has also been suggested to explain the inspissated nature of the secretions (Johansen et al, 1968). Thus in those patients with residual pancreatic function secretin will not effect a flow of water and bicarbonate (Hadorn et al, 1968).

Autonomic nervous system. Disturbance of autonomic control of secretion has been argued as a possible aetiological basis of the condition (Farber, 1942; Roberts, 1959; Dische et al, 1962; Holzel et al, 1962), overstimulation or imbalanced stimulation of secretory glands being a possible mechanism for explaining concentrated secretions.

In animal models overstimulation of salivary glands and experimental alterations in autonomic nervous activity have produced changes in the glands and the secretions which closely resemble features of CF glands and secretions (Grand, 1969; Mangos et al, 1969). Recent work with rats on chronic reserpine treatment is particularly interesting in this regard (Martinez et al, 1975a, b). The authors describe morphological changes in the submaxillary glands and in other exocrine secretory tissue (pancreas and intestinal mucosa) as well as alterations in electrolyte and carbohydrate content in these secretions similar to those in CF. These workers argue convincingly that this animal model could be a useful tool in the study of the pathogenesis of CF and in possible pharmacological approaches to the correction or improvement of the exocrine secretory process.

There is no clinical evidence for a generalised disturbance of the autonomic nervous system and minor observed differences in such things as pupillary reactivity may or may not be primary (Rubin et al, 1963; Esterley et al, 1968).

Investigation of mucopolysaccharide metabolism using tissue culture systems. In some but not all tissue culture studies using CF fibroblasts or lymphocytes, total acid mucopolysaccharides (AMPS) have been suggested to be increased (Matalon and Dorfman, 1968) but there is no pathological evidence for this in the tissues of patients with CF nor any striking abnormalities in the concentration of AMPS in the urine (Shwartz and Pallavicini, 1967; Kollberg, Lundblad and Ekbohm, 1973). Fibroblasts and white cells in culture from patients and parents have been found by some workers to show metachromatic staining (Danes and Bearn, 1968, 1969; Danes, 1973). This work is not readily repeatable by others (Reed et al, 1970) and the finding is relatively non-specific (Milunsky and Littlefield, 1960; Taysi et al, 1969) but has raised interesting speculation as to whether there are several genetic varieties of CF (Danes et al, 1969; Nadler et al, 1969).

Electrolyte changes in secretions. The sweat electrolyte abnormality is present from birth and throughout life, being unrelated either to severity of the disease or to whether other organs, such as pancreas or lungs, are grossly involved. Sodium, chloride and potassium levels are raised, but there is no evidence for change in calcium levels or other solutes, or for a change in sweating rates (Emrich et al, 1968). No morphological changes in the sweat glands have been recorded.

The composition of precursor fluid in the sweat coil is said to be normal but a defect of resorption of electrolytes in the duct has been postulated and good evidence provided (Sutcliffe, Style and Schwarz, 1968; Schulz, 1969).

Sweat from CF patients has been found to contain a 'factor' which will inhibit sodium resorption in animal salivary glands (Mangos and McSherry, 1968), or in normal human sweat glands (Kaiser, Drack and Rossi, 1971).

Secretions from small salivary glands in the buccal mucosa show marked changes in electrolyte content (Blomfield et al, 1973b) while that from the parotid and submaxillary glands demonstrates lesser changes (Wiesmann, Boat and di Sant'Agnese, 1972).

Pancreatic secretions in patients with partial pancreatic deficiency have been shown to have very low bicarbonate levels and a poor volume and bicarbonate response to i.v. secretin (Hadorn et al, 1968). The response of the kidney to secretin in this regard has also been said to be abnormal (Bretscher et al, 1974).

There is little real evidence at present which links the Na, Cl and K abnormalities of serous secretions with the abnormal characteristics of mucous or zymogen-containing secretions. However data regarding circulating or secreted 'factors' which may be cilio-inhibitory or cause alterations in ductular electrolyte absorption may provide an answer. For instance, Martinez et al (1975b) showed in their chronically reserpinised rats similar alterations in electrolyte concentrations in salivary secretion to those in CF and at the same time the appearance of a previously absent cilio-inhibitory 'factor'.

Cystic fibrosis humoral factors. Spock et al (1967) have demonstrated a 'factor' in the serum of CF patients that iniates 'dyskinesia' in the ciliary epithelium of rabbit tracheal explants and a 'factor' has been reported in CF sweat and saliva that inhibits sodium transport in animal salivary glands (Mangos and McSherry, 1967; Mangos, McSherry and Benke, 1967). This has led others to search for serum factors and factors in other secretions (Bowman, McCombs and Lockhart, 1970; Cherry et al, 1971; Beratis et al, 1973) and to test the effect of CF serum in experimental situations in relation to ion and membrane transport (Brown et al, 1971; Benke, Erbstoeszer and Pitot, 1972; Duffy and Shwartz, 1972; Taussig and Gardner, 1972; Morin, Desjeux and Authier, 1973). It is claimed that a ciliary inhibiting factor is produced by cultured lymphocytes (Conover et al, 1973a), is associated with the presence of metachromasia in cultured fibroblasts (Danes, 1973) and is present in cultures from heterozygote cells (Conover et al, 1973b).

Efforts have been made to develop simple assay systems of the ciliary inhibiting factor using a variety of lower animal forms with ciliated epithelium but results have been inconsistent and confusing (Bowman et al, 1970; Conover et al, 1973b) and this has led to considerable disagreement as to the importance of 'factors'. However it would appear that there is something in CF homozygote serum, and possibly in the serum of heterozygotes, that is heat labile, non-dialysable, and elutes on Sephadex or DEAE columns with IgG (Bowman et al, 1970) which has an effect on cilial movement in the experimental situation and probably on membrane transport. Its molecular weight, earlier thought to be in the region of 150 000 to 200 000, is possibly much less being in the region of 1000 to 10 000 (Wilson, Jahn and Fonseca, 1973). It is not certain whether the 'factor' observed in saliva or sweat of CF patients is the same as that in serum; but if it is and if the 'factor' produced by 'overstimulated' salivary glands in the experimental animal is also similar, support may be given to the suggestion that this 'factor' is a normal substance produced in excess (Martinez et al, 1975b) and appearing in the serum by an overflow phenomenon. Further work must be directed towards an understanding of the normal secretory mechanisms in exocrine glands and the changes in composition of the secretions in relation to various forms of stimulation especially those related to the autonomic nervous system.

Calcium binding properties of CF body fluids. CF serum has been found to have greater calcium binding properties by some (Fitzpatrick, Landon and James, 1972; Brown et al, in preparation) but not all investigators (Smith et al, 1972). A relationship of IgG to this calcium binding property has been observed. The ciliary inhibiting factor is also related to IgG but it is not IgG itself. As has been stated earlier, the calcium content of some CF exocrine secretions is raised and calcium forms complexes with the macromolecular content to render the secretion precipitable. Gibson et al (1971) have suggested an hypothesis linking calcium in secretions to the abnormality of mucus and sweat but it is not entirely convincing. However it would seem that there must be some link between circulating 'factors', sweat and salivary 'factors', IgG, calcium binding properties of serum and secretions, and the abnormal qualities of secretions and the ion transport differences in CF.

There is no doubt that chemical identification of the elusive 'factor' would be a significant advance in clarifying a link between these various observations. A good assay system based on chemical structure would be of advantage especially if it could be shown to identify the heterozygote, aid in diagnosis of the homozygote and effect antenatal and neonatal screening. Wilson et al (1975) have suggested a chemical assay and further elaboration and confirmation of their findings will be of importance.

Other lines of enquiry. Recently essential fatty acid metabolism has come under scrutiny in CF, but although serum (Watts et al, 1975) and cell membrane (McEvoy, 1975) deficiencies can be demonstrated there is no convincing evidence of a primary defect in their handling. A recent hypothesis (Rivers and Hassam, 1975) suggested a deficiency in fatty acid desaturating enzyme activity but other work disproves this (Watts et al, 1975).

Because of the relationship of *polyamines* to salt balance across membranes recent enquiry has been made into their metabolism but no convincing evidence of abnormality in CF has been revealed (Lundgren, Farrell and di Sant'Agnese, 1975; McEvoy and Hartley, 1975).

The behaviour of kallekrein-like substances in exocrine secretions is also being studied (Rao, Posner and Nadler, 1972; Rao and Nadler, 1975).

It can be seen that the riddle of cystic fibrosis is yet to be solved. When it is, hopefully we may be able to care more effectively for these children and young adults. Until then the disease taxes to the full the skill, patience and persistence of the doctor who provides continuing lifelong supervision of prophylactic and palliative treatment; it makes similar demands on the patients and their families.

REFERENCES

Addington, W. W., Cugell, D. W., Zelkowitz, P. S., O'Flynn, M. E. & Embry, S. (1971) Cystic fibrosis of the pancreas—a comparison of the pulmonary manifestations in children and young adults. *Chest*, **59**, 306–311.
Allan, J. D., Mason, A. & Moss, A. D. (1973) Nutritional supplementation in treatment of cystic fibrosis of the pancreas. *American Journal of Diseases of Children*, **126**, 22–26.
Allan, J. L., Townley, R. R. W. & Phelan, P. D. (1974) Family response to cystic fibrosis. *Australian Paediatric Journal*, **10**, 136–146.
Alderson, P. O., Secker-Walker, R. H., Strominger, D. B., Markham, J. & Hill, R. L. (1974) Pulmonary deposition of aerosols in children with cystic fibrosis. *Journal of Pediatrics*, **84**, 479–484.
Andersen, D. H. (1938) Cystic fibrosis of the pancreas and its relation to celiac disease. A clinical and pathological study. *American Journal of Diseases of Children*, **56**, 344–399.
Anderson, C. M. (1972) Pancreatic enzyme replacement in the treatment of cystic fibrosis. *Prescriber's Journal*, **12**, 45–49.
Anderson, C. M. & Burke, V. (1975) *Paediatric Gastroenterology*. Oxford: Blackwell Scientific Publications.
Anderson, C. M. & Goodchild, M. C. (1976) *Cystic Fibrosis. Manual of Diagnosis and Management*. Oxford: Blackwell Scientific Publications.
Anderson, C. M. & Freeman, M. (1960) Sweat test results in normal persons of different ages compared with families with fibrocystic disease of the pancreas. *Archives of Disease in Childhood*, **35**, 581–587.
Barclay, R. P. C. & Shannon, R. S. (1975) Trial of artificial diet in treatment of cystic fibrosis of pancreas. *Archives of Disease in Childhood*, **50**, 490–493.
Benke, P. J., Erbstoeszer, M. & Pitot, H. C. (1972) Transport of labelled compounds in control and cystic fibrosis cells in vitro. *Lancet*, **1**, 182–184.
Beratis, N. G., Conover, J. H., Conod, E. J., Bonforte, R. J. & Hirschhorn, K. (1973) Studies in ciliary dyskinesia factor in cystic fibrosis. III. Skin fibroblasts and cultured amniotic fluid cells. *Pediatric Research*, **7**, 958–964.
Berry, H. K., Kellogg, F. W., Hunt, M. M., Ingberg, R. L., Richter, L. & Gutjahr, C. (1975) Dietary supplement and nutrition in children with cystic fibrosis. *American Journal of Diseases of Children*, **129**, 165–171.
Blomfield, J., Dascalu, J., van Lennep, E. W. & Brown, J. M. (1973a) Hypersecretion of zymogen granules in the pathogenesis of cystic fibrosis. *Gut*, **14**, 558–565.

Blomfield, J., Warton, K. L. & Brown, J. M. (1973b) Flow rate and inorganic components of submandibular saliva in cystic fibrosis. *Archives of Disease in Childhood*, **48**, 267–274.
Boat, T. F., Wiesman, U. N. & Pallavicini, J. C. (1974) Purification and properties of the calcium precipitable protein in submaxillary saliva of normal and cystic fibrosis subjects. *Pediatric Research*, **8**, 531–539.
Bodian, M. (1952) *Fibrocystic Disease of the Pancreas. A Congenital Disorder of Mucus Production-Mucosis*, London: William Heinemann.
Bowman, B. H., McCombs, M. L. & Lockhart, L. H. (1970) Cystic fibrosis: characterisation of the inhibitor to ciliary action in oyster gills. *Science*, **167**, 871–873.
Bretscher, D., Schneider, A., Hagmann, R., Hadorn, B., Howald, B., Lüthi, C. & Oetliker, O. (1974) Response of renal handling of sodium and bicarbonate to secretin in normals and patients with cystic fibrosis. *Pediatric Research*, **8**, 899.
Brimblecombe, F. S. W. & Chamberlain, J. (1973) Screening for cystic fibrosis. *Lancet*, **2**, 1428–1431.
Brown, P. M., Hallenbeck, G. A., Soule, E. H. & Burgert, E. O., Jr (1960) Cystic fibrosis with fecal retention and intussusception in late stages: report of three cases. *New Englana Journal of Medicine*, **263**, 544–546.
Brown, G. A., Oshin, A., Goodchild, M. C. & Anderson, C. M. (1971) Inhibition of sugar transport by plasma from cystic fibrosis patients. *Lancet*, **2**, 639–640.
Brown, P. M. & Wilson, N. D. (1961) Tumor of the cecum with cystic fibrosis of the pancreas. *American Journal of Surgery*, **101**, 236–238.
Brune, W. T., Cornell, T. R., Lacey, J. A. & Whisler, K. E. (1974) One year screening study for cystic fibrosis with the BMC test in sixteen thousand newborn infants. 1975 *Cystic Fibrosis Club Abstract*, **13**, 20, Atlanta, Georgia: National Cystic Fibrosis Research Foundation, 3379 Peachtree Road, NE.
Burton, L. (1973a) Caring for children with cystic fibrosis. *The Practitioner*, **210**, 247–254.
Burton, L. (1973b) Cystic fibrosis—a challenge to family strength. *Health Visitor*, **46**, 186–189.
Burton, L. (1975) *Family Life of Sick Children*. London: Routledge & Kegan Paul Ltd.
Chang, N., Levison, H., Cunningham, K., Crozier, D. N. & Grossett, O. (1973) An evaluation of nightly mist tent therapy for patients with cystic fibrosis. *American Review of Respiratory Disease*, **107**, 672–675.
Chernick, W. S., Barbero, G. J. & Parkins, F. N. (1961) Studies on submaxillary saliva in cystic fibrosis. *Journal of Pediatrics*, **59**, 890–898.
Chernick, W. S. & Barbero, G. J. (1967) Reversal of submaxillary alterations in cystic fibrosis by guanethedine. *Modern Problems of Pediatrics*, **10**, 125–134.
Chernick, W. S., Eichel, H. J. & Barbero, G. J. (1964) Submaxillary salivary enzymes as a measure of glandular activity in cystic fibrosis. *Journal of Pediatrics*, **65**, 694–700.
Cherry, J. D., Roden, V. J., Rejent, A. J. & Dorner, R. W. (1971) The inhibition of ciliary activity in tracheal organ cultures by serum from children with cystic fibrosis and control subjects. *Journal of Pediatrics*, **79**, 937–942.
Conover, J. H., Beratis, N. G., Conod, E. J., Ainbender, E. & Hirschhorn, K. (1973a) Studies on ciliary dyskinesia factor in CF. II. Short-term leucocyte cultures and long-term lymphoid lines. *Pediatric Research*, **7**, 224–228.
Conover, J. H., Bonforte, R. J., Hathaway, P., Paciuc, S., Conod, E. J., Hirschhorn, K. & Kopel, F. B. (1973b) Studies in ciliary dyskinesia factor in CF. I. Bioassay and heterozygote detection in serum. *Pediatric Research*, **7**, 220–223.
Cooperman, E. M., Park, M., McKee, J. & Assad, P. J. (1971) A simplified cystic fibrosis scoring system. *Canadian Medical Association Journal*, **105**, 580–582.
Craig, J. M., Haddad, H. & Shwachman, H. (1957) The pathological changes in the liver in cystic fibrosis of the pancreas. *American Journal of Diseases of Children*, **93**, 357–369.
Danes, B. S. (1973) Association of cystic fibrosis factor to metachromasia of the cultured cystic fibrosis fibroblast. *Lancet*, **2**, 765–767.
Danes, B. S. & Bearn, A. G. (1968) A consistent abnormality in fibroblasts of patients with cystic fibrosis and in heterozygous carriers. *Journal of Clinical Investigation*, **47**, 24a.
Danes, B. S. & Bearn, A. G. (1969) Cystic fibrosis of the pancreas. A study in cell culture. *Journal of Experimental Medicine*, **129**, 775–793.
Danes, B. S., Foley, K. M., Dillan, S. D. & Bearn, A. G. (1969) Genetic study of cystic fibrosis of the pancreas using white blood cell cultures. *Nature*, **222**, 685–686.

Danks, D. M., Allan, J. & Anderson, C. M. (1965) A genetic study of fibrocystic disease of the pancreas. *Annals of Human Genetics*, **28**, 323–356.
Denton, R. (1960) Bronchial obstruction in cystic fibrosis: rheological factors. *Pediatrics, New York*, **25**, 611–620.
Di Sant'Agnese, P. A. & Andersen, D. H. (1959) Cystic fibrosis of the pancreas in young adults. *Annals of Internal Medicine*, **50**, 1321–1330.
Di Sant'Agnese, P. A. & Blanc, W. A. (1956) A distinctive type of biliary cirrhosis of the liver associated with cystic fibrosis of the pancreas. *Pediatrics, New York*, **18**, 387–409.
Di Sant'Agnese, P. A. & Talamo, R. C. (1967) Pathogenesis and physiopathology of cystic fibrosis of the pancreas. Fibrocystic disease of the pancreas (mucoviscidosis). *New England Journal of Medicine*, **277**, 1287–1295, 1343–1352, 1399–1408.
Di Sant'Agnese, P. A., Darling, R. C., Perera, G. A. & Shea, E. (1953) Abnormal electrolyte composition of sweat in cystic fibrosis of the pancreas. Clinical significance and relationship to the disease. *Pediatrics, New York*, **12**, 549–563.
Dische, Z., Pallavicini, C., Cizek, L. H. & Chien, S. (1962) Changes in the control of the secretion of mucus glycoproteins as possible pathogenic factor in cystic fibrosis of the pancreas. *Annals of the New York Academy of Sciences*, **93**, 526.
Duffy, M. J. & Schwartz, V. (1972) Cystic fibrosis and membrane transport. *Lancet*, **2**, 136–137.
Editorial (1973) Developments in cystic fibrosis research. *Lancet*, **2**, 307–308.
Emrich, H. M., Stoll, E., Friolet, B., Colombe, J. P., Richterick, R., & Rossi, E. (1968) Sweat composition in relation to rate of sweating in patients with cystic fibrosis of the pancreas. *Pediatric Research*, **2**, 464–478.
Esterley, N. B., Canolino, S. J., Alter, B. P. & Brusilow, S. W. (1968) Pupillatonia, hyporeflexia and segmental hypohidrosis: autonomic dysfunction in a child. *Journal of Pediatrics*, **72**, 852.
Farber, S. (1942) Experimental production of achylia pancreatica. *American Journal of Diseases of Children*, **64**, 953–954.
Feather, E. A. & Russell, G. (1970) Sputum viscosity and pulmonary function in cystic fibrosis. *Archives of Diseases in Childhood*, **45**, 807–808.
Feigelson, J., Pecau, Y., Cathelineau, L. & Navarro, J. (1975) Additional data on hepatic function tests in cystic fibrosis. *Acta paediatrica, Stockholm*, **64**, 337–342.
Fitzpatrick, D. F., Landon, E. J. & James, V. (1972) Serum binding of calcium and the red cell membrane in cystic fibrosis. *Nature New Biology*, **235**, 173–174.
Gayton, W. F. & Friedman, S. B. (1973) Psychosocial aspects of cystic fibrosis. A review of the literature. *American Journal of Diseases of Children*, **126**, 856–859.
Gibson, L. E., Matthews, W. J., Minihan, P. T. & Patti, J. A. (1971) Relating mucus calcium and sweat in a new concept of cystic fibrosis. *Pediatrics, New York*, **48**, 695–710.
Goodchild, M. C., Insley, J., Rushton, D. I. & Gaze, H. (1974a) Cystic fibrosis in 3 Pakistani children. *Archives of Disease in Childhood*, **49**, 739–741.
Goodchild, M. C., Sagaró, E., Brown, G. A., Cruchley, P. M., Jukes, H. R. & Anderson, C. M. (1974b) Comparative trial of Pancrex V Forte and Nutrizyme in treatment of malabsorption in cystic fibrosis. *British Medical Journal*, **3**, 712–714.
Goodchild, M. C., Banks, A. J., Drolc, Z. & Anderson, C. M. (1975) Liver scans in cystic fibrosis. *Archives of Disease in Childhood*, **50**, 813–815.
Goodchild, M. C., Murphy, G. M , Howell, A. M., Nutter, S. A. & Anderson, C. M. (1975) Aspects of bile acid metabolism in cystic fibrosis *Archives of Disease in Childhood*, **50**, 769–778.
Goodchild, M. C., Edwards, J. H., Glenn, K. P., Grundey, C., Harris, R., Mackintosh, P. & Wen zel, J. A search for linkage in cystic fibrosis. *Journal of Medical Genetics* (in press).
Gracey, M. & Anderson, G. M. (1969) Cystic fibrosis of the pancreas in adolescence and adulthood. *Australasian Annals of Medicine*, **18**, 91–101.
Gracey, M., Burke, V. & Anderson, C. M. (1969a) Assessment of medium-chain triglyceride feeding in infants with cystic fibrosis. *Archives of Disease in Childhood*, **44**, 401–403.
Gracey, M., Burke, V. & Anderson, C. M. (1969b) Treatment of abdominal pain in cystic fibrosis by oral administration of n-acetyl cysteine. *Archives of Disease in Childhood*, **44**, 404–405.

Gracey, M., Burke, V. & Anderson, C. M. (1970) Medium chain triglycerides in paediatric practice. *Archives of Disease in Childhood*, **45**, 445–452.

Grand, R. J. (1969) Control of protein synthesis in rat parotid gland in vitro. *Federation Proceedings*, **28**, 273.

Grand, R. J., Talamo, R. C., Di Sant'Agnese, P. A. & Shwartz, R. H. (1966) Pregnancy in cystic fibrosis of the pancreas. *Journal of the American Medical Association*, **195**, 993–1000.

Green, M. N. & Shwachman, H. (1968) Presumptive tests for cystic fibrosis based on serum protein in meconium. *Pediatrics, New York*, **41**, 989–992.

Gugler, E., Pallavicini, J. C., Swerdlow, M. & Di Sant'Agnese, P. A. (1967) Role of calcium in submaxillary saliva of patients with cystic fibrosis. *Journal of Pediatrics*, **71**, 585–588.

Gurry, D. L. (1975) Management of children with cystic fibrosis, Letter to editor. *Australian Paediatric Journal*, **11**, 89–90.

Hadorn, B., Johansen, P. G. & Anderson, C. M. (1968) Pancreozymin-secretin test of exocrine pancreatic function in cystic fibrosis and the significance of the result for the pathogenesis of the disease. *Australian Paediatric Journal*, **4**, 8–22.

Hall, B. D. & Simpkiss, M. J. (1968) Incidence of fibrocystic disease in Wessex. *Journal of Medical Genetics*, **5**, 262–265.

Holsclaw, D. S., Grand, R. J. & Shwachman, H. (1970) Massive hemoptysis in cystic fibrosis. *Journal of Pediatrics*, **76**, 829–838.

Holzel, A., Schwarz, V., Torkington, P. & Greville-Williams, G. E. (1962) Mucoviscidosis and autonomic nervous system. *Lancet*, **1**, 822.

Huang, N. N., Macri, C. N., Girone, J. & Sproul, A. (1970) Survival of patients with cystic fibrosis. *American Journal of Diseases of Children*, **120**, 289–295.

Hunton, D. B., Long, W. K. & Tsumagari, H. Y. (1966) Meconium ileus equivalent: an adult complication of fibrocystic disease. *Gastroenterology*, **50**, 99–106.

Jensen, K. G. (1962) Meconium ileus equivalent in a fifteen-year-old patient with mucoviscidosis. *Acta paediatrica, Uppsala*, **51**, 344–348.

Johansen, P. G., Anderson, C. M. & Hadorn, B. (1968) Hypothesis. Cystic fibrosis of the pancreas. A generalised disturbance of water and electrolyte movement in exocrine tissues. *Lancet*, **1**, 455–460.

Kaiser, D., Drack, E. & Rossi, E. (1971) Inhibition of net sodium transport in single human sweat glands by sweat of patients with cystic fibrosis of the pancreas. *Pediatric Research*, **5**, 167–172.

Kaplan, E., Shwachman, H., Perlmutter, A. D., Rule, A., Khaw, K. T. & Holsclaw, D. S. (1968) Reproductive failure in males with cystic fibrosis. *New England Journal of Medicine*, **279**, 65–69.

Kissane, J. M. & Smith, M. G. (1967) *Pathology of Infancy and Childhood*. St Louis: Mosby Company.

Knudson, A. G., Jr, Wayne, L. & Hallett, W. Y. (1967) On the selective advantage of cystic fibrosis heterozygotes. *American Journal of Human Genetics*, **19**, 388–392.

Kollberg, H., Lundblad, A. & Ekbohm, G. (1973) Studies in cystic fibrosis. Urinary excretion of hexosamine, sialic acid and fucose. *Acta paediatrica scandinavica*, **62**, 279–288.

Kramm, E. M., Crane, M. M., Sirken, M. G. & Brown, M. L. (1962) A cystic fibrosis pilot survey in three New England states. *American Journal of Public Health*, **52**, 2041–2057.

Kulczycki, L. L. & Schauf, V. (1974) Cystic fibrosis in Blacks in Washington, DC. *American Journal of Diseases of Children*, **127**, 64–67.

Lapey, A., Kattwinkel, J., Di Sant'Agnese, P. A. & Laster, L. (1974) Steatorrhea and azotorrhea and their relation to growth and nutrition in adolescents and young adults with cystic fibrosis. *Journal of Pediatrics*, **84**, 328–334.

Levy, I. J. (1966) Spontaneous pneumothorax: treatment based on analysis of 170 episodes in 135 patients. *Diseases of the Chest*, **49**, 529–537.

Lillibridge, C. B., Docter, J. M. & Eidelman, S. (1967) Oral administration of n-acetyl cysteine in the prophylaxis of meconium ileus equivalent. *Journal of Pediatrics*, **71**, 887–889.

Lloyd-Still, J. D., Khaw, K. T. & Shwachman, H. (1974) Severe respiratory disease in infants with cystic fibrosis. *Pediatrics, New York*, **53**, 678–682.

Lorin, M. I., Denning, C. R. & Mandel, I. D. (1972) Viscosity of exocrine secretions in cystic fibrosis: sweat, duodenal fluid and submaxillary saliva. *Biorheology*, **9**, 27–32.

Lundgren, D. W., Farrell, P. M. & Di Sant'Agnese, P. A. (1975) Polyamine alterations in blood of male homozygotes and heterozygotes for cystic fibrosis. *Clinica Chemica Acta*, **62**, 357–362.
McCollum, A. T. & Gibson, L. E. (1970) Family adaptation to the child with cystic fibrosis. *Journal of Pediatrics*, **77**, 571.
McCrae, W. M. (1974) Management of cystic fibrosis. In *Modern Trends in Paediatrics*, 4, ed. Apley, J. London: Butterworths.
McCrae, W. M., Cull, A. M., Burton, L. & Dodge, J. (1973) Cystic fibrosis—parents' response to the genetic basis of the disease. *Lancet*, **1**, 141–143.
McEvoy, F. A. (1975) Essential fatty acids and CF. *Lancet*, **2**, 236.
McEvoy, F. A. & Hartley, C. B. (1975) Polyamines in cystic fibrosis. *Pediatric Research*, **9**, 721–724.
McKendrick, T. (1962) Sweat sodium levels in normal subjects, in fibrocystic patients and their relatives and in chronic bronchitic patients. *Lancet*, **1**, 183–186.
Mandel, I. D., Eriv, A., Kutscher, A., Denning, C., Thompson, R. H., Kessler, W. & Zegarelli, E. (1969) Calcium and phosphorus levels in submaxillary saliva. *Clinical Pediatrics*, **8**, 161–164.
Mangos, J. A. & McSherry, N. R. (1967) Sodium transport: inhibitory factor in sweat of patients with cystic fibrosis. *Science*, **158**, 135–136.
Mangos, J. A. & McSherry, N. R. (1968) Studies on the mechanism of inhibition of sodium transport in cystic fibrosis of the pancreas. *Pediatric Research*, **2**, 378–384.
Mangos, J. A., McSherry, N. R. & Benke, P. J. (1967) A sodium transport inhibitory factor in the saliva of patients with cystic fibrosis of the pancreas. *Pediatric Research*, **1**, 436–442.
Mangos, J. A., McSherry, N. R., Benke, P. J. & Spock, A. (1969) Studies on the pathogenesis of cystic fibrosis: the isoproterenol treated rat as an experimental model. In *Proceedings of 5th International CF Conference*, Cambridge, ed. Lawson, D. Bromley: Cystic Fibrosis Research Trust, 5 Blyth Road, Bromley, Kent.
Marks, B. L. & Anderson, C. M. (1960) Fibrocystic disease of the pancreas in a man aged 46. *Lancet*, **1**, 365–367.
Martinez, J. R., Adelstein, E., Quissell, D. & Barbero, G. J. (1975a) The chronically reserpinised rat as a possible model for cystic fibrosis. I. Submaxillary gland morphology and ultrastructure. *Pediatric Research*, **9**, 463–469.
Martinez, J. R., Adshead, P. C., Quissell, D. & Barbero, G. J. (1975b) The chronically reserpinised rat as a possible model for cystic fibrosis. II. Composition and cilio inhibitory effects of submaxillary saliva. *Pediatric Research*, **9**, 470–475.
Matalon, R. & Dorfman, A. (1968) Acid mucopolysaccharides in cultured fibroblasts of cystic fibrosis of the pancreas. *Biochemical and Biophysical Research Communications*, **33**, 954.
Mearns, M. B. (1972) Treatment and prevention of pulmonary complications of cystic fibrosis in infancy and early childhood. *Archives of Disease in Childhood*, **54**, 5–11.
Meyerowitz, J. H. & Kaplan, H. B. (1967) Familial responses to stress: the case of cystic fibrosis. *Social Science and Medicine*, **1**, 249–266.
Milunsky, A. & Littlefield, J. W. (1969) Diagnostic limitations of metachromasia. *New England Journal of Medicine*, **281**, 1128–1129.
Mitchell-Heggs, P. F. & Batten, J. C. (1970) Pleurectomy for spontaneous pneumothorax in cystic fibrosis. *Thorax*, **25**, 165–171.
Morin. C. L., Desjeux, J. F. & Authier, L. (1973) Effect of saliva and serum from patients with cystic fibrosis on intestinal uptake of amino acids in rat. *Biomedicine*, **19**, 133.
Motoyama, E. K., Gibson, L. E. & Zigas, C. J. (1972) Evaluation of mist tent therapy in cystic fibrosis using maximum expiratory flow volume curve. *Pediatrics, New York*, **50**, 299–306.
Nadler, H. L., Swae, M. A., Wodnicki, J. M. & O'Flynn, M. E. (1969) Cultivated amniotic fluid cells and fibroblasts derived from families with cystic fibrosis. *Lancet*, **2**, 84–85.
Oppenheimer, E. H. & Esterly, J. R. (1969) Observations on cystic fibrosis of the pancreas. V. Developmental changes in the male genital system. *Journal of Pediatrics*, **75**, 806–811.
Prosser, R., Owen, H., Bull, F., Parry, B., Smerkinich, J., Goodwin, H. A. & Dathan, J. (1974) Screening for cystic fibrosis by examination of meconium. *Archives of Disease of Childhood*, **49**, 597–601.

Rao, G. J. S. & Nadler, H. L. (1975) Deficiency of arginine esterase in cystic fibrosis of the pancreas. Demonstration of the proteolytic nature of the activity. *Pediatric Research*, **9**, 739–741.

Rao, G. J. S., Posner, L. A. & Nadler, A. L. (1972) Deficiency of kallekrein activity in plasma of patients with cystic fibrosis. *Science*, **177**, 610–611.

Reddy, C. R. R. M., Devi, C. S., Anees, A. M., Murthy, D. P. & Reddy, G. E. (1969) Cystic fibrosis of the pancreas in India. *Journal of Pediatrics*, **75**, 522–523.

Reed, G. B., Bain, A. D., McCrae, W. M. & Scott, F. M. (1970) Cellular metachromasia in cystic fibrosis. *Journal of Pathology*, **101**, 251–257.

Rizk, V. E. & Kissane, J. M. (1959) 'Adult' mucoviscidosis. *American Journal of Medicine*, **27**, 483–493.

Rivers, J. P. W. & Hassam, A. G. (1975) Hypothesis. Defective essential-fatty-acid metabolism in cystic fibrosis. *Lancet*, **2**, 642–643.

Roberts, G. B. S. (1959) Fundamental defect in fibrocystic disease of the pancreas. *Lancet*, **2**, 964–965.

Rosenlund, M. L. & Lustig, H. S. (1973) Young adults with cystic fibrosis. *Annals of Internal Medicine*, **78**, 959–961.

Rubin, L. S., Barbero, G. J., Chernick, W. S. & Sibinga, M. S. (1963) Pupillary reactivity as a measure of autonomic balance in cystic fibrosis. *Journal of Pediatrics*, **63**, 1120.

Ryley, H. C., Neale, L., Brogan, T. D. & Bray, P. T. (1974) Plasma proteins in meconium from normal infants and from babies with cystic fibrosis. *Archives of Disease in Childhood*, **49**, 901–904.

Schulz, I. J. (1969) Micropuncture studies of sweat formation in cystic fibrosis patients. *Journal of Clinical Investigation*, **48**, 1470–1477.

Schwartz, R. H. & Pallavicini, J. C. (1967) Immunological and chemical studies of cystic fibrosis and normal urinary glycoprotein of Tamm and Horsfall. *Journal of Laboratory and Clinical Medicine*, **70**, 725–735.

Shwachman, H. & Holsclaw, D. S. (1969) Complications of cystic fibrosis. *New England Journal of Medicine*, **281**, 500–501.

Shwachman, H. & Khaw, K. T. (1972) Cystic Fibrosis. In *Pediatric Therapy*, ed. Shirkey, H. C., 4th edn, p. 573. St Louis: Mosby.

Shwachman, H. & Kulczycki, L. L. (1958) Long-term study of 105 patients with cystic fibrosis. *American Journal of Diseases of Children*, **96**, 6–15.

Shwachman, H., Kulczycki, L. L. & Khaw, K. T. (1965) Studies in cystic fibrosis: a report on sixty-five patients over 17 years of age. *Pediatrics, New York*, **36**, 689–699.

Shwachman, H., Redmond, A. & Khaw, K. T. (1970) Studies in cystic fibrosis: report of 130 patients diagnosed under 3 months of age over a 20-year-period. *Pediatrics, New York*, **46**, 335–343.

Shwachman, H., Kowalski, M. & Khaw, K. T. (1974) 70 patients with cystic fibrosis over 25 years of age—a new outlook. In *Cystic Fibrosis Club Abstract* 13, No. 3, Atlanta: National Cystic Fibrosis Research Foundation, 3379 Peachtree Road, NE.

Shwachman, H., Lebenthal, E. & Khaw, K. T.(1975) Recurrent acute pancreatitis in patients with cystic fibrosis with normal pancreatic enzymes. *Pediatrics, New York*, **55**, 86–95.

Siassi, B., Moss, A. J. & Dooley, R. R. (1971) Clinical recognition of cor pulmonale in cystic fibrosis. *Journal of Pediatrics*, **78**, 794–805.

Smith, Q. T., Shapiro, B. L., Hamilton, M. J. & Warwick, W. J. (1972) Lack of differences in serum binding of calcium in cystic fibrosis, carriers and controls. *Nature New Biology*, **240**, 56.

Spock, A., Heick, H. M. C., Cress, H. & Logan, W. S. (1967) Abnormal serum factor in patients with cystic fibrosis of the pancreas. *Pediatric Research*, **1**, 173–177.

Stephan, U., Busch, E.-W., Kollberg, H. & Hellsing, K. (1975) Cystic fibrosis detection by means of a test-strip. *Pediatrics, New York*, **55**, 35–38.

Sturgess, J. M. (1969) A new pattern of sputum viscosity. In *Proceedings of the 5th International Cystic Fibrosis Conference*, ed. Lawson, D., p. 368–385. Bromley: Cystic Fibrosis Research Trust, 5 Blyth Road, Bromley, Kent BR1 3RS.

Sutcliffe, C. H., Style, P. P. & Schwarz, V. (1968) Biochemical studies of sweat secretion in cystic fibrosis. *Proceedings of Royal Society of Medicine*, **61**, 297.

Taussig, L. M. & Gardner, J. D. (1972) Effects of saliva and plasma from cystic fibrosis patients on membrane transport. *Lancet*, **1**, 1367–1369.
Taussig, L. M., Lobeck, C. C., Di Sant'Agnese, P. A., Ackerman, D. R. & Kattwinkel, J. (1972) Fertility in males with cystic fibrosis. *New England Journal of Medicine*, **287**, 586–589.
Taussig, L. M., Kattwinkel, J., Friedewald, W. T. & Di Sant'Agnese, P. A. (1973) A new prognostic score and clinical evaluation system for cystic fibrosis. *Journal of Pediatrics*, **82**, 380–390.
Taysi, K., Kistenmacher, M. L., Punnett, H. H. & Mellman, W. J. (1969) Limitations of metachromasia as a diagnostic aid in pediatrics. *New England Journal of Medicine*, **281**, 1108–1111.
Tomashefski, J. F., Christoforidis, A. J. & Abdullah, A. K. (1970) Cystic fibrosis in young adults. An over-looked diagnosis with emphasis on pulmonary function and radiological patterns. *Chest*, **57**, 28–36.
Tucker, A. S., Stern, S. S., Pitman, E. & Perrin, V. (1973) Intussusception in older children— a complication of cystic fibrosis. *Annales de radiologie*, **16**, 173.
Turk, J. (1964) Impact of cystic fibrosis on family functioning. *Pediatrics, New York*, **34**, 67–71.
Tyson, R. T., Schuster, S. R. & Shwachman, H. (1968) Portal hypertension in cystic fibrosis. *Journal of Pediatric Surgery*, **3**, 271–277.
Warton, K. L. & Blomfield, J. (1971) Hydroxyapatite in the pathogenesis of cystic fibrosis. *British Medical Journal*, **3**, 570–571.
Warwick, W. J. & Pogue, R. E. (1969) Computer studies in cystic fibrosis. In *Proceedings of 5th International CF Conference*, Cambridge, ed. Lawson, D., pp. 320–330. Bromley: Cystic Fibrosis Research Trust, 5 Blyth Road, Bromley, Kent BR1 3RS.
Watts, R., Taylor, S., Postuma, R. & Smalley, C. A. (1975) Letter to *Lancet* **2**, 983.
Weber, A. M., Roy, C. C., Morin, C. L. & Lasalle, R. (1973) Malabsorption of bile acids in children with cystic fibrosis. *New England Journal of Medicine*, **289**, 1001–1005.
Webster, R. & Williams, H. (1953) Hepatic cirrhosis associated with fibrocystic disease of the pancreas: clinical and pathological reports of 5 patients. *Archives of Disease in Childhood*, **28**, 343–350.
Whitman, V., Stern, R. C., Bellet, P., Doershuk, C. F., Liebman, J., Boat, T. F., Borkat, G. & Matthews, L. W. (1975) Studies on cor pulmonale in cystic fibrosis. I. Effects of diuresis. *Pediatrics, New York*, **55**, 83–85.
Wiesmann, U. N., Boat, T. F. & Di Sant'Agnese, P. A. (1972) Flow rates and electrolytes in minor-salivary-gland saliva in normal subjects and patients with cystic fibrosis. *Lancet*, **2**, 510–512.
Wilson, G. B., Fudenberg, H. H. & Jahn, T. L. (1975) Studies on cystic fibrosis using isoelectric focusing. I. An assay for detection of cystic fibrosis homozygotes and heterozygote carriers from serum. *Pediatric Research*, **9**, 635–640.
Wilson, G. B., Jahn, T. L. & Fonseca, J. R. (1973) Demonstration of serum protein differences in cystic fibrosis by isoelectric focusing in thin-layer polyacrylamide gels. *Clinica Chemica acta*, **49**, 79–91.
Wiser, W. C. & Beier, F. R. (1964) Albumin in the meconium of infants with cystic fibrosis. A preliminary report. *Pediatrics, New York*, **33**, 115–119.
Wright, S. W. (1969) Racial variation in the incidence of cystic fibrosis. In *Proceedings of 5th International Cystic Fibrosis Conference*, ed. Lawson, D., pp. 91–101. Bromley: Cystic Fibrosis Research Trust, 5 Blyth Road, Bromley, Kent BR1 3RS.
Zuelzer, W. W. & Newton, W. A. (1949) The pathogenesis of fibrocystic disease of the pancreas: a study of 36 cases with special reference to the pulmonary lesions. *Pediatrics, New York*, **4**, 53–69.

INDEX

Abetalipoproteinaemia, 41
Absorption, 73
  alcohol, 149, 163
  bile acids, 76
  fat, 27, 74
  sites, 75
Achalasia, 17
Acid
  perfusion test, 13
  reflux test, 13
Aflatoxin, 284
Alcohol
  absorption, 149
  cirrhosis of the liver, 156
  fatty liver, 153
  folic acid, 164
  gastric secretion, 160
  hepatitis, 155
  liver injury, 152, 158
  metabolism, 149
  oesophagus, 159
  pancreas, 165
  small intestine, 162
  steatonecrosis, 155
  vitamin B_{12}, 164
Alcohol dehydrogenase, 151
Alpha-1 antitrypsin
  deficiency, 271
  function, 270
  genetics, 270
Anthracene laxatives, 128
Antral G-cell hyperplasia, 57, 58
Apudoma, 50
Arteritis, 111

Bacterial overgrowth
  bile acids, 203, 211
  cholylglycine breath test, 208
  diarrhoea, 216
  Ehlers–Danlos syndrome, 114
  fat absorption, 40
  intestinal resection, 79
Bile, 219
Bile acids
  absorption, 31, 76, 201

Bile aids—*continued*
  body pool, 31, 220
  cholestasis, 204
  cirrhosis of the liver, 205
  cystic fibrosis, 304
  deconjugation, 201, 208
  deficiency, 38, 78
  diarrhoea, 214
  gallstones, 218
  laxatives, 133
  malabsorption, 209
  micelles, 30, 74, 199
  serum levels, 202
  sulphation, 201, 204, 207
Bile salts, *see* Bile acids
Biliary atresia, 238, 274
  aetiology, 275
  definition, 275
  diagnosis, 277
  liver transplantation, 281
  management, 279
Biliary obstruction, 204
Bilirubin metabolism, in neonate, 261
Bulk laxatives, 131

Carcinoid syndrome, 59
  diagnosis, 62
  flushing, 60
  treatment, 63
Carcinoid tumours, 60
Castor oil, 133
Cathartic colon, 134
  radiology, 137
Chenodeoxycholic acid, 30, 200
Cholecystokinin
  alcohol, 161, 168
  fat absorption, 30, 37
  lower oesophageal sphincter, 9
  saline cathartics, 129
Cholegenic diarrhoea, 215
Cholestasis, 204
Cholestyramine, 39, 79, 90, 217, 218, 279, 281
Cholic acid, 30, 200
Cholylglycine breath test, 29, 79, 207

Chylomicrons, 34, 75
Cimetidine, 59
Cirrhosis of the liver, 156, 158
 alcoholic hepatitis, 155
 alpha-1 antitrypsin deficiency, 271
 bile acid metabolism, 205
 biliary atresia, 276, 280
 cystic fibrosis, 291, 304, 314, 319
 haemodynamic measurements, 233
 portasystemic shunts, 239
 steatosis, 154
Cystic fibrosis, 297
 aetiology, 322
 alimentary system, 299, 317
 bile acid metabolism, 217, 304
 electrolytes in secretions, 325
 fibroblast culture, 324
 genital tracts, 307
 incidence, 297
 inheritance, 298
 liver disease, 273
 management, 314
 pathogenesis, 299
 prognosis, 313
 psychological aspects, 319
 respiratory system, 307, 315
 screening procedures, 321
 sweat glands, 308
 transfer of care, 320
Coeliac disease, 40, 213
Congenital hepatic fibrosis, 238
Connective tissue disorders, 96
Coronary–caval shunt, 247
CRST syndrome, 106
Cutis laxa, 114

Deoxycholic acid, 30, 201
Dermatomyositis, 107
Detergent laxatives, 132

Ehlers–Danlos syndrome, 113
Elemental diet, 84
Endoscopic retrograde cholangio-pancreatography (ERCP), 178
 abdominal pain, 182
 complications, 179
 pancreatic cancer, 183
 relapsing pancreatitis, 181
Endoscopic sphincterotomy, 192
Enterohepatic circulation, 76, 199, 222
Ethanol, *see* Alcohol
Exchange transfusion, 265

Faecal fat
 measurement, 28
 origin, 27
Fat, absorption, 27, 74, 199
 chylomicrons, 34

Fat absorption—*continued*
 intracellular mechanisms, 33
 luminal phase, 29
 mucosal phase, 32
 stomach, 29
Fat malabsorption
 abetalipoproteinaemia, 41
 alcohol, 165
 bacterial overgrowth, 40, 211
 bile acid deficiency, 38
 cirrhosis of the liver, 204
 coeliac disease, 37, 40
 cystic fibrosis, 302, 317
 diagnosis, 28
 gastric emptying, 37
 ileal disorders, 214
 intestinal lymphatic obstruction, 41
 intestinal resection, 39, 78
 pancreatic insufficiency, 39, 169
 scleroderma, 104
 systemic lupus erythematosis, 101
Fructosaemia, 269

Galactosaemia, 269
Gallstones
 bile acid metabolism, 218
 ERCP, 182
 intestinal resection, 78, 83
 metabolic defects, 221
Gastric inhibitory polypeptide, 67
Gastrin
 alcohol, 161
 gastrinoma, 57
 intestinal resection, 79
 lower oesophageal sphincter, 4, 7, 18
 radioimmunoassay, 56
 rheumatoid arthritis, 97
 structure, 55
Gastrinoma
 acid secretion, 54
 fat malabsorption, 40
 management, 59
 serum gastrin, 55, 57
Gastritis, alcoholic, 161
Gastro-oesophageal junction, 1
Gastro-oesophageal reflux, 3, 18
 endoscopy, 12
 manometry, 12
 medical treatment, 10
 radiology, 12
 scleroderma, 103
 surgical treatment, 14
Giant cell arteritis, *see* Temporal arteritis
Glucagon
 lower oesophageal sphincter, 9
 structure, 67
Glucagonoma, 69

Henoch–Schönlein purpura, 112

Hepatic
   collagen metabolism, 159
   encephalopathy, 233, 241, 247, 282
   portoenterstomy, 279
   steatosis, 153
   vein obstruction, 251
Hepatitis
   alcoholic, 155
   chronic active, 206
   infants, 267, 276
Hepatitis B antigen
   infants, 268
   polyarteritis, 108
   temporal arteritis, 111
Hiatus hernia
   scleroderma, 103
   sliding, 3
Homocystinuria, 114
Hormone-secreting tumours, 49
   pathology, 50
Hydroxylation of cholesterol, 200, 204, 221
Hyperbilirubinaemia
   conjugated, 267
   unconjugated, 261
      exchange transfusion, 265
      management, 263
      phenobarbitone, 266
      phototherapy, 265
Hypersplenism, 247
Hypoglycin, 284

Ileal disease
   cholylglycine breath test, 209
   diarrhoea, 214
   malabsorption, 214
Ito cell, 159

Kernicterus, 264

Lactoferrin, 169
Lactulose, 134
Laxative
   abuse, 65, 134
      management, 140
      pathology, 138
      radiology, 137
   action, 128
   anthracine derivatives, 128
   bile acids, 133
   bulk, 131
   castor oil, 133
   consumption, 124
   dangers, 141
   detergents, 132
   lactulose, 133
   polymethane cathartics, 130
   saline cathartics, 129
Lithocholic acid, 201, 206

Lower oesophageal sphincter, 4
   control, 5, 7
   relaxation, 7
   rheumatoid arthritis, 98
   scleroderma, 103

Mallory's hyaline, 156
Meconium ileus, 305
Meconium ileus equivalent syndrome, 305, 318
Medium-chain triglycerides, 75, 85, 88, 317
Melanosis coli, 138
Mesocaval shunt, 243, 290
Microsomal ethanol oxidising system, 151
Micelles
   bile acid, 30, 74, 199
   mixed, 31, 74, 199

Oesophageal manometry
   achalasia, 17
   gastro-oesophageal reflux, 12
   scleroderma, 19, 103
   spasm, 20
Oesophagus, cancer, 159
   spasm, 10, 20
   stricture, 10, 12, 16, 103
   varices, 235, 289
Omentopexy, 250
Oxalic acid
   absorption, 42
   intestinal resection, 79

Pancreas
   arteriography, 187
   cancer, 183, 189
   cystic fibrosis, 299, 317
   cytology, 189
   enzymes
      ERCP collection, 191
      fat absorption, 30, 74
   function tests, 187
   insufficiency, 39, 169, 302, 312
   scanning
      isotope, 185
      ultrasonic, 186
Pancreatic cholera, 64
   diagnosis, 65
   management, 67
Pancreatitis
   chronic calcifying, 165
   ERCP, 179, 181, 185
Papillary manometry, 194
Phenylmethane cathartics, 130
Phototherapy, 265
Physiological jaundice, 261
Polyarteritis nodosa, 108
Polysaccharide laxatives, 131

Portacaval shunt,
  arterialised, 249
  end-to-side
    complications, 241
    emergency, 242
    prophylactic, 239
    therapeutic, 240
  metabolic disorders, 251
  side-to-side, 242
Portal hypertension, 232
  angiography, 288
  childhood, 286
  cystic fibrosis, 291, 304, 319
  parenchymal, 238, 276
  postparenchymal, 251
  preparenchymal, 235, 241, 289
  splenic venography, 288
Portal vein thrombosis, 289
  children, 235
  cirrhosis of the liver, 250
Portal venous pressure, 233
Portarenal shunts, 244
Portasystemic shunts, 231
  children, 235, 290
  cirrhosis of the liver, 239
  complications, 241
  cystic fibrosis, 319
  haemodynamic measurements, 233
  hepatic encephalopathy, 233
  indications, 235
  types, 236
Pseudoxanthoma elasticum, 112
Pulseless disease, *see* Takayasu's disease

Rectal prolapse, 113
Reye's syndrome, 282
  aetiology, 283
  management, 285
  pathology, 283
Rheumatoid arthritis, 96
  gastritis, 96
  liver dysfunction, 99
  malabsorption, 98
  peptic ulcer, 96
  vasculitis, 98

Saline cathartics, 129
Scleroderma, 19, 103
  liver dysfunction, 106
  pneumatosis intestinalis, 105
  small intestine, 104

Secretin
  lower oesophageal sphincter, 8
  structure, 67
Serotonin, 62
Schistosomiasis, 239
Sjögren's syndrome, 96, 99
Small bowel,
  bypass, 83
  resection, 73
    clinical course, 81
    compensatory adaptation, 80
    gastric hypersecretion, 91
    management, 84
    primary effects, 77
    secondary effects, 79
Splanchnic circulation, 232
Splancho-thoracic shunt, 249
Splenectomy, 288, 290
Splenopexy, 250
Splenorenal shunt, 245, 290
  selective (distal), 248
Stagnant loop syndrome, *see* Bacterial overgrowth
Steatorrhoea, *see* Fat malabsorption
Streptozotocin, 59, 64, 69
Systemic lupus erythematosus, 100
  acute abdomen, 101
  fat malabsorption, 101
  liver dysfunction, 102

Takayasu's disease, 111
Temporal arteritis, 111
Transhepatic cholangiography, 180
Transplantation, liver, 281

Umbilical vein shunt, 250
Unstirred layer, 31
Uridine diphosphoglucuronyl transferase, 262

Vagotomy
  diarrhoea, 217
  fat absorption, 6, 37
  lower oesophageal sphincter, 3
Vasoactive intestinal peptide, 64, 66
  structure, 67
Verner–Morrison syndrome, *see* Pancreatic cholera

WDHA syndrome, *see* Pancreatic cholera
Wegener's granuloma, 111

Zollinger–Ellison syndrome, *see* Gastrinoma